OPEN WINDOW

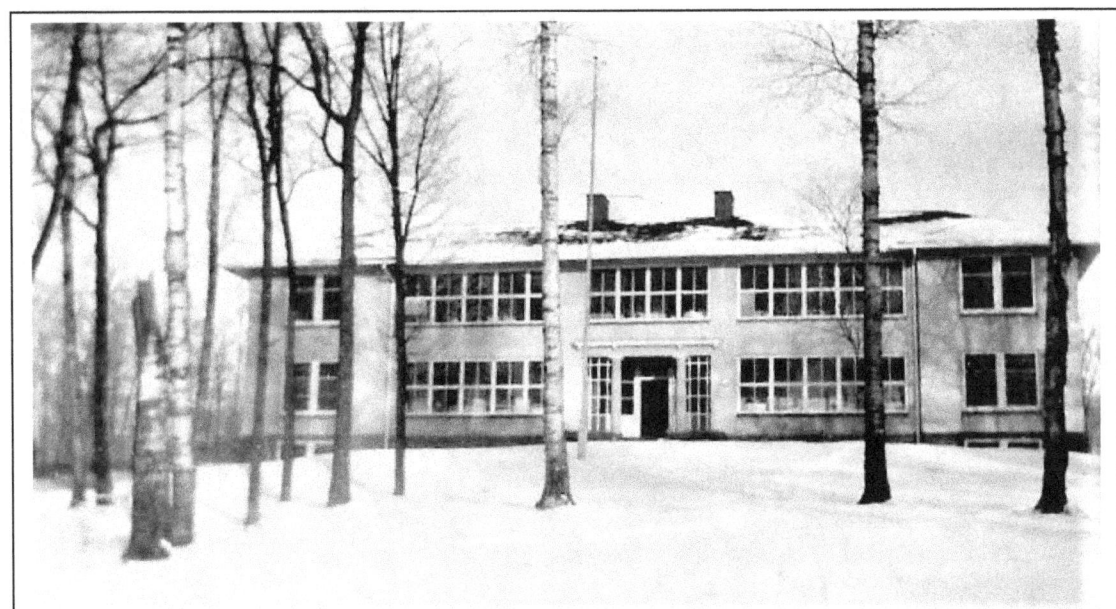

The Lake Julia TB Sanatorium
A Community Created by Tuberculosis
James Ghostley collection

OPEN WINDOW

The Lake Julia TB Sanatorium

A Community Created by Tuberculosis

*While attention is focused
on Coronavirus 19 (COVID-19),
tuberculosis still infects
one person in four in the world.*

By Pat Nelson

Copyright 2020 by Pat Nelson—All rights reserved.

It is illegal to reproduce, duplicate, or transmit any part of this document in either electronic means or printed format. The recording of this publication is strictly prohibited.

Every effort has been made to accurately depict life as it was at the Lake Julia Tuberculosis Sanatorium and in the surrounding area and to provide accurate information. Because I was not present to witness most of the dialogues and scenes in this book, many of which occurred more than 100 years ago, I depended on interviews and research. Some language has been used in a historical context even though other terminology may be more acceptable or more common today. I have presented the facts as I understand them. Some creative license was necessary to tell these stories.

I have made every effort to ensure that the information in this book was correct at press time. However, I do not assume and hereby disclaim any liability to any party for any loss, damage, or disruption caused by errors or omissions, whether such errors or omissions resulted from negligence, accident, or any other cause.

This book is not a substitute for the medical advice of licensed physicians. The reader should consult a physician in matters relating to his or her health.

Cover-photo Credits
Lake background: Shutterstock
Art Holmstrom at the Sanatorium window: Art Holmstrom collection
Author photo: Bob Nelson

"We shall not cease from exploration, and the end of all our exploring will be to arrive where we started and know the place for the first time."
T. S. Elliot

Table of Contents

Section One: My Journey 11
    Chapter 1 Leaving Minnesota 11
    Chapter 2 Returning for a Visit 19
    Chapter 3 Why Me? 27

Section Two: The Fight Against TB 31
    Chapter 4 What is Tuberculosis? 31
    Chapter 5 State and County Sanatoriums 35
    Chapter 6 Lake Julia Sanatorium's First Years 37
    Chapter 7 Dr. Laney Makes Changes 45
    Chapter 8 The Lomen Sisters 51

Section Three: Dr. Mary Chapman Ghostley 59
    Chapter 9 The Unstoppable Mary 59
    Chapter 10 Love Letters 65
    Chapter 11 Growing Closer 71
    Chapter 12 Mary Takes a Break with Family 79
    Chapter 13 Four Young Doctors 85
    Chapter 14 Dr. Mary Relocates 89
    Chapter 15 Dr. Mary's Bold Changes 97
    Chapter 16 Dr. Mary's Friend Ober 107

Section Four: My Family 111
    Chapter 17 My Mother's Path to the San 111
    Chapter 18 My Father's Rocky Road 117
    Chapter 19 Marriage and Family 121
    Chapter 20 Leaving the Dairy—but not Forever 127
    Chapter 21 Bernice Bakke, Laundress 137

Section Five: The Holmstrom Family 143
    Chapter 22 Family History 143
    Chapter 23 Getting Down to Business 147

Chapter 24 The Job Search 149

Chapter 25 Another Son 153

Chapter 26 Art Holmstrom, Student 157

Chapter 27 The Summer Job 159

Chapter 28 Illness Strikes 161

Chapter 29 Sanatorium Admittance 167

Chapter 30 Meeting the Neighbors 175

Chapter 31 Treatment Begins 179

Chapter 32 Roommates 183

Chapter 33 A Young Patient 189

Chapter 34 The History Lesson 193

Chapter 35 Patient Visitation Night 201

Chapter 36 A Change of Plans 203

Chapter 37 Passing the Long Hours 209

Chapter 38 Big Changes 221

Chapter 39 Continuing the Cure 229

Chapter 40 New Drugs 243

Chapter 41 After the San 247

Section Six: Story Without End 253

Chapter 42 Moving On 253

Chapter 43 Deja Vu 265

Chapter 44 My Surprise 271

Epilogue 272

About the Author 275

Recommended Reading About Minnesota 276

Gratitude 278

Reviews 279

How Reviews Work 280

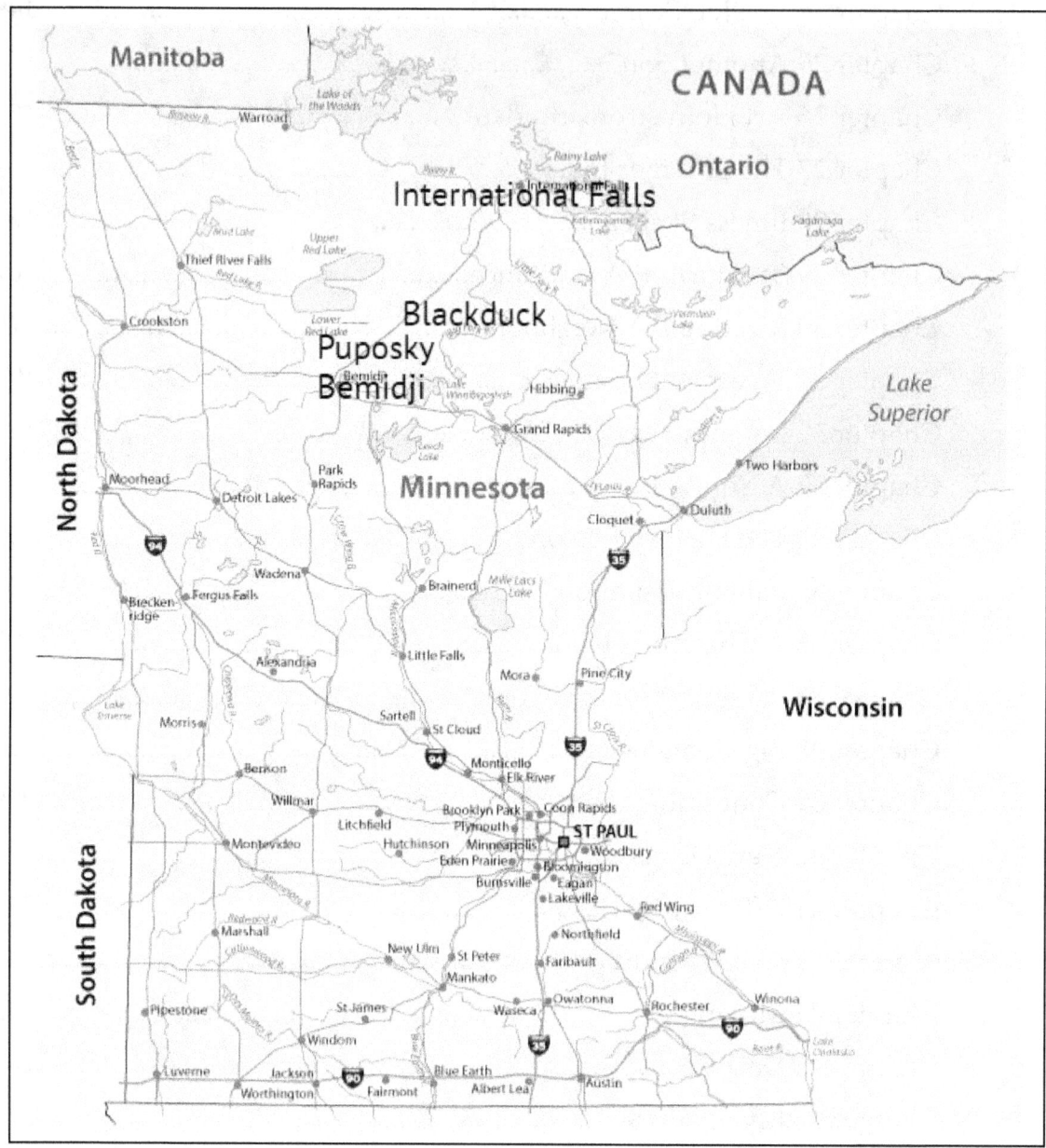

- **BEMIDJI, the first city on the Mississippi, is in North Central Minnesota.**
- BLACKDUCK is 24 miles northeast of Bemidji.
- INTERNATIONAL FALLS is 112 miles northeast of Bemidji.
- PUPOSKY is 13 miles north of Bemidji.
- RANIER is three miles east of International Falls.

Introduction

Real lives make up nonfiction narratives—that's what makes them so compelling. *Open Window* is several stories about the tight-knit community created by the Lake Julia Tuberculosis Sanatorium: stories about its doctors, patients, employees, and neighbors. It is a collective biography about its superintendent, Dr. Mary Ghostley; a young patient, valedictorian-hopeful Art Holmstrom and his family; and my parents, sanatorium employees Lee and Ella Hedglin.

Perhaps you have discovered, as I have, that some of your ancestors died of consumption, the White Plague, or TB. Those are all names for tuberculosis.

Most towns in this book are in Minnesota. The state name follows locations that are not in Minnesota. But whatever the state, or even country, after reading *Open Window,* you will know more about your ancestors and others who suffered from—and possibly died from—tuberculosis.

Today, fear of the Coronavirus Disease 19 causes widespread panic. Many of us forget about a far-more-prevalent disease, tuberculosis. TB has never been far away, and today, **one person in four** in the world carries the disease, even without exhibiting symptoms. The next time you are in a large group, silently look through the crowd and count off: "one, two, three, **four,** one, two, three, **four."** The statistics are frightening.

Those who test positive for the disease without having its active form are said to have latent tuberculosis, and until tuberculosis becomes active, it is not contagious. People with latent tuberculosis are infected, but they do not have symptoms, and they do not feel sick. Ten percent of people with latent tuberculosis will likely develop the active form of the disease and will then be capable of transmitting it to others.[1] Today, there is a treatment for those with latent TB, and most can take medicine to keep it from turning into the active form. [2]

---

[1] www.CDC.gov
[2] World Health Organization

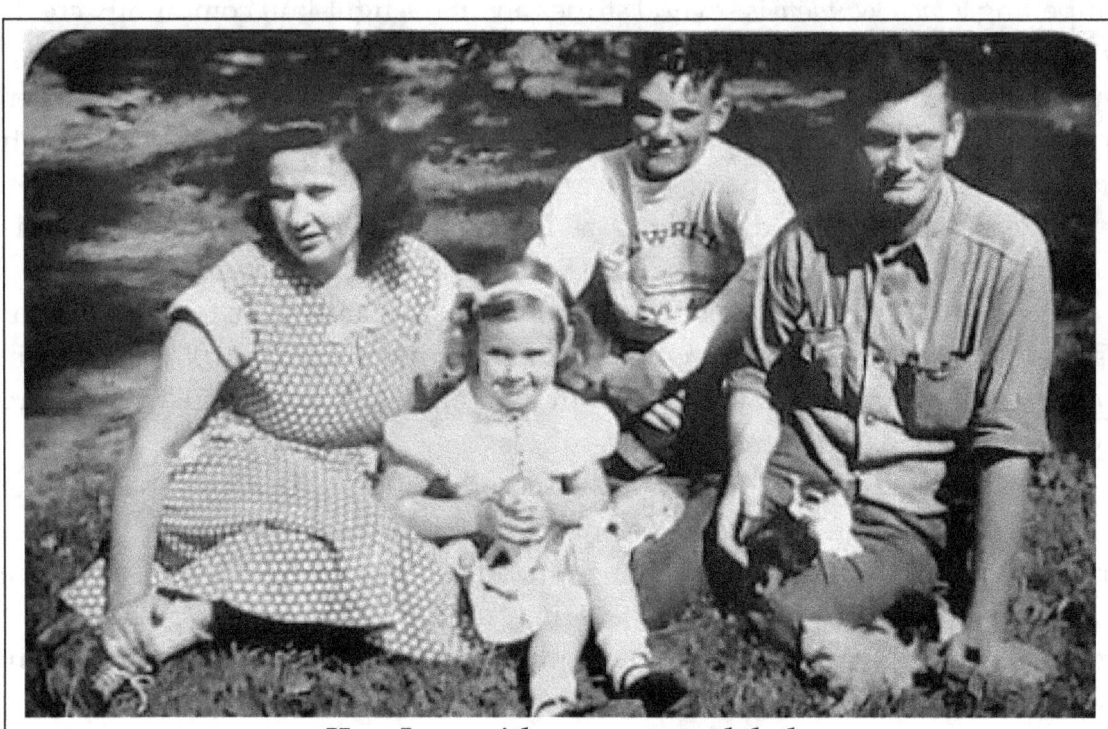

*Here I am with my mom and dad
and my brother Lloyd
before Dad left Minnesota for Washington in 1951.
We collected these cuddly kittens from the barn for the photo.
Ella Hedglin collection*

Section One: My Journey

Chapter 1
Leaving Minnesota

My mother, Ella Hedglin, my two brothers, their friend, and I piled into a 1939 Buick with a leaky radiator and drove from Sauk Centre, Minnesota, to Longview, Washington. It was June 1952. We had recently moved from the Lake Julia Tuberculosis Sanatorium in Puposky, and then we had to move again. I had just completed kindergarten, and my brother Lloyd had finished his junior year of high school. His friend Dean came along to help drive and to seek both adventure and a job. My oldest brother, Jim, was on leave from the Navy. Nine months earlier, my father, Lee Hedglin, had moved to Longview, Washington, to take a job with Weyerhaeuser, then the world's largest pulp, paper, and lumber mill.

I didn't take up much room in the cramped car, but I had to stretch if I wanted to see out the windows unless I sat on Mama's lap. As we drove away from Sauk Centre, I held my favorite paper doll along with an envelope containing a few of her well-worn cutout dresses, grateful that I hadn't sold them in the moving sale along with most of my other toys. Mama had only

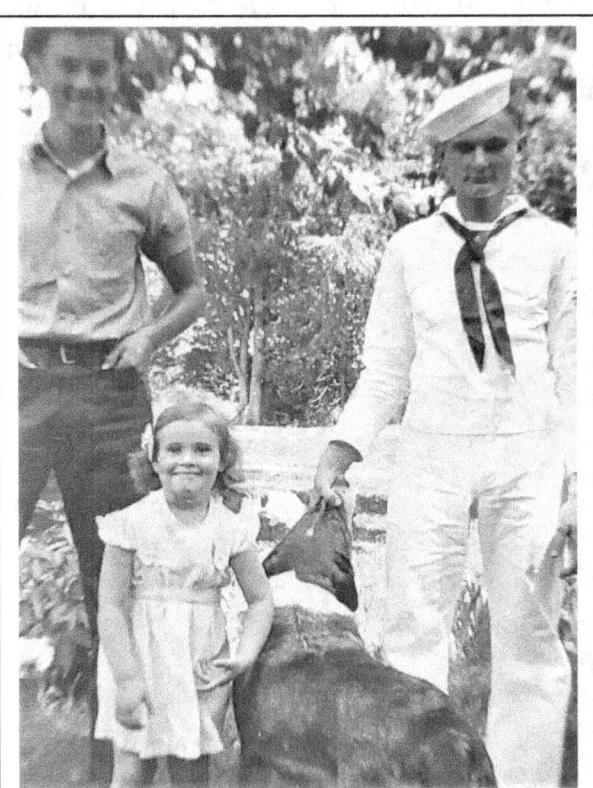

*My brother Lloyd, me, my brother Jim, and my dog, Ring
before moving to Washington
Ella Hedglin collection*

packed a few small treasures for the move, like the framed picture of me with a bunch of barn kittens and her favorite set of salt and pepper shakers.

As we drove away, I tried to hide the tears that trickled down my cheeks as I thought about the day I'd had to give away my constant companions—my dog, Ring, and the lamb I called Lambie. Oh, how I had sobbed when I returned home from kindergarten and found that they were gone. But Mama said that's what had to happen if I wanted to see my daddy. I asked if we would return, but Mama said, "No."

Mama gathered all the eggs from the coop before we left, and she sold them along the way for travel money. We had a little more room in the car once those eggs were gone.

Lloyd, 17, was the man of the family in Daddy's absence. Jim, 20, and Lloyd's friend Dean took turns driving the barely reliable Buick. I remember frequently stopping along the roadside to fill the radiator, and we carried one of those canvas bags filled with water in case we ran low.

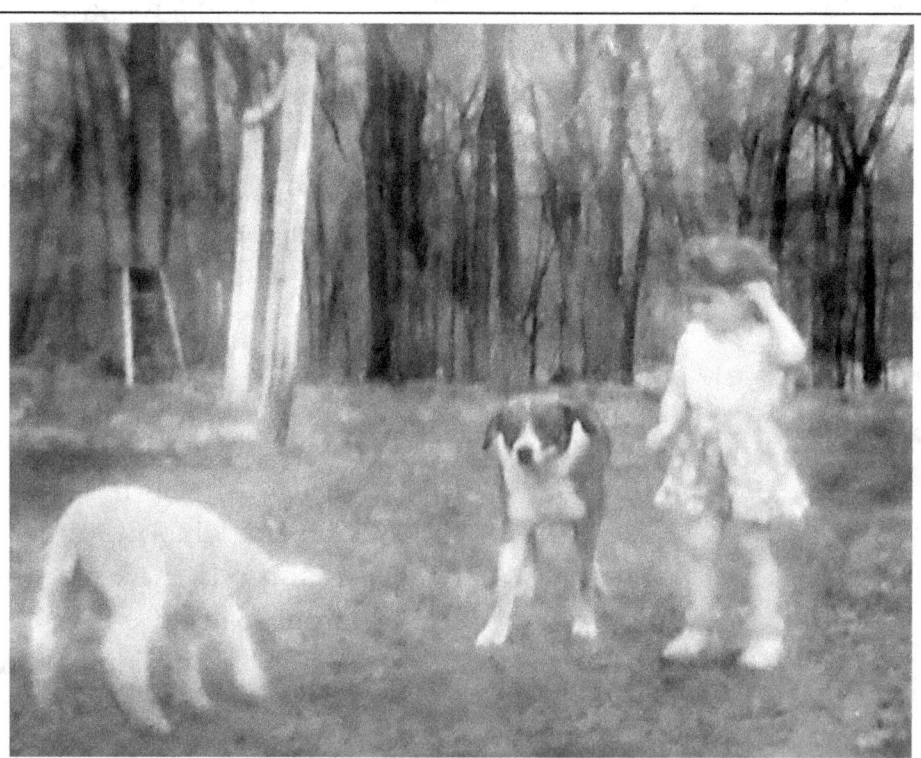

Here I am with my pets, Lambie and Ring, around 1950.
I had to leave them when we moved to Washington.
Ella Hedglin photo

On the way, we approached a flooded section of road, and Mama was afraid we wouldn't be able to drive through the water. Lloyd stopped the car, took off his shoes and socks, rolled up his pant legs, and waded into the cold, murky water to be sure it wasn't too deep for our car. He decided we could get through, and we were all relieved when we reached the other side of the flooded area.

Lloyd was Mama's hero. He was my hero, too. When we lived in Sauk Centre, he would carry me on his shoulders to the school-bus stop, and he would meet me at my kindergarten classroom after school. Before that, we lived in Puposky, where we made snowmen together or sledded in winter, and we played along the shores of Lake Julia in summer.

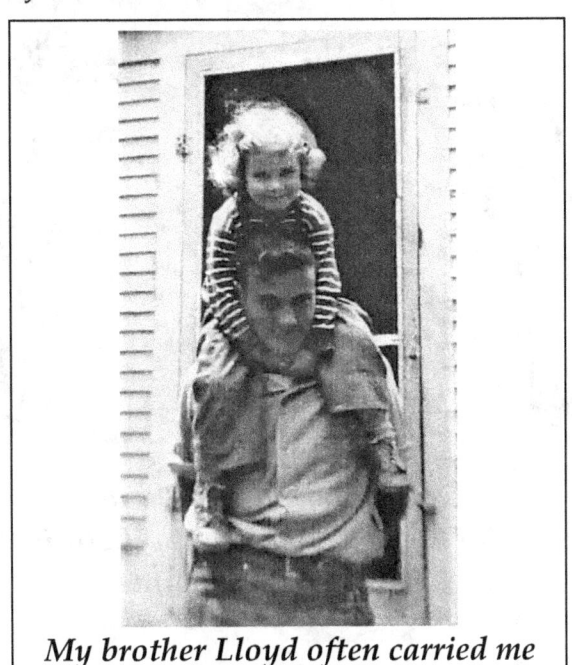

My brother Lloyd often carried me on his shoulders.
Ella Hedglin photo

My family had lived at several places around Puposky, close to both Mud Lake and Lake Julia, before moving to Sauk Centre.

The name Puposky (Papushkwa) is from the Native Ojibwe language, and it means "the end of the shaking land," referring to the Red Lake Bog.[3] Mud Lake occupied about 3 square miles but was too shallow to use for recreation, so residents swam and boated at Lake Julia instead. However, Mud Lake had

---

[3] Puposky Centennial Booklet, 2005

bountiful crops of wild rice, and that rice attracted ducks, making it a popular place to hunt.

The distance between the beautiful Lake Julia, 43-feet deep in places, and the shallow Mud Lake is less than a mile. The Continental Divide passes along the south end of Lake Julia, once thought to be the source of the Mississippi River.

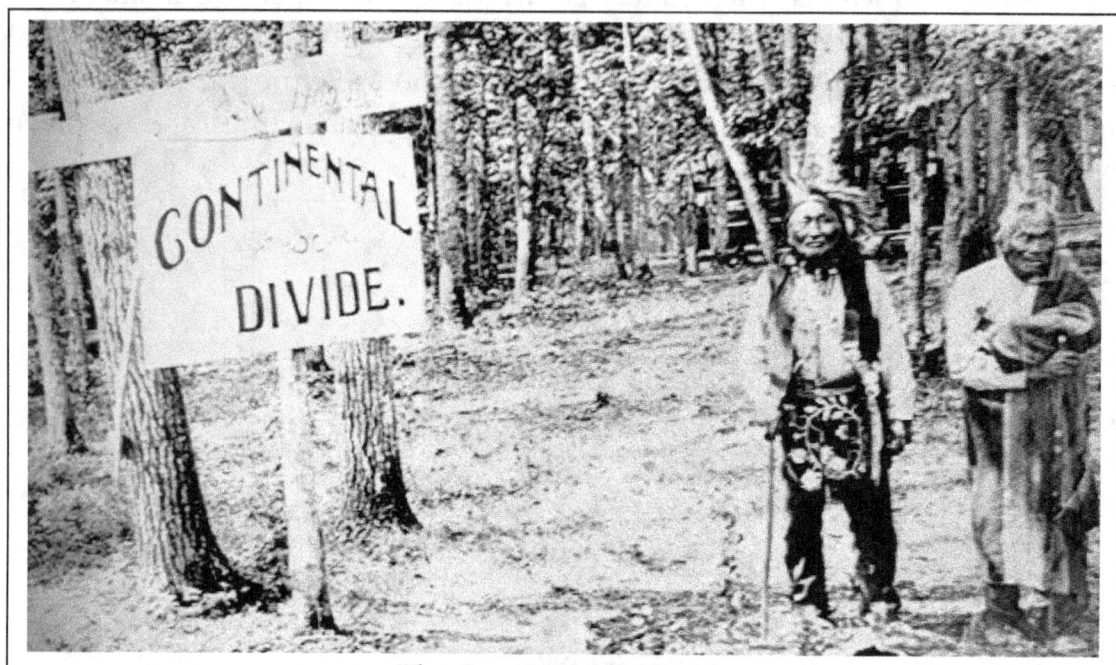

The Continental Divide
Courtesy of the Beltrami County Historical Society
Bemidji, Minnesota

The Lake Julia Tuberculosis Sanatorium sits on Lake Julia's north shore. Most people just called the place the San. Both of my parents moved to Puposky in the early 1930s to work there, and that's where they met. Dad worked as a janitor, and Mom was a maid before transferring to the kitchen. The San was one of the few places where folks in the area could find a job, and although the work came with health risks, it came with many benefits—a wage, a warm place to sleep, plenty of food, and free medical care—things that became especially important during the Depression. The San employed residents around Puposky for nearly 40 years, and it created a tight community made up of its employees, patients, and neighbors.

When my parents met, Mom had just moved into the basement next door to the San in what some employees called "the nursing home." It was not a nursing home for the elderly, but was lodging for the nurses and other female employees.

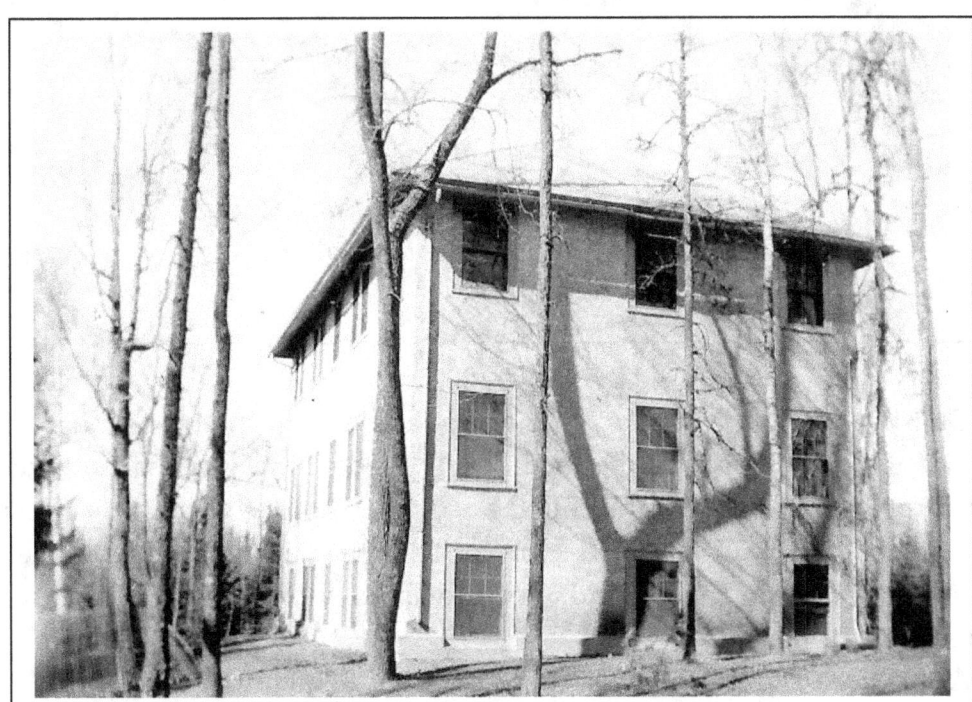

The Nurses' Home, called the "nursing home" by some
Art Holmstrom collection

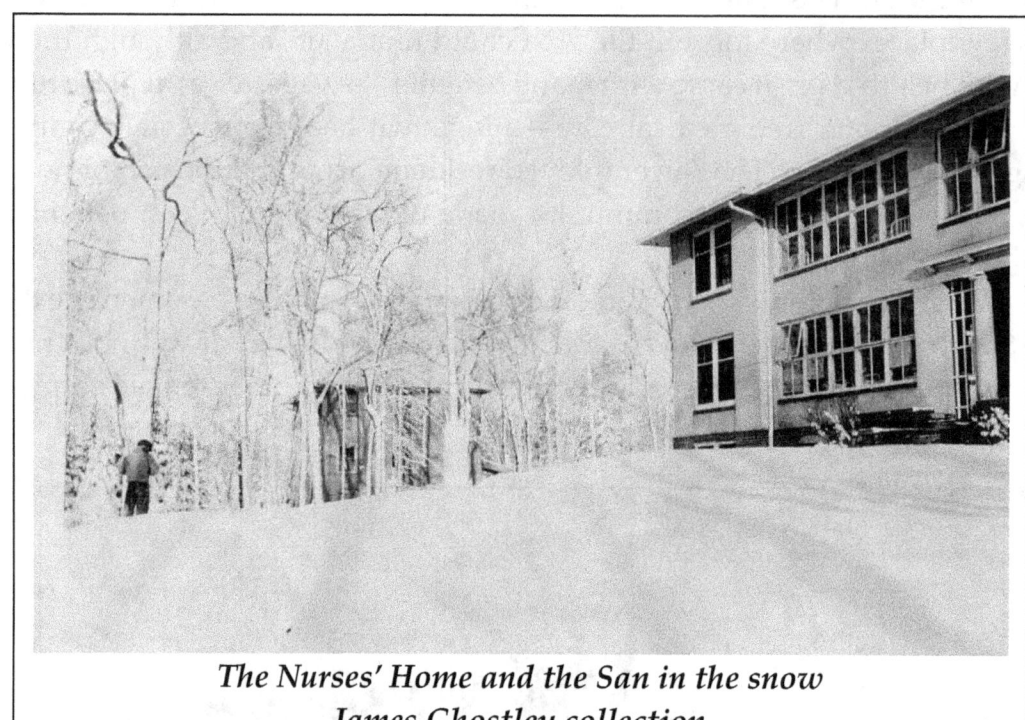

The Nurses' Home and the San in the snow
James Ghostley collection

Dad lived in the basement of the San, along with the other male workers. Lung patients filled the hospital, so no one smoked inside. Dad had smoked since he was barely a teenager, and he rolled his cigarettes to save money. He smoked at the corner of the building with some of the other employees, and they left a telltale pile of butts on the ground. There was no such thing in those days as a "smoke-free campus."

After Mom and Dad married and had their first child, my brother Jim, they lived at and operated the nearby San Dairy, the farm that provided the Sanatorium with plenty of fresh milk, butter, and eggs. The San Dairy, like the San, sat on the shores of Lake Julia.

According to Patsy Maher Schwartz, who grew up in Puposky, 2000-year-old Native American artifacts were discovered at the lake's outlet. That is where

San employees held a wedding shower for my parents and where many locals picnicked and swam.

Dr. Mary, who was the superintendent when my parents worked at the San, loved picnics and planned them often. I remember going to a community picnic at the Puposky school when I was only 3 years old. That was the first place I ever tasted soda pop. I recall sliding down a metal slide on the playground, and just a few feet beyond its bottom was a washtub filled with big chunks of ice and the most beautiful bottled beverages in bright, fruity colors ... orange, green, red, and purple.

We left Puposky for Sauk Centre so Dad could earn more money, then Dad left for Washington State because there were prospects of not only more money but of a long-term position.

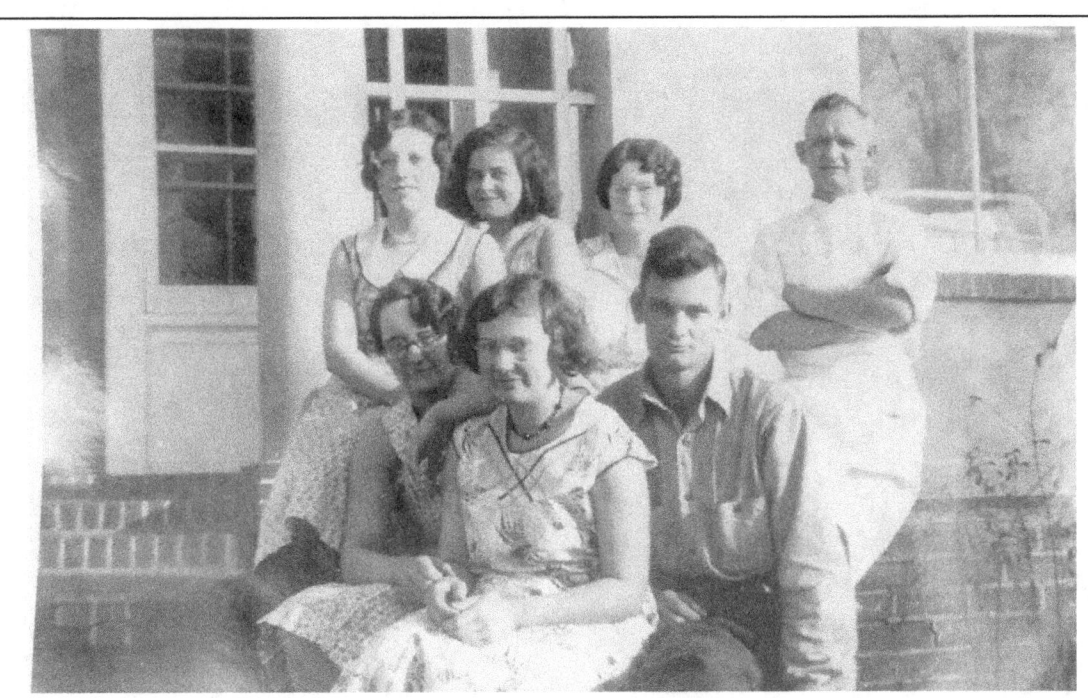

Front row: Myrtle Webster;
my mother, Ella Hedglin; my father, Lee Hedglin
Back row: Wanda Rice, Emily Stanek, Violet Allen, Adolf Becker
Ella Hedglin collection

18

Chapter 2
Returning for a Visit

After we moved to Washington, I didn't return to Minnesota for 28 years, not until 1980, when my mother asked me to accompany her to a family reunion at her birthplace, Fergus Falls. The trip would also include a visit to Bemidji, in North Central Minnesota, then on to nearby Puposky to see the Lake Julia Tuberculosis Sanatorium that had closed at the end of 1952. Bemidji was the first city on the Mississippi. It sits on the southwest shore of the 11-square-mile glacially formed Lake Bemidji.

I wasn't interested in taking a trip back to my first home. I didn't feel any attachment to the place. *What would I do while my mother looked at a crumbling old hospital that had closed years earlier,* I wondered. For my entire life, my parents had talked about *Dr. Mary this* and *Dr. Mary that.* Whenever I'd had a cough, a sniffle, or a fever, Mom had first asked herself, *What would Dr. Mary do?* When I helped Mom wash dishes at home, she had me run such hot water that I could barely touch it. Why? Because that's how Dr. Mary would have wanted it. I'd heard far too much about the San and Dr. Mary! But Mom wanted me to accompany her, and I did want to see my cousins. Finally, I agreed to go.

We rented a car in Fergus Falls and left from the reunion to visit Bemidji and Puposky. My Aunt Bernice, the widow of my mother's brother Norman, and two of their adult children—my cousins Barbara Madsen and Paul Grande, who lived in South Dakota—accompanied us. Bernice had also worked at the San, so I was sure she and Mom would talk nonstop about the place.

Just outside Bemidji, we passed signs for Lake Itasca, the actual source of the Mississippi River. Next, we came to Lake Bemidji, where I recognized the enormous statues of Paul Bunyan and Babe, the Blue Ox. I remembered standing next to them once when I was a child, bundled in heavy brown leggings, a wool hat, and my winter coat and mittens, staring in awe at the size of the giant statues while the frigid winter air bit my cheeks.

As we continued to drive through Bemidji, Mom and Aunt Bernice reminisced. My cousin Barbara commented that she could almost see the hands of the clock turn backward as our mothers shared memories.

We next drove to the Greenwood Cemetery, where my aunt and my mother hoped to locate the graves of some friends and relatives. I wanted to see the headstone of my Grandma Anna, my father's mother. Even though I had contacted the cemetery in advance to learn where I might find her, I searched for Grandma's grave for several minutes without luck.

I walked up and down, row after row, reading each headstone. *Where was Anna Maude Hedglin?* When I reached the sidewalk, I turned and proceeded down another long row. Back and forth, I walked through fresh-smelling newly mown grass as cut blades of green plastered themselves to the toes of my shoes. Finally, I became discouraged and decided to head back to the comfort of the air-conditioned car. I turned to motion to my family, and as I did, I spotted my grandmother's grave. She had a perfect resting place near the Chief Bemidji memorial—the monument for the Indian chief who had been well-liked and respected by many in the area. According to my father, his mother had had many Indian friends. Dad's family lived at the edge of the Red Lake Indian Reservation in Maple Ridge Township. The Indians harvested Grandma's high-bush cranberries for half the pickings. I bent down and brushed dried grass from her granite headstone, and instead of cold granite, I felt Grandma's warmth.

Grandma Anna died when my dad was barely a teenager. Still, I felt close to my grandmother, probably because Dad always spoke fondly of her. As a child, I imagined myself curled up in her ample lap, and although we never met, I wrote about my love for her.

On the drive toward Puposky, on a road bordered by birch, tamarack, and Jack pine trees, we came to the one-room former Turtle Lake School at Buena Vista, where my dad had attended school. I pulled into the parking area.

My grandmother died on July 18, 1922, just after my father completed seventh grade. After that, there was no money for him to attend school. Standing in front of that old schoolhouse, so close to my dad's history, made me miss him even more than usual. I remembered him telling me he had pumped water before school, and he had carried wood to heat the building.

A cast-iron water pump stood in the schoolyard, and I pictured Dad as a young boy, bringing the handle up, then forcing it down to fill a bucket with water for his teacher. I could almost hear a rusty squeal followed by the slosh of water. I gripped the handle, then brought my fingers to my nose and deeply inhaled the metallic odor.

When I noticed a piece of siding dangling below the schoolhouse by just a thin fiber, I tugged at it and stuffed it into my pocket. I suddenly needed to know more about my family's time in Minnesota. I ran my thumb over the weathered strip of wood. Its deep grooves reminded me of my dad's work-worn fingernails, and a lump of emotion pressed at my throat.

We drove on past the Buena Vista Ski Lodge, a bump on the right that was small compared to the ski slopes I often visited on Oregon's Mount Hood. Soon after that, Mom and Bernice excitedly pointed to the left. "That's it! That's it!" shrieked my mother. "That's Lake Julia, and that's where Daddy taught the boys to swim!"

Bernice chuckled. "Even though he didn't know how to swim himself!"

Moments later, we approached the old Lake Julia Tuberculosis Sanatorium. Vines wound through rusted metal and held open the once-fancy entrance gates. Bernice nodded to the right as we drove past a log house. "That's where Dr. Mary lived."

We parked between the small log house and the imposing San. It felt good to get out of the car and stretch. I gazed at the large building, then out at the calm lake, at the view the patients would have had and the one I'd had as a child when I'd helped Daddy deliver milk. He'd taken it in the kitchen door. I couldn't go inside, so I had waited in the truck while he took the milk to the walk-in refrigerator. On those days, I had stared at the open windows of the San, imagining life inside. Whenever I'd glimpsed a patient, I had turned away quickly as if I could catch the disease just by looking. Once, a patient waved, but I was too shy to wave back.

On the day of our return visit, the sky was blue, and the lake was glassy. Chalky birch trees stood tall, and memories sprouted like Dr. Mary's prized hollyhocks awakening after a long winter. Silent emotion filled my chest. I had returned home.

Bernice chattered excitedly. "I remember, like yesterday, when Dr. Mary came to the house to ask me to work." Then, a puzzled look crossed her face. "Where's our nursing home?"

Mom pointed. "It should be right there, but someone built that house right where it used to stand!"

My mother turned and climbed the steps to the San's massive front doors. A bulky chain held them shut. She tugged anyway, but they did not budge. As she cupped her hands against the glass and peered through grimy windows, I joined her.

"That's the dining room, just beyond this entrance. It's where your brother Lloyd performed in the Luther League play, 'The Bashful Birdie,' for the 'up patients' … you know, the ones who didn't have to stay in bed and were no longer considered contagious."

I remembered the photo, taken by a patient, of my handsome brother as he and the other cast members smiled at the camera. As a parent myself, I wondered if I would have allowed my children to perform there. But everyone in the community except the preacher, the postmaster, and the store owner had worked at the San, and they knew that no contagious patients would be in the audience.

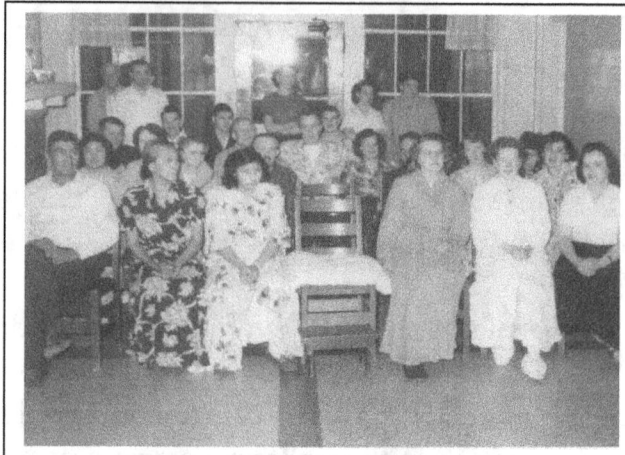

"Up-patients" watch a play.
Art Holmstrom photo

Mom and I turned from the doors as we heard Bernice speak from the nearby pathway: "Oh, there's Lovers' Lane." When Norman and Bernice had held hands and walked along that path, they hadn't thought about the heartache inside those walls—the illness and death. All they had thought about was each other.

Tears moistened Bernice's eyes. We cousins glanced at each other. For the first time, I pictured my aunt not as a middle-aged woman but as a carefree young adult walking hand in hand with Norman. I thought about the importance of my teen and young-adult memories, and finally, I understood. It was here that our parents had lived those years that bridged childhood and adulthood, dependence and independence—and those first experiences of falling in love.

"I still remember when Norman was hauling cordwood for the San," Mom commented to Bernice. "You saw him walk by the window, and when you heard someone say he was my brother, you came straight to the kitchen to ask me to introduce you."

"Oh, I did!" Bernice exclaimed. "And I already had a boyfriend at the time!"

"That's right, I'd forgotten," Ella remarked.

"Yes, and my parents liked my boyfriend better than I did. They weren't too happy when I started going with Norman. When I left the San to move back to Aberdeen, South Dakota, they thought that would end the relationship, but we sure fooled them!

"I remember that when the paychecks came out," Bernice reminisced, "a bunch of us would go to Bemidji to a movie or shopping. Norman and I did that often. He liked to ice skate and roller skate. I didn't know how to do either one and was afraid to learn, but I went along and watched."

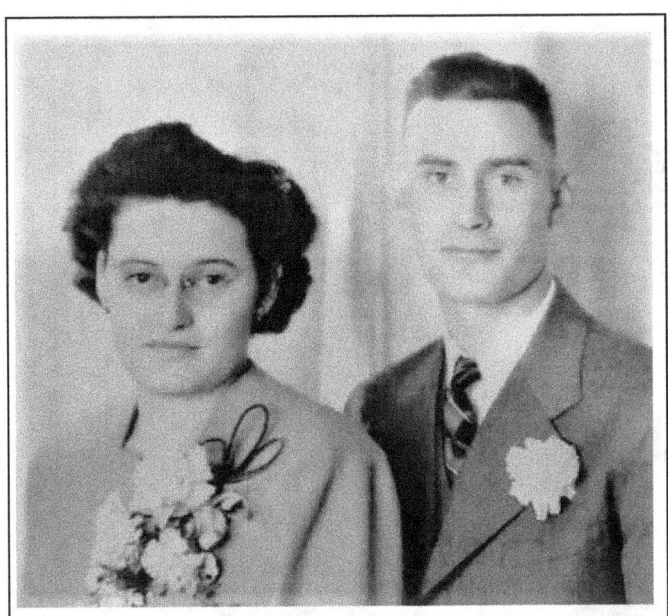

Bernice Bakke weds my uncle Norman Grande
Bernice Grande collection

"I remember you telling me how cold you got just standing there while he skated!" Ella exclaimed.

"Yes! And I remember one time in the spring when the roads were muddy. We got stuck in a ditch, and someone pulled us out. It seems like we were always getting stuck or changing a flat tire. Oh, those were the days!"

Mom and I walked down the San steps, then she turned to her left and pushed through tall weeds to get to a basement window. She gasped. "Oh, there's Daddy's little bed!" she exclaimed. There, in the dark basement where my father had slept when he was a janitor at the San, were the springs and iron frame of a small bed.

Even though chains secured the San's doors, they hadn't stopped Mom and Bernice from unlocking their memories and sharing them with their children. We cousins no longer found the San boring. We wanted to know more.

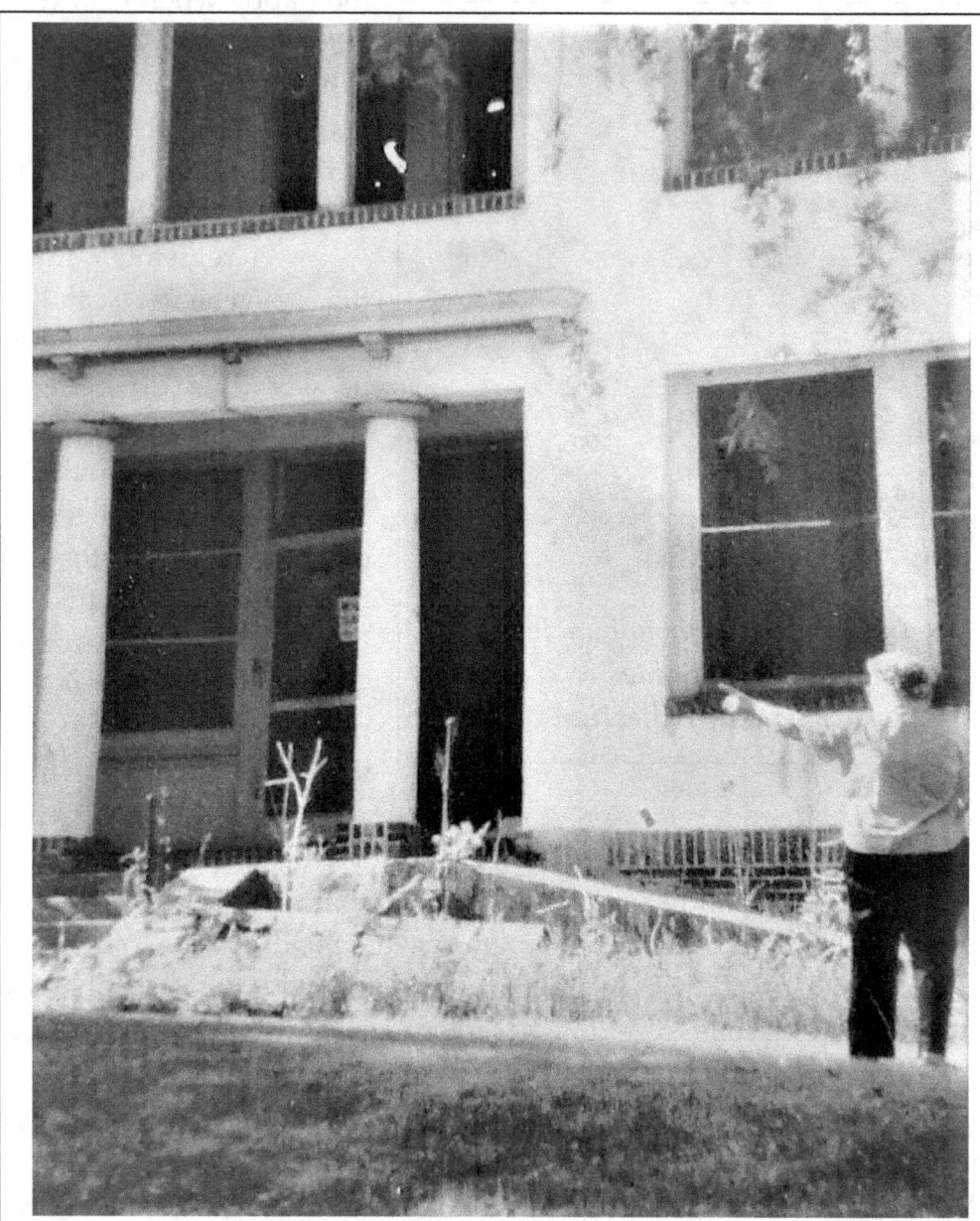

My aunt Bernice Grande looks over the vacated San in 1980.
Pat Nelson photo

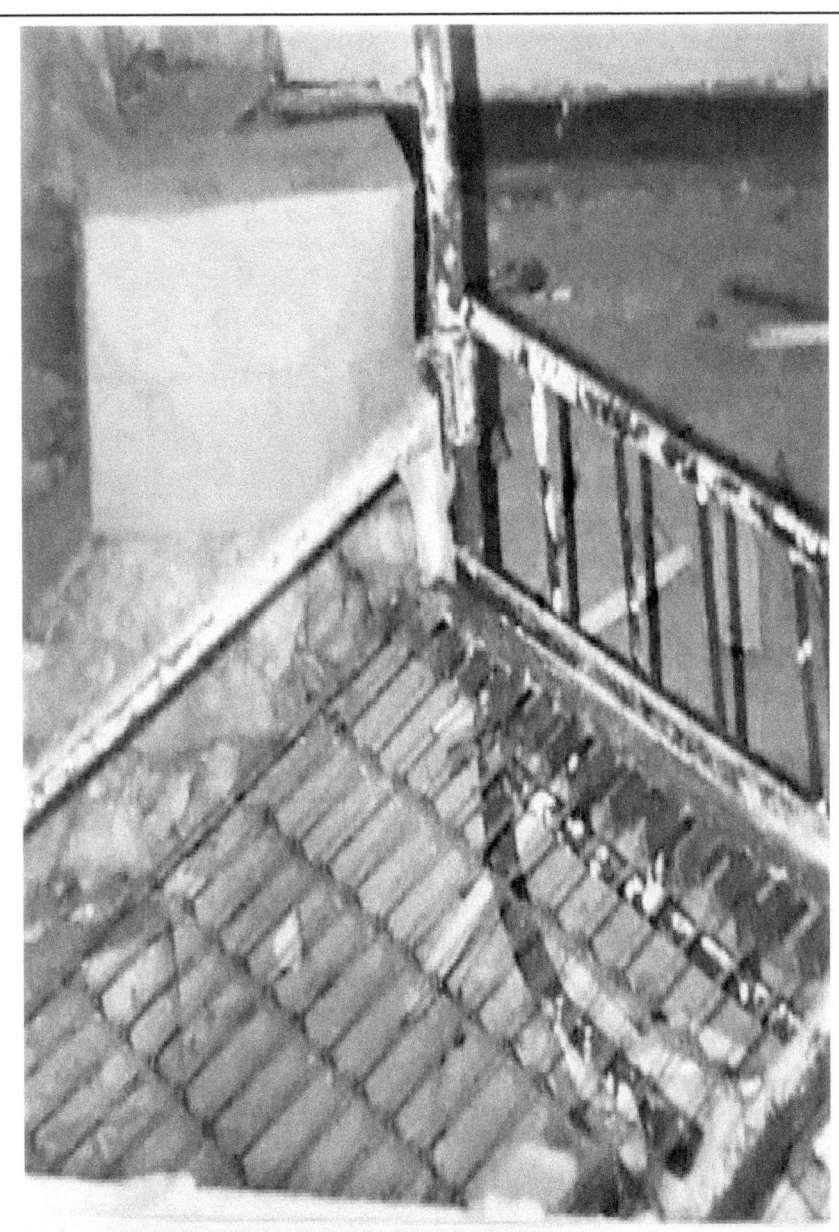
My mother spotted this old bed frame through the basement window

Chapter 3
Why Me?

I moved from Puposky when I was only 4 years old, so you might be surprised that people often contact me for information about the Lake Julia Tuberculosis Sanatorium.

Following my visit to the San with my mother in 1980, I wanted my children to see the place too. After all, they didn't know anything about the years that I'd lived in Minnesota.

It was because of my daughter-in-law, Laura Ellsworth, that this desire became a reality. Laura had received a kidney transplant from her father in 1999. After her recovery, she participated in the U.S. Transplant Games, athletic competitions for organ recipients. In July 2004, my family—my son, Steve Ellsworth (Laura's husband); my daughter, Susan Rose; my grandchildren, Max and Chelsea Rose; and my husband, Bob, and I—traveled to St. Paul to watch Laura compete. After the Transplant Games, we drove to Bemidji and Puposky so that I could introduce my family to my first home. Our first stop in Bemidji was to show the grandchildren Paul Bunyan and Babe the Blue Ox. Chelsea, age 4, made us laugh by calling them "Tall Bunyan and the Blue Box."

This time, I arrived in Puposky filled with excitement to see the San. The owner allowed me to take my family inside, and I proudly showed the place off like it was my own.

We stayed at the Birchmont Lodge on Lake Bemidji. While there, I visited Jim Ghostley and his wife, Connie, who lived nearby. Jim's mother, Dr. Mary Ghostley, was the San's superintendent when my parents worked there. Jim and his sister, Cathie, grew up in the log house next to the San.

Each time I visited Jim and Connie over the years, I learned more about the place. I told Jim I would like to write a book about his mother and the San, but he looked skeptical. "Everyone always says they're going to write a book about my mother, but no one ever does it."

The stories of Dr. Mary and the San had always been a part of my life, and I enjoyed writing. I vowed to be the one who would follow through. On two later trips to Minnesota, I researched at the Minnesota History Center in St. Paul. I returned home with copies of the patient and employee records plus other information about the Lake Julia Tuberculosis Sanatorium.

I spent several days at the Beltrami County History Center in Bemidji, scanning newspaper articles and searching for information.

When the History Center created a "Doctor, Doctor" display, the director asked if I would like to contribute something, so I created a photo book titled *Ghostley Images* about the San and Dr. Mary Ghostley. A copy is available to view at the Beltrami History Center, 130 Minnesota Ave. SW, Bemidji, MN 56601 under call number F612.B39 G4 2010 and catalog No. 2010.102. All other copies of the book are in private collections.

On one visit to Bemidji, Jim Ghostley suggested that my husband and I drive to International Falls to meet former San patient Art Holmstrom. International Falls, located on the Rainy River, across from Fort Francis, Ontario, in Canada, is known as the Icebox of the Nation, with winter temperatures frequently being the lowest in the contiguous states, and averaging 109 days a year below freezing. The town was first known as Koochiching, an Ojibwe word meaning "neighboring lake and river." The name change occurred in 1903 because of the river serving as a border between the United States and Canada.

The next day, Bob and I drove there and met Art and his wife, Edith. It was the first of several visits, during which I recorded Art's fascinating story and copied photos from his San scrapbook. Later, Edith mailed original letters to me that Art had written while he was a patient, as well as correspondence between Dr. Mary and both Art's father and his former doctor.

On my next trip to Bemidji, I located Anneliese Petersen—Annie—who was Art's girlfriend when they were patients at the San. I drove her to International Falls for a long-overdue reunion with Art. They had not seen each other for more than 60 years. The drive gave us an excellent opportunity to talk about her San experiences.

I interviewed former employees, patients, and neighbors of the San. I studied the patient records and found that some of my relatives had been patients or employees, or both.

In 2005, Bob and I went to Puposky to attend its centennial celebration. The little village turned 100 on my birthday, September 26. The gathering allowed me to interview many people whose families had been part of the Puposky community when the San was in operation—families that had socialized, worked, and raised their children alongside each other.

When we returned to the Minneapolis area to fly home, my cousin David Grande helped me contact his aunt Teresa (Tres) Lomen Hansen, who had been both a patient and a nurse at the San. Two of her sisters had also been patients:

David's mother, Inga Lomen Grande, who became a nurse, and her sister Clara Lomen, who died at the San. David provided their two "memory books" from the San for use in this book. Good wishes, poems, and friendly messages from patients fill the pages.

Several individuals with connections to the San contacted me. These contacts provided me with additional information, letters, photos, and memories. Others contacted me with questions about their family members who I was often able to find listed in the patient or employee records.

One time when I visited Minnesota, I wanted to retrace Dr. Mary's steps. I hoped to see the places she had lived and worked and to visit the cabin she had so loved at Rainy Lake. I rented an apartment at Tara's Wharf in Ranier, and when I visited Dr. Mary's cottage, I let my daydreams float across the water as I imagined her frequent swims to the rock in the distance. I also enjoy swimming, and as I focused on "her rock," I wished for warmer water so that I could swim to it as she had.

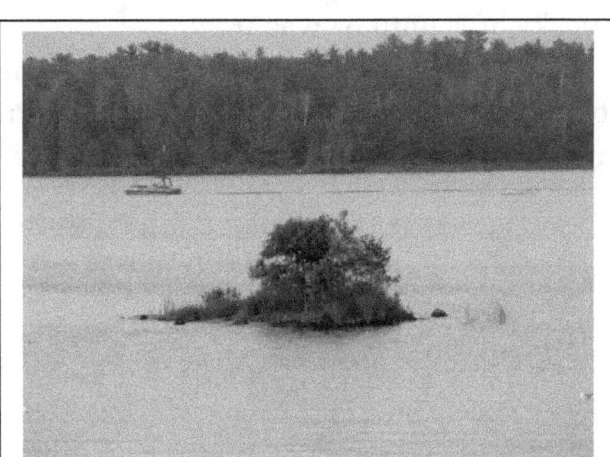

Mary liked to swim to the rock in front of her Birch Point cabin in Ranier. Pat Nelson photo

I visited Blackduck, where Dr. Mary and her husband, Fred, had first practiced medicine, and I searched the history center there for information.

In International Falls, where Dr. Mary had worked with doctor-friends Elizabeth and Robert Monahan at the Northwestern Hospital, I found the hospital's former location as well as other places Dr. Mary had lived. I visited descendants of Elizabeth and Robert Monahan in Ranier.

On the evening before my return to Bemidji, I was at Dr. Mary's cabin with her granddaughter Barbara when Barbara's father, Jim Ghostley, called. He sounded excited. "Guess what I found in the attic. I have the letters that my mother and her future husband wrote to each other in 1906 while they were in med school!"

I, too, was excited. When I left International Falls, I drove to Jim's house in Bemidji and spent my last evening in Minnesota making copies of the precious letters. The correspondence allowed me, finally, to hear Mary's and Fred's voices.

Little did I know when I started this project that my mother would still be telling me about Dr. Mary and the San. I was surprised to find that the source of information closest to home was in my deceased mother's boxes of family history, stored just feet from my computer. In Mom's notes, she described her job at the San in detail, even writing how far up the wall she washed when she was a maid. Another source of information was my brother Lloyd, who had lived in the Puposky area until he was 16.

After several people had contacted me for information, I realized that even though I was only 4 years old when I left Puposky, I had become a voice for the San and a caretaker of its memories.

Section Two: The Fight Against TB

Chapter 4
What is Tuberculosis?

Tuberculosis (TB) is a life-threatening disease caused by *Mycobacterium tuberculosis*. Mycobacterium tuberculosis, once the leading cause of death in the United States, may have been around 3 million years, and it's still with us today. It is a disease that can infect patients of all ages, as it did 17-year-old Art Holmstrom, whose fascinating story is in Section Five.

TB can affect many parts of the body, such as the kidneys, the spine, the brain, the lymph nodes, or the eyes. When the disease affects the lungs, it is called pulmonary TB. When TB affects any other part of the body, it is called extrapulmonary TB. Doctors in Washington State speculated that it might have been a type of extrapulmonary TB, *tuberculosis of the eye*, that forced my father into early retirement when he lost his eyesight to a disease they could not positively identify.

Pulmonary tuberculosis can cause a victim to feel weak, to lose his or her appetite, and to lose weight. A victim might also cough up mucus and blood; have chills, fever, and night sweats; or other symptoms. Suspicious symptoms of the disease sent 17-year-old Anneliese Petersen (Chapter 30) to the Lake Julia Tuberculosis Sanatorium, where her brother, Karl, had already been a patient for eight years.

When a person with TB of the lungs coughs, sneezes, talks, sings, or spits, the germs are propelled, infecting others who inhale only a few of the harmful bacteria.[4]

Tuberculosis has gone by many names. The ancient Greeks called it phthisis; the English called it consumption; the ancient Romans called it tabes, and the ancient Hebrew called it schachepheth. Tuberculosis of the lymph nodes was called scrofula. Johann Schoenlein of Zurich began calling the disease tuberculosis in 1839. In 1861, Oliver Wendall Holmes called it the White Plague because it left its sufferers pale. It is commonly called TB, a shortened version of tubercle

---

[4] www.cdc.gov

bacillus.[5] It was probably introduced to Minnesota's Indigenous Peoples when the first white men came in 1659, or it may have been introduced to the area shortly after that by white fur traders. Unknowingly, in 1819, Army soldiers brought the tubercle bacilli—plural for tubercle bacillus—and settlers packed it along when they moved into the Minnesota Territory.

Even more of the contagious bacterium arrived around 1849 when the area was marketed as a favorable climate for sufferers of tuberculosis, drawing folks from Scandinavia, Germany, and the eastern part of the United States.

According to the United States census tables of 1860, one in every seven deaths in Minnesota was from tuberculosis. Hundreds of patients admitted to the Lake Julia Tuberculosis Sanatorium from 1916 to 1952 lost their lives to the disease. Patient Elida Josephson (Chapter 18), knowing she was losing the battle, handed out photos of herself so people would remember her. For some patients, like Elroy Ramstad (Chapter 32), who also had progressive diabetes, having an additional disease complicated treatment, and he died at the San.

From 1865 to 1867, a Frenchman, J. A. Villemin, proved the transmission of tuberculosis from man to animal as well as from animal to animal. In 1882, Dr. Robert Koch of Germany announced that he had isolated the tubercle bacillus. By following Koch's procedures, other doctors and scientists reproduced the results. For this discovery, Koch received the Nobel Prize in physiology.

By 1880, the rush of invalids to Minnesota dramatically slowed because once the Union Pacific Railroad opened, consumptives—those with tuberculosis—could travel to Arizona, Colorado, California, and New Mexico to seek better health. But many tuberculosis sufferers who had already become Minnesota residents stayed and continued to spread the disease.

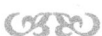

At the beginning of the 20th century, there were two known kinds of tubercle bacilli, the human and the avian. In 1906, Theobald Smith of Harvard University announced another, the bovine type, which caused the disease in cattle. Bovine tuberculosis could be transmitted from animal to human, so destroying tuberculous animals was encouraged. Cattle were monitored closely at Minnesota's tuberculosis-sanatorium farms like the one at Lake Julia, where my father worked.

---

[5] *Invited and Conquered*, Minnesota Public Health Association, 1949

By 1920, the foreign-born and their families made up 64% of Minnesota's population. Once the germs arrived from other parts of the world, it was impossible to send them back. The only option was to learn to control the disease. One way to do that was to educate the public.[6]

In the early 1900s, that effort had already begun. It was common to see men spit on the sidewalks. They often missed the spittoons in the saloons, causing both the germs in their phlegm and brown tobacco juice to travel from place to place on the soles of their shoes. A campaign encouraged people not to spit on the sidewalks, boardwalks, and floors. Some businesses posted signs, trying to stop the nasty practice. Others installed bricks stamped, "Don't Spit on Sidewalk."

Spittoons holding a germicide were made available in homes and public places to contain the dangerous sputum. People began boiling their handkerchiefs. Women started wearing their skirts shorter so that their clothing would not drag

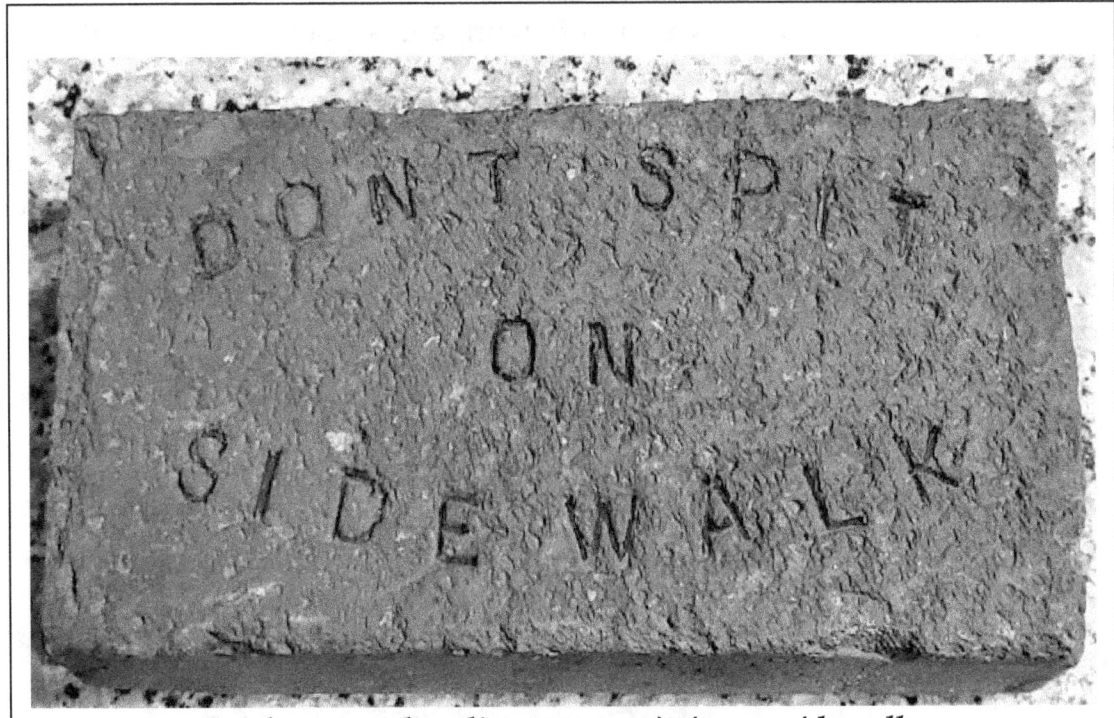

Brick stamped to discourage spitting on sidewalks
Pat Nelson photo

---

[6] *Invited and Conquered,* Minnesota Public Health Association, 1949

on dirty, sputum-tainted sidewalks, and men began shaving their beards to avoid harboring disease in their facial hair.

As the drive for sanitation grew, paper sputum cups and disposable handkerchiefs came into use in the sanatoriums because they could be destroyed by burning.[7]

Some families added porches to their homes to create separate quarters for tuberculous family members. But none of those measures were enough.

Those who lived in close quarters, such as in crowded households, the military, dorms, or prisons spread the disease when they released tiny, bacterium-laden droplets into the air.

⊗

Not all tuberculosis becomes active. When the infection is latent, the immune system prevents it from multiplying, keeping the germs suppressed. There are no symptoms of latent TB, and it is not contagious. But when immunity is compromised, the bacteria can begin to grow. Patient Art Holmstrom (Section 5) carried the disease around with him to work and school without knowing he had it, but until it became active, he did not spread the disease.

About one-fourth of the world's population has latent TB.[8] Ninety percent of those infected with Mycobacterium tuberculosis never develop the active form of the disease. But the other 10%, particularly those with weakened immune systems, such as children, those who have HIV, or persons undergoing chemotherapy, develop the active form of tuberculosis.[9] If it becomes active, it can be deadly.[10]

---

[7] *Invited and Conquered*, Minnesota Public Health Association, 1949
[8] World Health Organization
[9] *Scientific American*, March, 2009
[10] *Invited and Conquered*, Minnesota Public Health Association, 1949

Chapter 5
State and County Sanatoriums

In 1915, the Minnesota State Sanatorium Law provided that any county with the approval of a majority of the county commissioners could construct a hospital to remove tuberculous patients from the general population. Minnesota already had a state-run sanatorium at Walker, about 50 miles from Lake Julia.

Named "Ah-gwah-ching," which means "out of doors" in the Native Ojibwe language, the Minnesota State Sanatorium for Consumptives had already been in operation for nine years when the Lake Julia Tuberculosis Sanatorium opened. The State San sat on the south shore of Leech Lake and overlooked Shingobee Bay, about 3 miles south of Walker in Cass County.

Doctors hoped to find a way to eradicate TB. One doctor at Ah-gwah-ching thought tuberculosis was spread by touch, so he ordered his staff to wash all books and to iron all paper money. Unfortunately, his idea didn't stop the disease.[11] TB cannot live on surfaces and cannot be spread by touching something that a person with the disease has had contact with, but that was not yet known. People who spend a lot of time in close contact with someone who has TB are more likely to become infected.[12]

Self-sufficiency was the goal at the State San. It provided dairy products, vegetables, and electricity. That became the goal of the new county facility, the Lake Julia Tuberculosis Sanatorium, as well.

Ah-gwah-ching had a complete farm operation, and in the years 1932-35, its herd of registered Holstein cattle was the largest in Northern Minnesota. Holsteins had a lower fat content, which made the milk easier to digest. The farm had around 100 registered Holsteins and about 150 milking stock, and many farms in the area purchased their cattle from the Sanatorium, which named and numbered each cow. The Sanatorium farmed 600 acres for hay. On another 160 acres, it raised potatoes, corn, and the feed for its dairy cattle.[13]

---

[11] Minnesota History Center, Ah-gwah-ching Tuberculosis Sanatorium collection
[12] *Each Breath*, A blog by the American Lung Association, March, 2019
[13] *Invited and Conquered*, Minnesota Public Health Association, 1949

Indigenous patients were a federal responsibility. Tuberculous Indians in Minnesota first had their own hospital in Onigum in mid-November of 1924, where a school was converted into a sanatorium. There were few beds for Minnesota's Indian patients for the next 10 years, which resulted in tuberculosis spreading throughout the Native American population.

Around 1934, the Indian Building, paid for by the federal government, opened on an acre of land at Ah-gwah-ching. Even though this was a state institution, the federal government owned the Indian Building. Prospective patients arrived by school bus and nurses' cars to receive chest X-rays. Before long, the death rate from tuberculosis among the Indian population dropped by half. After a January 1935 fire, the 26 patients at Onigum transferred to Ah-gwah-ching.

Several times, Ah-gwah-ching reported that an Indian had run away from the institution to return to the reservation. The authorities knew the runaway patient had active tuberculosis, so they would take him back to Ah-gwah-ching and treat the disease from a jail in the basement. It was bad enough to have TB, but it must have been even worse to be jailed because of it. However, during winter, it may have been a blessing for those locked in the basement when they could not receive the fresh-air treatment.

Eventually, Indians, as citizens of the state, were eligible for admission to both county sanatoriums and the Ah-gwah-ching State Sanatorium.[14]

---

[14] *Invited and Conquered*, Minnesota Public Health Association, 1949

Chapter 6
Lake Julia Sanatorium's First Years

Mrs. Margaret Marston Neal was the first superintendent. Her husband, Dr. Homer Neal, joined her. A head nurse, a trained nurse, and a practical nurse assisted Mrs. Neal, and a doctor visited a couple of times a week. L. G. Guyer was the physician from July to November 1916, and M. Levy filled the position from December 1916 to August 1917.[15]

Dr. Neal, who had battled TB for years, could probably have been considered as the San's first patient since he arrived with his wife. However, he wasn't officially listed on the patient roster until his wife gave up her position as superintendent. While his wife was in charge, the couple lived upstairs in private quarters, and the doctor looked in on him as a courtesy to the Neals.

Therefore, 28-year-old Nels Saltness of Solway, rather than Dr. Neal, had the distinction of being the San's first patient. Saltness had emigrated from Norway in 1907 at age 19. Dr. Einer Johnson, one of the San's board members, sent Saltness to the San in July 1916, a day before the facility officially opened. He knew there was staff on hand to let Saltness in, and he wanted him to begin treatment as soon as possible. Saltness rode the train from Bemidji to Puposky, then a neighbor of the new sanatorium drove him the rest of the way.

Dr. Johnson and the rest of the board members decided to drive rather than take the train, and they also arrived a day early. Mrs. Neal was surprised when a nurse came to tell her that not only had the board members arrived, but so had Saltness. She entered a room full of strangers and didn't know which one was the patient.

Dr. Neal wanted a chess partner, so he taught Saltness the game. Neal told Saltness he had learned from a champion chess player from Kansas. After playing for three months, Saltness had still not won a game against the doctor, but one night he was finally close. They played until bedtime and planned to continue the next day. In the morning, Mrs. Neal put the board away because Dr. Neal was not

---

[15] Minnesota History Center, Lake Julia Tuberculosis Sanatorium, Ann Ethen Statistical Report

well, and she wanted him to rest. Saltness never did get to beat the doctor at a game of chess.[16]

When Dr. Levy left in August 1917, no doctor was willing to take over, so he continued to fill the position for two months until Dr. W. C. Jessen came on board. Jessen left after just two months.

☙❧

Treatment was harsh in the early years of TB sanatoriums. The San's exterior windows had no glass. Heavy canvas curtains kept out some of the snow. The facility's construction allowed air to flow throughout the building. The frigid wind that blasted off the lake pushed in the south windows and on through the interior window openings and hallways, then out the open windows on the north side of the San.

Patients were required to be outside as much as possible in the fresh air, even though they were ill. Northern Minnesota seemed to be perfect for "the cure," with pine forests, clean air, and cold winters. Patients wore stocking hats and heavy pajamas, both outdoors and inside.

The typical treatment for TB included enforced rest periods each afternoon and lots of fresh air. A healthy diet, physical and occupational therapy, and medication were also standard. Some patients received pneumothorax—the collapse of a lung by insertion of air or gas into the pleural cavity to allow the diseased lung to rest. Less commonly, physicians performed thoracoplasty. This procedure surgically collapsed the lung and wall of the chest permanently on the same side as the disease by the removal of ribs.

☙❧

Because Saltness could not get warm in the winter next to the open windows, he stuffed layers of newspaper under his mattress for insulation.[17] The papers were not enough to provide warmth, so in October 1917, after 459 days and four different San physicians—and even though he was still not strong—Saltness went home for a visit and decided not to return.[18] Although he did not go back for further care, he lived many more years, until June 10, 1978.

---

[16] Darlene Pearson, Puposky, Minnesota: Original Nels Saltness interview for *North Country History* by Hilda Rachuy

[17] Darlene Pearson, Puposky, Minnesota: Original Nels Saltness interview for *North Country History* by Hilda Rachuy

[18] Minnesota History Center, Lake Julia Tuberculosis Sanatorium, Patient Register

☙❧

During Saltness's stay, the San admitted two of my aunts. My father's half-sister Flora Long Mackaman, age 19, went into the San on July 18, 1916, as the third patient. The doctor discharged her for insubordination after only 12 days. Flora's sister Maude Long, age 17, was admitted on July 20, 1916, as patient number nine. She stayed 157 days and left to marry Harry Higbee.[19]

☙❧

A few months later, two young girls entered the San. Their parents, Johan and Amanda Nyman, had three children, Eva and John, who were both born in Sweden, and Mary, who was born on February 4, 1912, in Nymore, Minnesota.

In September 1916, 14-year-old Eva was admitted to the San, followed in May 1917 by little Mary.

Johan saved the letters Eva wrote to him from the Sanatorium, and his family members shared them with me. I have printed correspondence in this book in its original form.

"April 27, 1917

"I received your letter today and was glad to hear that mamma (mum) was a little bit better. Well I am feeling pretty good. Well you want to know about that gas. Well first they put something in my arm and then they make me get on top of the bed then they put a sheet over me, two towels, one over my face then they tell me not to cough and keep still, not to talk or anything and the doctor puts the gas in my side. But they don't give me chloroform for the stuff they put on my arm that takes away the pain then they put the gas in my left side. My side don't hurt as bad as you would think. This is all I can think of about the gas because I can't see what they use. Miss Kavanagh is writing this letter for me because my hand got tired and I couldn't write."

"Sunday, May 20, 1917
"Dear Papa,

"Mary was alright for a while when she was with me. But then when rest hour came the nurse told her she had to go to bed. Then nurse took her to the bathroom. Changed her clothes. Then after a while the youngest boy began teasing her til she began to cry. She cried a whole hour. Began to cry again in the afternoon. Then nurse came, sat a long time

---

[19] Minnesota History Center, Lake Julia Tuberculosis Sanatorium, Patient Register

trying to quiet her. Then she (nurse) sat down on bed and began to color. When Mary saw that, she was soon ready to help nurse. Then nurse left her and she kept on coloring. One of the ladies has sent some things cut out of magazines, paperdolls. She is playing with them. They don't let me have her. Mary came to me to show me what a lady had given her. Nurse saw her. Mary ran back. Then nurse said she must stay in bed. She is not sick at all. I think it is crazy."

"Monday

"Mary cries all the time. They will not let her be with me at all, not even for a little while, the poor thing is so lonesome. She don't know what to do, they make her stay in bed all the time. Well what can I do? It is impossible for me to do anything. I know how she feels for nurse has said to me get to bed. It is awful."

"June 12, 1917
"Dear Papa,

"Will thank you for the paper. They went ahead and opened my package downstairs and put the strawberries away. I got so mad. I want to open my own packages.

"Miss Wilson is leaving as soon as a nurse takes her place. We have two new nurses. The cook has left us. The new one gives us raw oatmeal, no salt in potatoes or gravy or soup. Papa take and make some bread sandwiches with brick cheese between sardines in olive oil, I am not allowed to have meat. Also send some pickles (sweet) don't be afraid to take that along when you come. Send two fat herrings also, please take that along and the nurse wants you to take a pair of black stockings up without holes for Mary, those white stockings were too small for her. I have had such poor meals that a rat could not get fat on the food."

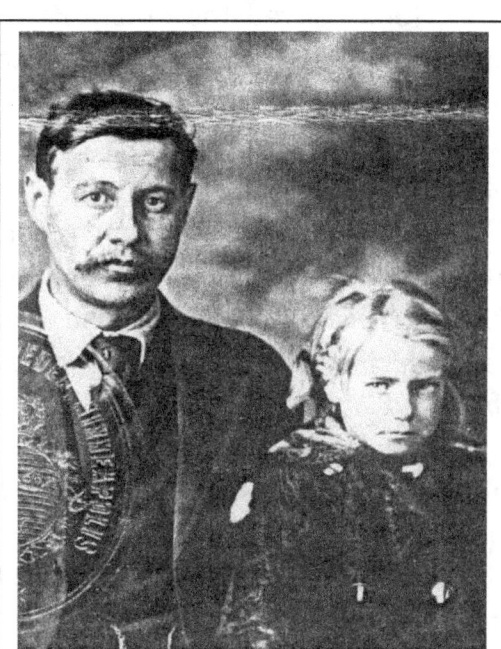

Johan and Mary Nyman's passport photo
Jessica Holm, Nyman family photo collection

The Nyman's stay in Minnesota was tragic. Their son drowned in Lake Bemidji the same year that Eva and Mary were admitted to the San. And Mrs. Nyman died on May 3, 1917. Mary was discharged on July 22, 1917. Sadly, her sister, Eva, died at the San a month later. That left only the father, Johan, and his youngest daughter, Mary.[20]

⊂₃₂⊃

The daily routine of Lake Julia was like that of Ah-gwah-ching, where, at 5 a.m., the night nurses handed out water basins and bedpans.

Each patient had a thermometer. The nurse would bring cotton balls or gauze soaked in rubbing alcohol to disinfect the instrument before and after each use. Those patients who were capable took their temperature themselves, then handed the thermometer to the nurse, who recorded the reading.[21] It was sometimes difficult for a patient to shake the mercury in the glass stick to a point below the normal temperature before placing the "temp stick" under his tongue. If the exertion were too much for the patient, the nurse would shake down the thermometer with a few practiced quick snaps of her wrist.

The patient kept a thermometer in a container on the bedside table to protect it from breaking, and the nurse collected the cotton or gauze so that it could be disposed of or burned.

After taking temperatures, it was time for each patient to dip a washcloth into the basin that waited on the bedside table, add a little soap from his soap dish, and wash his face and hands for breakfast. The water was warm when the nurse brought it into the room, but when the air was chilly, the water was often lukewarm or cold by the time the patient was ready to wash.

The lucky few who were well enough ate in the dining room. For the rest, breakfast trays arrived in the wards around 7 a.m. Those on complete bedrest had to be propped up by pillows, making eating awkward. Many patients spent restless nights, so after breakfast, nurses straightened sheets and blankets. If a bed was soiled, the patient would be transferred to a gurney while the nurse changed the bedding. Each patient got fresh sheets and blankets at least weekly. Occasionally, for comfort, mattresses were turned before remaking the bed.

---

[20] Jessica Holm, Nyman family collection
[21] Minnesota History Center, Ah-gwah-ching Tuberculosis Sanatorium collection

The Thermometer

Your such a fragile little thing
and slender as can be.
Sometimes I can't quite understand
How you mean so much to me
But I can't live without you.
Tho' I have often tried.
For life is not worth living without
You by my side.
Yet you cause me lots of worry
and cost me lots of cash.
Sometimes I'd like to grab you
and smash you all to smash.
But since I've got to have you
I'll try to never kick
For after all, you'll always be
My very own temp. stick.

Actual thermometer and poem from the 1936-37 San scrapbook of Mrs. Ray C. Shelton, from her hospitalization in a Texas sanatorium Scrapbook provided to me by Mrs. Shelton's family

Mornings were busy. After nurses straightened the beds, they gave each patient who did not have bathroom privileges a partial bath and a back rub, and they did the same in the evening. Patients got full bed baths weekly, but those with bathroom privileges bathed without assistance.

Finally, with the morning duties completed, there was time for patients to visit, write letters, work on crafts, or read. For some patients, those activities were too strenuous, so they lay quietly in bed. The doctor made rounds to check on patients, offer encouragement, and spend whatever time was needed to help the sickest patients, those in isolation.

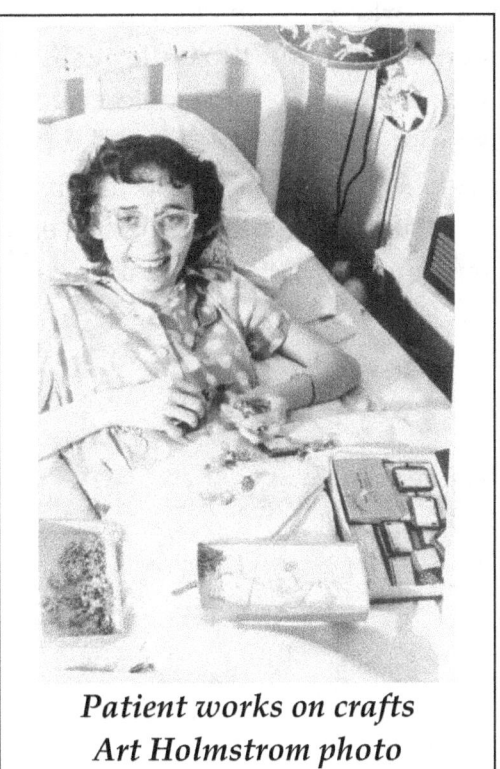

Patient works on crafts
Art Holmstrom photo

At the Lake Julia Tuberculosis Sanatorium, the doctor performed procedures such as artificial pneumothorax to aid in healing the lungs and additionally provided medical care to others in the community, simply because there was a need. The San did not initially have the equipment to take X-rays, so patients who needed them were transported to other medical facilities. Travel was not easy for the patients.

The doctor was often occupied and would miss some meals or eat on the go. Physicians could never count on regular meal times or work hours. For the patients, dinner—which I call "lunch"—was at noon, followed by rest time from 1-3 p.m. At 3 p.m., patients again received basins and washcloths. Suppertime—which I call "dinner"—was around 5 p.m. and then there was time for other activities until lights went out at 9 p.m. To help the patients relax for sleep, they were allowed to listen to their radios on headphones until 10 p.m.[22]

Nurses and doctors wore gowns when they worked with patients, and they often wore masks. They thoroughly and frequently washed their hands. Before going into the dining room, they changed uniforms so that they would not transfer

---

[22] Minnesota History Center, Ah-gwah-ching Tuberculosis Sanatorium Collection

germs. When they went for coffee or before going back onto the patient floors, they changed again. The doctor's evenings were busy with paperwork and visiting the sickest patients, sometimes spending the night at a patient's bedside.

Dr. Mary started her day early with quick rounds. Employees were already busy working in the kitchen and laundry, so she would stop by to check on them when she entered the building. Then she would have a quick bite to eat and do paperwork. Jim Ghostley described the mail sack that was frequently delivered to his mother by the little Puposky post office. "It was a huge canvas bag with brass buckles across the top and a belt that went through them. Chest X-rays from all over usually filled it. Doctors often mailed the X-rays to her to ask her opinion by a written report, then they took the credit."

Chapter 7
Dr. Laney Makes Changes

The swift turnover of doctors at Lake Julia continued. W. L. Mattick stayed from January through July 1918, then E. C. Davis was there for the next five months. When W. H. Fortin took over, it looked like the San finally had a doctor who planned to stay; but he arrived in December 1918 and left in May 1921. W. E. Byington was next, but he left after only five months. [23]

In 1920, the doctor's residence, a log house, was built, but no one moved in.

Dr. Neal, who had arrived with his wife, superintendent Margaret Neal, was officially admitted as a patient on February 24, 1920, by Dr. Fortin.[24] Soon after, Mrs. Neal left for Wisconsin to care for her ailing mother. She returned in the spring and rented a house in Puposky, but did not go back to her position as superintendent of the San.

The facility sorely needed a physician who would commit to staying, and it needed a new superintendent as well. That's when the board hired a physician to fill both roles. It was a turning point for the struggling San.

In October 1921, Dr. R. L. Laney, a recovered TB patient, arrived as superintendent, along with his wife, Joan. They were the first to occupy the log house that still stands. Dr. Laney earned $350 per month and later received a $50 increase. His wife, Joan, made $70 per month as a housekeeper.

Laney was anxious to put his many plans into effect. First, he had to deal with a typhoid epidemic.[25] On January 4, 1922, Dr. Homer Neal, who was still a patient at the San, died of typhoid fever. Then, in April, Laney diagnosed 13-year-old patient Agnes Lindstrom with typhoid fever. She had entered the San six months earlier. She died the day after Christmas of the same year. Alice Beck and Joseph Zeleznecker were admitted three days apart in June 1921. Both contracted typhoid fever. Laney discharged Zeleznecker on April 6, 1922, his right

---

[23] Minnesota History Center, Lake Julia Tuberculosis Sanatorium, Ann Ethen Statistical Report
[24] Minnesota History Center, Lake Julia Tuberculosis Sanatorium Patient Register
[25] Mnsans.com/lake_julia_sanatorium.html

foot paralyzed following his bout with typhoid. Beck contracted a severe case of the disease, and the doctor transferred her to the hospital on March 5, 1923.[26]

Laney had to do something. He examined the possibilities. Was the food supply contaminated? The water supply? The San had begun pumping lake water into the facility when the well malfunctioned. If the water was contaminated, Laney had to consider several possible causes. Was the sewage-disposal system polluting the lake? Was there a decaying animal in the water? Had contaminated trash been disposed of in Lake Julia?

The doctor finally traced the epidemic to a male patient who did not have active typhoid but who was a carrier. A carrier can shed the typhoid bacteria from stool, urine, or wounds. The disease can survive in the gallbladder, and even if it does not cause symptoms, it can infect others. To end the spread of typhoid through the water supply, Laney had two new wells drilled.[27]

One of Dr. Laney's young patients was Eriga Hallisch, who entered the San on May 4, 1925, at age 15. Eriga said, "The doctor blocked off one area in front of the San with chairs so that the girls could have privacy to sunbathe as part of their treatment." Sun therapy was called heliotherapy.[28]

Eriga had emigrated from Germany at age three with her parents, who settled south of the Falls in Ericsburg. She had a small spot of tuberculosis on the top of each lung. Eriga said this about her stay: "The windows were open all night for fresh air, and it was freezing."

Staying at the San was Eriga's first time away from home. "I had a lot of fun there," Eriga told me more than 80 years after her stay. You can read more about Eriga Hallisch in Chapter 43.

In the early days of the San, patients worked outside in the frigid winter weather, even when they had a fever. They often chopped wood. The San purchased toboggans from Bemidji Hardware, and the patients went sledding.[29] Outdoor activities were all, supposedly, to aid in recovery. Then patients went back to bed in their cold rooms next to open windows, even when the

---

[26] Minnesota History Center, Lake Julia Tuberculosis Sanatorium Patient Register
[27] *The Bemidji Pioneer*, John Eggers, October 1, 2017
[28] *The Bemidji Pioneer*, John Eggers, October 1, 2017
[29] Minnesota History Center, Lake Julia Tuberculosis Sanatorium, Expense Report

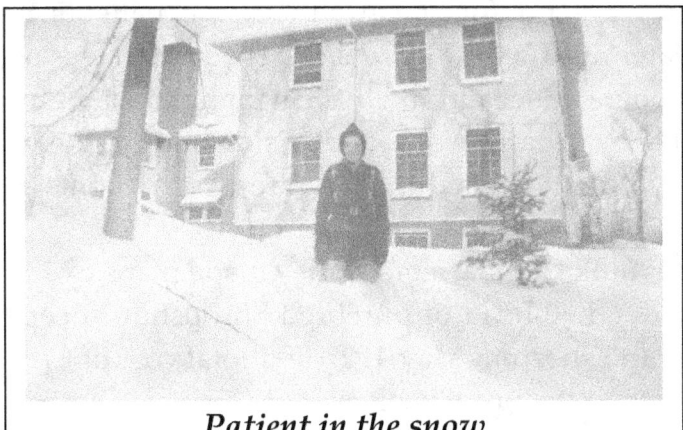

Patient in the snow
James Ghostley collection

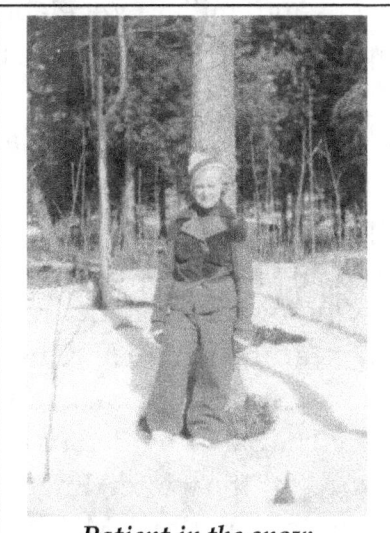

Patient in the snow
James Ghostley collection

temperatures were far below freezing. The cold was hard on employees, too, as they tended to patients in wards that felt like iceboxes.

In the spring, the San constructed a nurses' home for the female staff members, which provided more room in the sanatorium to house the growing number of patients.

ଓଞ୍ଚ

When Laney arrived, he planned to clear land and purchase livestock. Because his goal was to make the place self-sufficient, like Ah-gwah-ching, he convinced the board to purchase 120 additional acres.

He replaced an old icehouse with a modern garage that had offices upstairs. Workers cleared land for farming, and they built a greenhouse. Laney and his staff grew a vegetable garden, flower gardens, and hay crops. Flowers to provide pleasant surroundings for both patients and staff soon decorated the area that surrounded the San. In winter, the gardener kept walkways clear of snow, and he shoveled a path from the log house to the San.

Laney's hard work and vision meant the San eventually produced almost everything it needed to take care of its patients and employees. With 1,500 tomato plants, the San was able to sell tomatoes in Bemidji. It grew cabbage, cauliflower, beets, turnips, radishes, and lettuce to feed patients and staff. Additionally, it grew potatoes, rutabagas, and carrots and stored them in a reinforced concrete root house with removable bins. Laney also took responsibility for growing alfalfa, clover, and millet. Vegetables were good for the health of the patients and employees and were a necessity later during the Depression. The garden was near the public access to Lake Julia. To operate the laundry, the San pumped water from the lake near the root cellar. Laney's hard work and vision meant the San eventually produced almost everything it needed to take care of its patients and employees.

At that time, the San bought milk from farmers. Laney made plans to add a dairy herd, and he had already added 30 head of purebred Shropshire sheep to help clear the land. He registered the sheep in May 1927 at a total cost of $12. A new barn housed them, and Laney had the property fenced.

The San provided its heat, and in 1926, workers cut and laid down 650 cords of wood for the winter. Engberg's Electrical sold the facility a generating plant that year.[30] Rodney (Bob) Maher, neighbor and former San employee, told me, "The San initially burned wood but eventually had coal delivered by the railcar load. There were tracks with a spur down to the lake west of the San." The plant provided plenty of electricity to run the San and its outbuildings and houses, to pump water for the laundry, and to operate an X-ray machine, with energy to spare.

Laney realized that some homes were crowded or lacked ventilation and that some families either did not have enough food to provide proper nourishment, or they knew more about how to feed their hogs and cattle than how to feed their children. Undernourishment showed up often at clinics in Beltrami and the adjacent counties.

Examination of the malnourished children the San took in showed that some of them had tuberculosis. Laney hoped to establish a preventorium where undernourished children could receive treatment to build up resistance and avoid contracting the disease.

---

[30] Minnesota History Center, Lake Julia Tuberculosis Sanatorium, Expense Report

Laney never did open a preventorium, but he did start a school for children who were patients. The Beltrami County School Board provided supervision. Marie Garrison taught briefly in September 1925, then again for six months beginning in October 1926. She earned $50 per month.

Her 12-year-old daughter, Sylvia, had been admitted with asthma in June 1921 and was a patient for six months. Marie had been a patient twice, once in 1922 and again in 1923.[31] Many San employees had previously been patients.

Others who taught at the San were Isabel Quinn, 1927; Mabel Thorpe, 1928; and Mabel McGinty, 1928.[32]

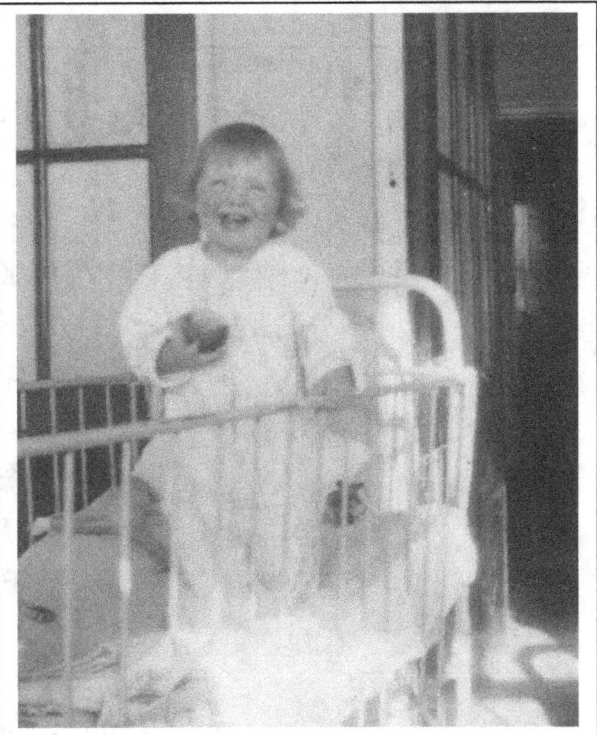

*A young child at the San
James Ghostley collection*

The community supported Laney's ambitious work. Because there was no outside entertainment for the patients, the *Bemidji Sentinel* and *Bemidji Pioneer* donated radios and earphones for every bed. Patients liked to listen to the Bemidji Boys' Band concerts and other broadcasts.

Nurses and patients learned sewing, dressmaking, and other handicrafts from an instructor who spent three weeks training them. Learning crafts not only helped the patients keep busy, but it taught them skills that they could use to get a job when they left.[33]

Dr. Laney got the San off to a good start, but then he notified the board that he planned to resign. It wasn't easy, however, to find a replacement.

---

[31] Minnesota History Center, Lake Julia Tuberculosis Sanatorium, Patient Register
[32] Louis Marchand, *A History of the Rural Schools of Beltrami County*, 2006
[33] *North Country History*, Vol. 4, No. 48, Hilda Rachuy

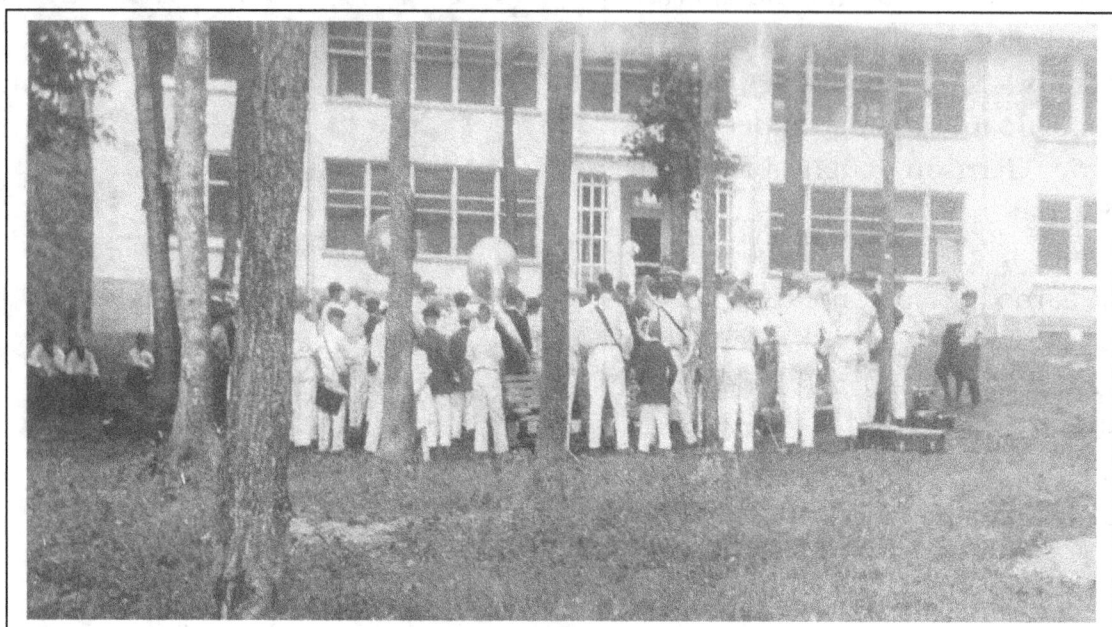

*The Bemidji Boys' Band
entertaining the patients
James Ghostley collection*

Chapter 8
The Lomen Sisters

It wasn't uncommon for several members of the same family to be stricken with tuberculosis. Three of the daughters of T. J. and Anna Lomen of Solway—Clara, Inga, and Teresa (Tres)—were admitted to the San with the disease between 1925 and 1928.[34] During that time, patients had memory books, like autograph books, which they passed around to write encouraging greetings to each other. The memory books of both Clara and Inga became family keepsakes.

Clara Lomen went into the San on August 2, 1925, at age 19. Her sister Inga Lomen was admitted on March 4, 1927, also at age 19.

Clara died at the San September 7, 1927, at age 21. Clara's and Inga's sister Tres entered the San on May 6, 1928, at age 18. Even though Clara died at the San, Tres said, "I wasn't afraid because I didn't believe I had TB." Tres went home Christmas Day, 1928, after 234 days.[35]

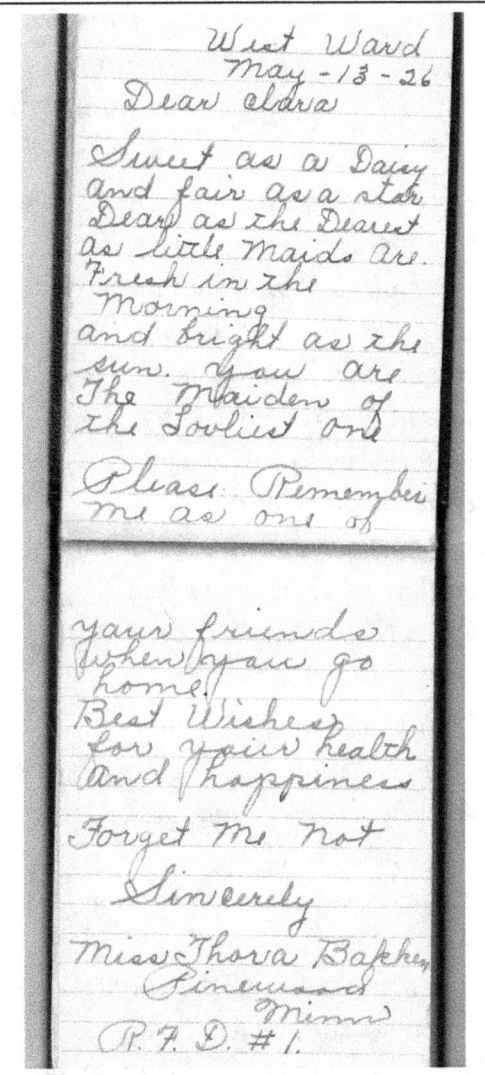

Thora Bakken, formerly a patient and then a nurse and X-ray tech at the Lake Julia Tuberculosis Sanatorium. Clara Lomen's memory book, David Grande collection

---

[34] Minnesota History Center, Lake Julia Tuberculosis Sanatorium, Patient Register
[35] Minnesota History Center, Lake Julia Tuberculosis Sanatorium, Patient Register

**Clara wrote this in
her own memory book:**

"Nothing's richer, brings more joys
Than friendships true and sweet
And in this book I wish to find
The names of friends I chance to meet."

☙❧

"April 5, 1926, North Porch
Dear Clara,
Your smile as I pass your doorway
Makes my day much brighter;
Your cheerful, kindly, helping words
Make my heart seem lighter
Pleasure I've felt in knowing you,
Perhaps I have no sign.
Your friendship lives close to my heart.
For always – Friend 'o Mine
Nevis, Minn. 'Red' Thorpe"

☙❧

"Dear Clara:
Clara was a dark-haired girl
With cheeks of red, and eyes of brown.
Who set our hearts in a whirl
And never was seen with a frown.

From me to you, a friend-ship true
Hath tenderly wended its way.
And in years to come, when I am blue
I will think of my San friend, & then be gay.
To one of the sweetest girls I know
These true blue lines I dedicate,
Hoping that when from the San you go,
On <u>me</u> you will sometimes meditate.
Clara L. Olson, Blackduck, Minn."

ଚ୬୧୦

"April 5, 1926 North Porch
In your book of memories
I'll be glad to take part,
For I wish to be remembered
By one as true as your 'dear heart'

Forget not our confidential task sublime
You told your experiences
And I told mine.
And you would say, 'O, don't hurry away.'
I'd answer, 'Don't you know the bell rang
I can't stay.'

Remember how the cure we took with the rule
We'd obey the Doctor and nurses
Like the teacher at school,
To chase T.B. is our main work.
And in this nothing we must shirk.

Clara dear I expect we'll be together here
For some time but when we leave the San,
And leave our bugs behind
Send your letter to this place & <u>me</u> it will find –
Mrs. E. R. Wall, Park Rapids, Minn."

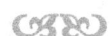

"I'm thinking of you dear,
As every day I do
For knowing you has made
The whole world over new.
May every day's joyous cheers,
Make your day glad all thru
As mine are all the year
With happy tho't of you
**Your Swede Sister of Rebeccahs,
Louise Bostrom, Eveleth, Minn., Lodge no. 224, Bootsie"**

○₈○

"Dear Clara,
Will write a few lines in your memory book. I expect to go home soon, and I want you to remember me. Of all the Dear Friends I met at the San, I will always remember your cheerful face, always a smile no matter how sick you are and never a frown. I hope it won't be long before you will be well and can go home. I wish you happiness and perfect health.
Your Friend Mrs. K. Tuttle,
Bagley, Minn."

○₈○

"May 9, 1926
Just being happy is a fine thing to do;
Looking on the bright side rather than the blue;
Sad or sunny musing is largely in the choosing.
And just being happy is brave work and true.
Please remember me as one of your friends.
Pearl Seado, Bemidji, Minn."
(This was during Pearl's second admission. She later became a nurse at the San.)

○₈○

"How well I remember the first time I seen you, you were just a little girl with eyes so bright. Neer did we dream that at the 'San' we would be. Happy we'll be when we can go to our homes once more and work and play like we used to. O, won't it be fun. Een work will seem like pleasure. But when you to your home do go, remember me as a friend.
Mrs. Mary Waldron, Wilton, Minn."

○₈○

"North Porch, June 7, 1926
Out of the troubles I have had have come my richest friendships here. Kind hands have helped to bear my care, kind words have fallen on my ear; An' so I say when trouble comes I know before the storm shall end that I shall find my bit of care has also brought to me a friend. I'm wishing you the best-est of everything, my dear, and please remember and drop me a line.
Friend Mae Frazer, Big Fork, Minnesota"

And a long note from her sister Inga:
"If the sun persists in shining
Tho' the body's feeling blue,
If the leaves turn red and golden
Tho' the rain is falling too;
If the water keeps on sparkling
Tho' the reeds obstruct the view;
If your friends all keep on smiling
Tho' their aches and pains they rue –
Why, what's the use of worrying?
I wouldn't if I were you!

If the doctor persists in teasing,
'Stead of answering what you ask
If your one little <u>pint</u> of milk
Seems just like a <u>cask</u>;
If you get uncomfortable hot
When you lay in the sun and bask, -
Why just remember this, my dear –
That very thing's <u>your task</u>.

If you got too many callers
When you merely want <u>some</u>;
If they were all entire strangers,
Why the thing you should have done
Was just to make each one feel
As if he was 'the one,'
And you were glad <u>he</u> came
Tho' none of the others had come.
If you're tired of eating cabbage,
Apricots, peaches & ham
Why, you'd better be tickled to pieces
That you're eating what you am.
Of course some pork would taste good
And maybe some strawberry jam,
But I'll bet if <u>you</u> were the poor old cook,

You'd feel like saying, 'Dam!'

Of course I'm not so hardboiled
As my verses seem to say –
What I really mean to tell you
In an optimistic way
Is to follow Doctor's orders
And to pray to God each day.
"I.A.L." (Inga Adelia Lomen, Clara's sister)

Inga had worked as a teacher. After her May 9, 1927 release from the San,[36] she took nurses' training at Nopeming Tuberculosis Sanatorium near Duluth, then worked at Lake Julia Sanatorium.

Inga's mother died in November 1929, so she quit her job to go home and take care of her younger siblings. When two of her younger sisters took over the household duties, Inga worked as a nurse at Ah-gwah-ching Sanatorium.

While working at Lake Julia, Inga met my uncle, Louis Grande, who had replaced my father as a janitor at the San. Louis and Inga later married, making Inga my aunt. She was one of many of my relatives who were employees or patients at the San.

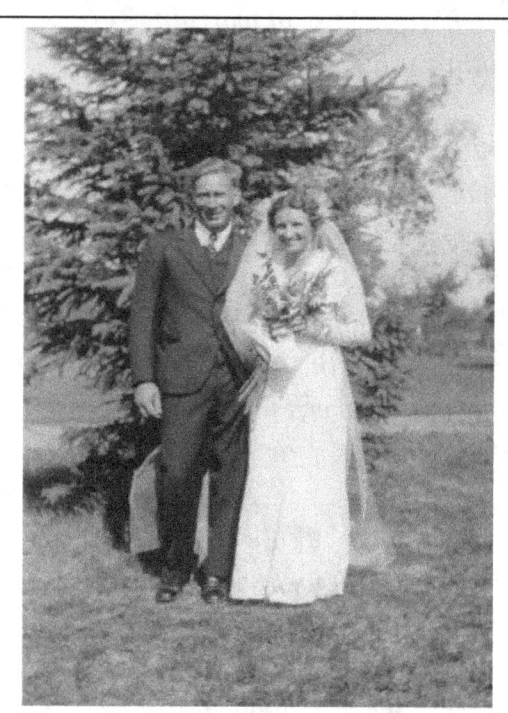

My uncle Louis Grande weds former San patient Inga Lomen.
Ella Hedglin collection

---

[36] Minnesota History Center, Lake Julia Tuberculosis Sanatorium, Patient Register

When I visited Tres Lomen, she told me about the time she had spent at the San: "Inga suggested that I, too, take nurses' training. I trained one year at Nopeming Sanatorium, as Inga had done. I wanted to complete the three-year nursing course at the hospital, but because I'd had TB and had a spot on one lung,

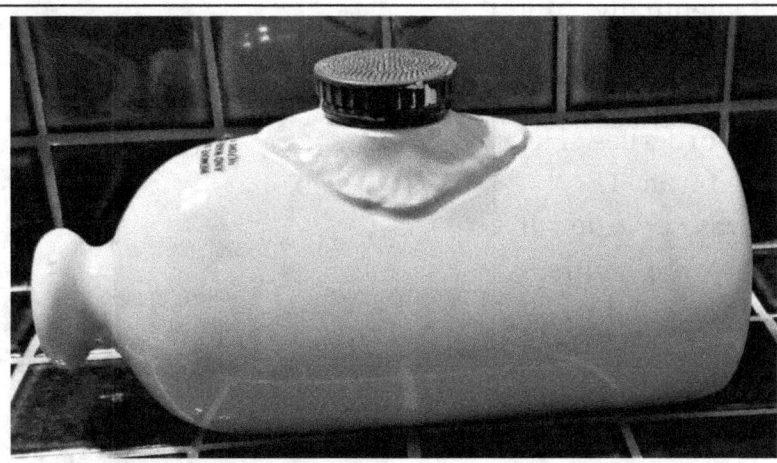

A stoneware "pig" like those used at the San, filled with hot water to warm the patients
Pat Nelson photo

I was not allowed to work in a hospital; I could only work as a nurse in a TB sanatorium. I went to work at Lake Julia in October 1930 as a floor nurse earning $60 per month.[37] Even though I had not been allowed to take the three-year nursing program at the hospital, I did the same work as an RN, including dispensing medications.

"Twice per shift," Tres said, "nurses were required to carry heavy trays of glazed vessels filled with hot water to warm the patients in their beds. The containers were called 'pigs.' The snout-like handles on the jugs gave them a pig-like appearance, hence their name." San records showed that the San purchased the stoneware jars from the same place it bought milk bottles, Merrill, Greer & Chapman.

---

[37] Minnesota History Center, Lake Julia Tuberculosis Sanatorium, Patient Register

"When people died at the San," Tres said, "we nurses had to 'get them ready.' That," she said, "included washing the deceased patients and plugging their openings with cotton.

"The pay was better at Nopeming, so eventually, my friends talked me into working there. That's where I met Arne Lien, one of the orderlies. He, too, had recovered from TB.

"There was a rule at Nopeming that the nurses couldn't date other employees. The head nurse reprimanded me. I said, 'What I do on my own time is my own business.' I decided that must have been OK because the staff gave me a wedding shower, and the head nurse attended."

Like many of the patients who had recovered from TB, Tres Lomen lived a long life, passing away at 101.

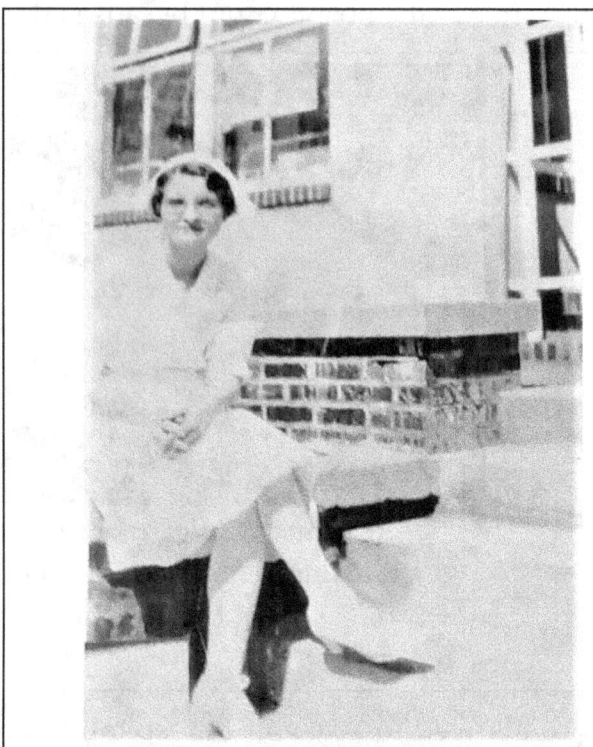

Tres Lomen
Ella Hedglin collection

Section Three: Dr. Mary Chapman Ghostley

Chapter 9
The Unstoppable Mary

Mary Madison Chapman was born on August 1, 1881, in Frost Village, Quebec, Canada, the second child of Catherine Ross and John Chapman. Anna was the oldest child. Then there were siblings Mary, Margaret (Peggy), Don, Henry, and Merrill. Their father, a farmer and railroad worker, had moved the family to South Dakota in the 1890s, where they bought a small farm. Later they moved to Minnesota, near Glencoe.[38]

As Mary reached adulthood, she turned heads with her slender waist and long, shiny hair that she often wore pinned up on her head or topped with a stylish hat. She was beautiful, smart, courageous, and confident.

Mary's parents had taught her not to let unreasonable ideas and stereotypes keep her from reaching her goals. Her father loved to tell her about another John Chapman, better known as Johnny Appleseed, who planted apple nurseries everywhere he went. Mary didn't see why she, too, could not make a name for herself by doing something great, and she refused to let being a female stop her.[39]

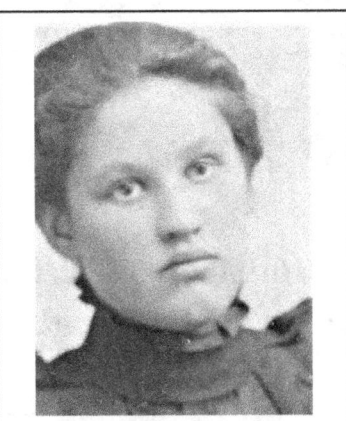

Mary Madison Chapman
James Ghostley collection

---

[38] James Ghostley interview
[39] James Ghostley interview

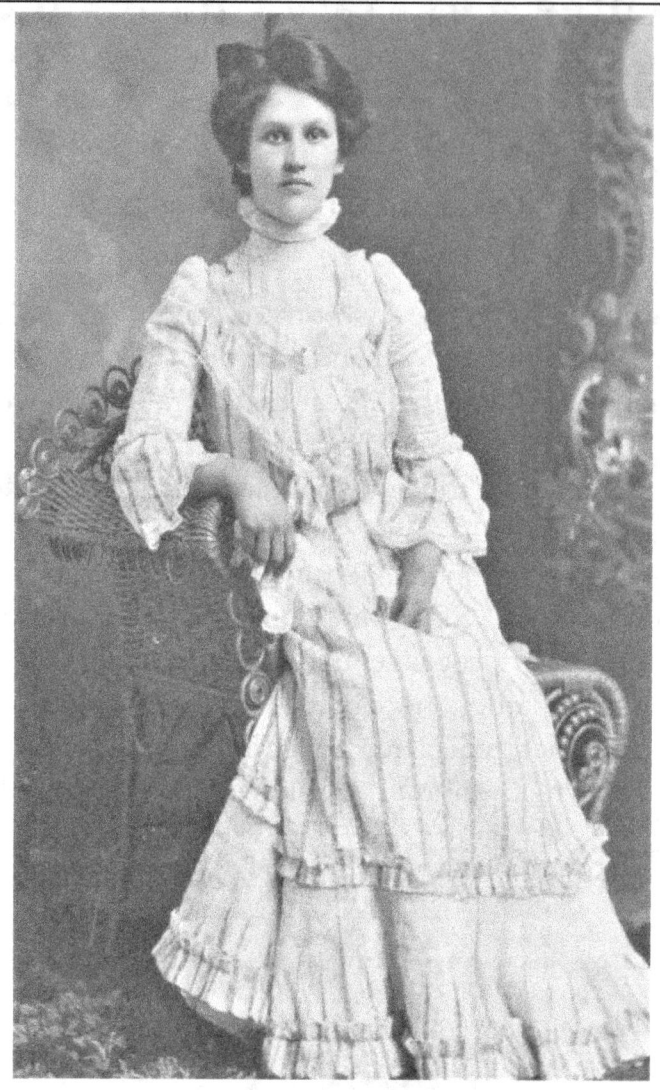

The beautiful Mary Madison Chapman
James Ghostley collection

Mary's parents believed in the value of a good education. At a time when many could not graduate from high school, Mary not only graduated but also went on to receive her teaching certificate.

She taught school at Glencoe, and during that time, her brother Henry became ill. She wished she could do something to help him, and that's when she became interested in health care. She decided to save the money she earned

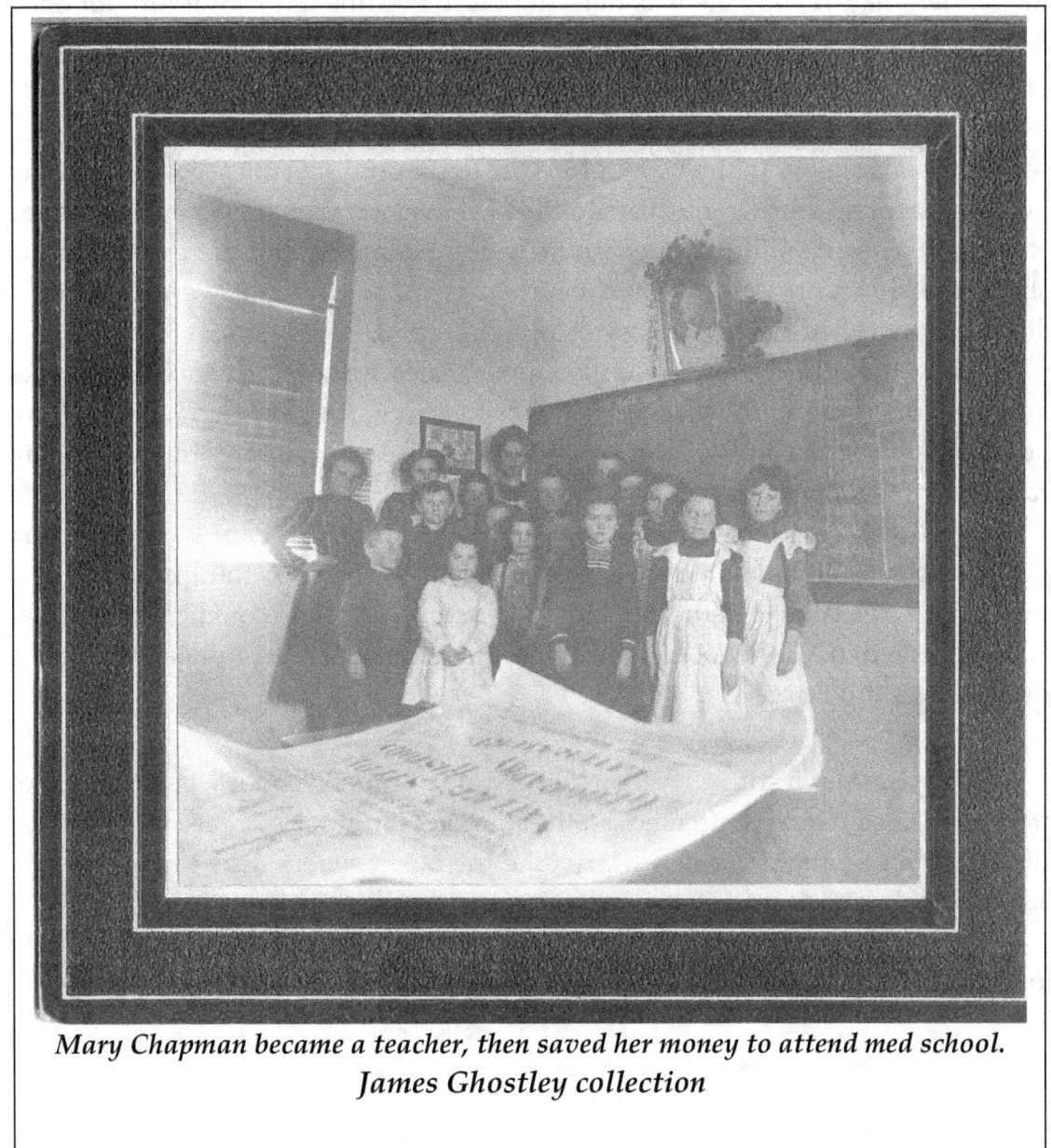

Mary Chapman became a teacher, then saved her money to attend med school. James Ghostley collection

teaching to attend medical school, even though she knew people would fuss about a woman wanting to become a doctor.

In 1906, when Mary had saved enough money, she enrolled at Hamline University in St. Paul to pursue her goal. Word spread quickly. It couldn't have been easy for her to endure the ridicule of townspeople. She heard comments like, "Mary Chapman, you're a witch!" and, "Girls shouldn't study medicine!" The rude words reminded her of earlier days when some people had criticized her independent nature, but she was determined to become a doctor. "I'm not one to let *talk* bother me," she told her brothers.[40]

◦°◦

Hamline was Minnesota's oldest university and one of the first coeducational colleges in the U.S. In 1854, its first home was the second floor of the Red Wing general store in the Territory of Minnesota, which became a state four years later. When Hamline opened, there were 73 students, but there was no actual college division until 1857. In the beginning, most students were children or adolescents enrolled in the primary or preparatory departments.

Even though it was unpopular for females to gain advanced education, Hamline's first graduating class, in 1859, consisted entirely of two women, Emily and Elizabeth Sorin. They were not only Hamline's first graduates but also the first graduates of any college or university in Minnesota.

The Red Wing location closed in 1869. Hamline's St. Paul location opened in September 1880, but in 1883, University Hall burned to the ground. Eleven months later, the college dedicated a new structure. In 1895, a medical department was established in Minneapolis when Hamline took over the Minneapolis College of Physicians and Surgeons.[41]

◦°◦

Mary caused a stir in 1906 on her first day of med school when she walked into a class filled mostly with men. At the sound of laughter, her face radiated heat, but she didn't let that stop her. Mary, like the Sorin sisters, was unwilling to let society hold her back, and she was determined to follow in their footsteps.

Mary disregarded those who thought she shouldn't be there. Soon the other students saw how capable and determined she was, and most accepted her.

---

[40] James Ghostley interview
[41] Hamline.edu/history

The beautiful Mary, with her dark hair, hazel eyes, and strong determination, immediately captivated one male student. His name was Fred Ghostley, and he was from Anoka, in Hennepin County. He was born Frederick James Ghostley on July 8, 1888, to Frank Ghostley, from England, and Catherine Tucker Ghostley, a Minnesota native.

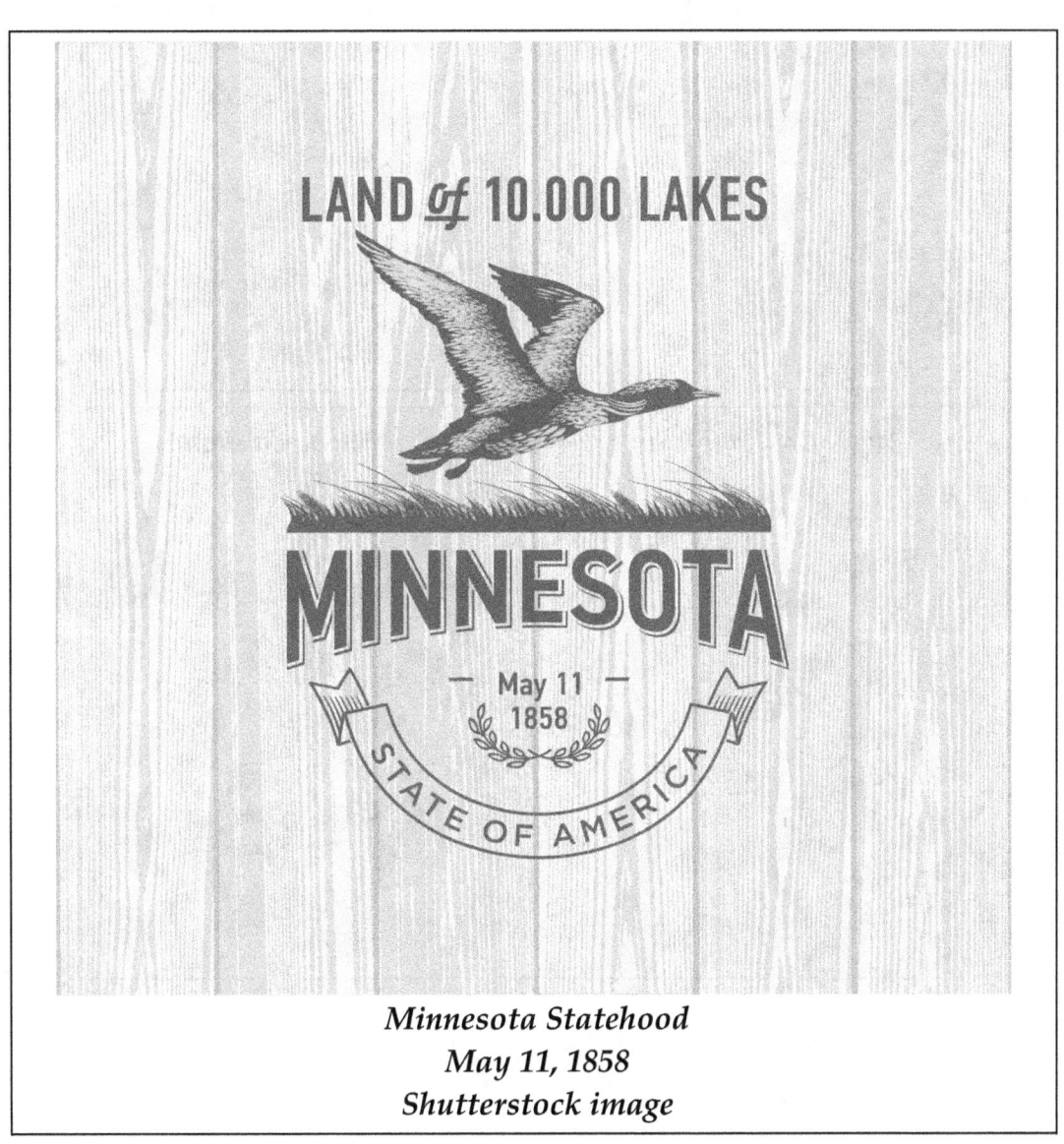

Minnesota Statehood
May 11, 1858
Shutterstock image

April 11, 1906, from Mary Chapman to Fred Ghostley

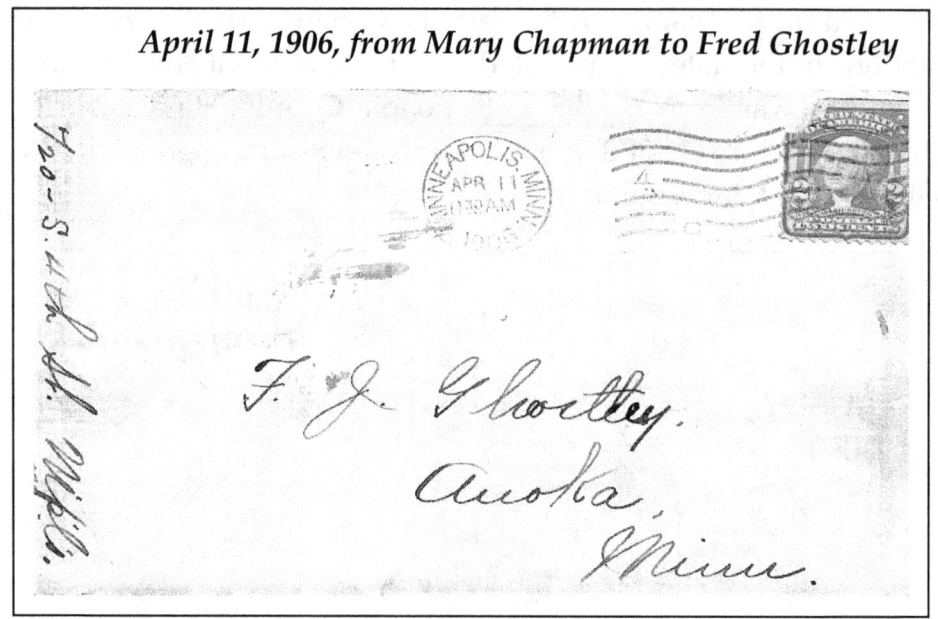

August 2, 1906 from Fred Ghostley to Mary Chapman

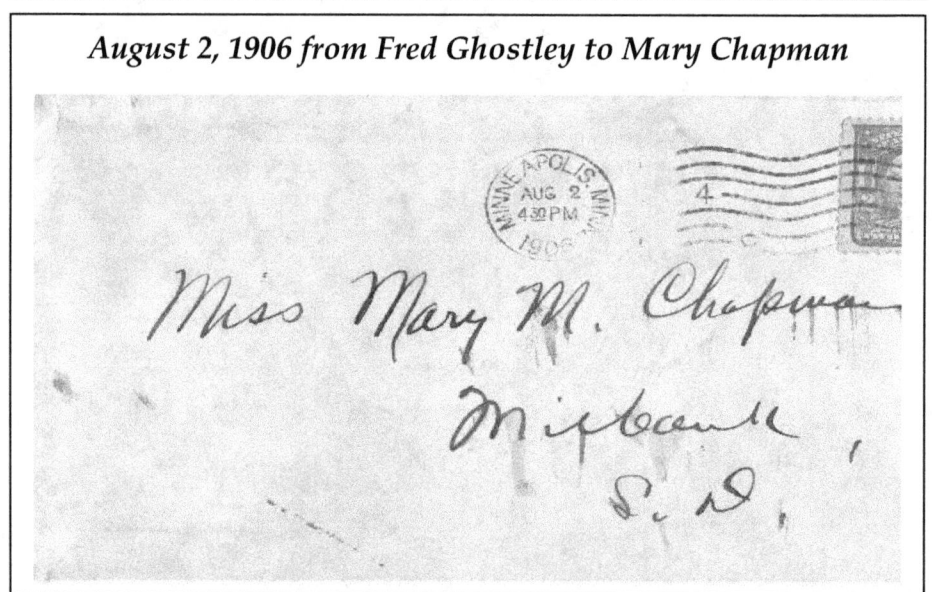

Chapter 10
Love Letters

Soon Mary and Fred began to write letters to each other whenever they were apart, and after a short time, they fell in love.

It's this correspondence that allows me to hear the voices of Mary Chapman and Fred Ghostley nearly 115 years later. Grammar, word usage, and spelling change over time, as you may notice in their letters.

The missives began when Fred Ghostley came down with an illness and decided to leave school to recover at home in Anoka. Mary missed Fred, and she wrote her first letter to him on April 10, 1906. In the letter, "ever-honest-Mary" confessed that she had sat up in front near classmate Beardsley, Fred's roommate, during a quiz and had cheated for the first time. However, she didn't feel too much remorse, as she later enjoyed watching baseball from an upper window on campus for an hour.

I was interested in reading about things Mary did in her spare time. She wrote about the time she and her friend Mrs. Monahan went into the damp, wooded areas at Minnehaha to collect bloodroot, a spring wildflower long known as a Native American cure-all. They planned to gather the roots

Excerpt from Mary's letter to Fred
James Ghostley collection.

and rhizomes for medicinal uses. The juice was known to be good for coughs and sore throats, as well as being beneficial for skin conditions. In case they got hungry, they planned to fill their pockets with bread and butter.

"*Professor Dunn told us that we are the most brilliant class he has ever had,*" Mary proudly reported in her letter.

She didn't want Fred to get behind on his schoolwork, so she told him that she and classmate Mr. Baird had made him "*a regular art gallery of slides*" in his absence. "*It may puzzle you to decide whether they are calves foot jelly, lemon pies or embryology specimens,"* Mary teased, *"but to a genius of your penetration that will be mere play."*

Fred replied promptly on April 12, *"The servant of the U.S. could not have brought me a happier and better message. The absent member feels very grateful to you for making specimens for him."*

During Fred's recuperation, he read *Autobiography of a Quack* by Dr. S. Weir Mitchell; *Light of Asia* by Sir Edwin Arnold; and *Law of the Land* by a naturalist and former editor of *Field and Stream.* He was a voracious reader and often quoted from works he had read.

He believed he was getting better, and that the influenza was gone, but he still had a bad cough and nasal and bronchial catarrh. He hoped to return to school Sunday, and he had plans to call Mary that day. He signed the letter formally: *"Very Sincerely Yours, Fred J. Ghostley."*

Fred again wrote on the 22nd. Since talking to Mary by phone Friday, he had read over the muscles. *"The various muscles of the back seem to attach to so many different places from the transverse processes of the upper six dorsal vertebrae to the transverse processes of the cervical vertebrae from the 2nd to the 6th inclusive."* He didn't yet feel that he knew them well enough.

He had missed the Phi Rho Sigma banquet two weeks prior but wasn't sure he cared. Even though he was a member of a Greek fraternity, he did not approve of secret societies.

Common sense told Fred he would see Mary the next day, and he had received her letter the day before. Still, he was lonesome, so he spent a pleasant hour writing her.

He wrote on May 6, *"I feel about all right except my throat is sore, and I have simple Erythema (a rash caused by gastro-intestinal infection) which itches. My excess of temperature is all gone. Expect to get down tomorrow afternoon."*

On May 21, Fred was again ill with a temperature of 101. He returned home, where he saw the doctor. By afternoon, he did not have a fever, and the doctor told him he would be all right in a day. He expressed to Mary that Anoka was a miserable town to him: *"No place will ever seem good without you, 'dear.'"* The relationship continued to blossom as he called Mary *"Honey"* and signed the letter, *"With love, Your aff. Fred."*

His frequent illnesses sometimes brought his spirits down, and he left this note: *"In the event of my death I want a ring (value $100) to be given to Mary M. Chapman."* Signed: *"F. J. Ghostley."* Had he purchased a ring for Mary? There was no further mention of the ring in his letters.

Fred had read 45 pages of *Evolution of Man*. He hoped to see Mary the next day.

For the first time in his letters, he called Mary *"Little Girl,"* which became his pet nickname for her.

Note from Fred in the event of his death
James Ghostley collection

He complained about the brassy phonograph across the street. It gave off *"sound waves with large amplitudes."* He didn't think anyone should force their neighbors to *"join their war dance."*

After spending a few days back in Minneapolis, Fred was again in Anoka on June 4. Mary wrote that she had forgotten her key and had locked herself out the night before. He wished he had been there to help her.

When she received his letter, Mary realized she liked his nickname for her, *"Little Girl,"* so, in her next one, she playfully called him *"Little Boy."* She took the teasing one step further: *"How does the infant feel about his exams?"*

"Dear little mother, she's lonely but won't admit it," Mary wrote. *"Margaret will be with her from this time on, so she won't mind my being away. I fancy I soon will be getting a homesick spell and packing a little box for the 'Land of the Dacotahs' before long."* She signed the letter, *"Lovingly yours, Mary—720 S. 4th St."*

Fred next wrote that *"no place will ever seem good without you 'dear.' You don't know how much good it did me to see you this morning."*

He wrote again on June 6. *"The walking is not as good as it was last week, of course. Up here, I am compelled to go all by my lonesome. Last week in Minneapolis—well, you know how well I liked my company. You worried me talking about packing your trunk so soon. Don't you run off for 2 or 3 weeks anyway. If you really intend to go soon, I shall probably come down Sunday morning, for I want to see you sometime, at least, before you leave.*

"Only because I believe the crooked marks which I make upon the paper make the letter of value to you do I dare to write you on this 'Frat' paper. Truly, I do not like to use it. It seems that I am ostentatious. I do not wish to publish the fact that I am a Phi Rho Sigma member. However you know that I do not. I can't find any other paper; and I must write to you this morning. I received your letter 3-K Wednesday evening—and the last one yesterday. It is needless for me to tell you that I was glad to hear from you—always am, and you know it."

He wrote more the same day: "And my dear Woman, we shall see many things from the same viewpoint. I shall put my arm around you and press you close to my side, and we shall lovingly and tenderly show each other what the other does not see. For I know that I love you; and I know that you love me; and I know that we both look for the best."

Mary teased Fred in her letter of June 7, trying to make him jealous. She had just attended graduation ceremonies. "Mr. Taft was an usher. We had an excellent seat, rest assured. Mr. Grover sat on my right. We held hands between acts."

She promised not to go home without giving Fred due warning. After signing the letter, "Lovingly," she wrote, "That's foolish sentiment, is it not? I forget that I ought to be sensible and that you carry my effusions around carelessly and might easily lose them."

Fred wrote on June 8: "I am lonesome for you most of the time. I see your face, hear your voice, and think of you in most everything. Dear Heart, know that I love you better than all else in the world."

He offered quotes from Omar and Plato, then continued, "Mary, I love you because of some inward spiritual thing, your kind soul and smart womanly face. I carry your letters around with me, but not carelessly. If anybody ever troubled to read any of my correspondence—events would be unpleasant."

Mary promptly responded, "I received your letter tonight, and you don't know how happy it made me.

"Was I the least bit lonely for you? Ah, so often, I think of you, and it seems to me I would give just anything to have you put your arm around me and look down at me in your dear, kind way."

Fred next wrote Sunday, the 10th. "When I am outdoors all day and entirely removed from thots of books, study and writing it is very hard to write at all connected. Even now, the dog is trying to push the tablet off my knees so that I will pet him. (I am sitting down on the grass under some trees.) I have had a very good time the last 3 or 4 days and think I have grown stronger too."

Fred left his home in Anoka at 2:30 p.m. Friday for the three-hour ride to the family farm with a cousin. The corn was barely coming up. Some wasn't even planted yet because of water standing in the fields. The wettest, one of about 20 acres, had been planted to potatoes and was nearly underwater.

That night, he had gone to bed listening to a wolf chorus accompanied by *"a lone, chilly, creeping sensation"* which passed slowly up his spinal column and into his cerebrum, described by him as sounding like the wind sighing thru the pine in a snowstorm.

He awoke Saturday, milked two cows, ate breakfast, planted seeds, then got a small load of corn with the team and wagon in the afternoon.

Sunday morning, he fished in the river, though the water was high. Then, he shot his Winchester rifle for a while.

Fred returned to the river after dinner. Even though his friend, Mr. Hines, caught fish and he did not, Fred gained knowledge of fish anatomy by dissecting out the heart, gills, and large blood vessels of a large dogfish.

He wrote to Mary about superstitions he had heard. One Dutch fellow told him that when the minnows were thick along the shore, the fish would bite. He guessed that this time, the moon must not have been in the right quarter because the fish were not biting. Another man insisted that even though his horse had cataracts, it could see during certain phases of the moon. Fred found that some people only installed fence posts on certain days, and others would choose the best days to butcher, believing the pork would be "more solid." *"It is astonishing the amount of superstition and ignorance prevalent among our common classes."*

On his first day at the farm, he felt *"as lame as an old man of 70 years."*

He ended the letter with this postscript: *"I picked some wild roses walking out to the mail box. I have put 2 or 3 in the letter, but they will not be fresh when they arrive."*

HAMLINE UNIVERSITY
College of Medicine

Dear Mary,—

Everything is of relative value in the world of perfection. Yet—this world of the heart is the highest spiritual ideal world. I have been thinking about you. I feel that I want to speak to you. It is an affair of the heart, too. I find that I do not have anything to write you today

Excerpt, letter from
Fred Ghostley to Mary Chapman
James Ghostley collection

Chapter 11
Growing Closer

On June 20, Fred wrote with a pencil because he had left his pen in Minneapolis for repair. He had read the novel *Faith Doctor* by Eggleston.

Fred was lonely, and he poured out his feelings. *"Dear Heart, I am happy when I am with you. With you I find happy contentment and peace of heart. If it is possible, I love you better every day. Mary, you are all and you are everything to me. I can not get along without you. We must have each other, Dear heart. We should work lovingly hand in hand thru eternal time."*

When Mary wrote on June 21, she told Fred, *"I used to be a 'mopey,' peevish little thing much given to the sulks and possessing less amenable traits than now ... if possible.*

"You have my sincere sympathy inasmuch as Dr. A. heartlessly deprived you of all your pet ailments. You still have recourse to the idea that either you or he is non compos mentis," (not of sound mind).

She wrote again later the same day, saying, *"Yes I know you wanted to stay and I did wish you could, too. I was selfish enough tonight to wish you would come down and work when I read your letter; but I did not wish it long. You know and I do too, that you are far better off where you are. We could not see very much of each other, anyway, and the country is a better place than a stuffy city drugstore to get well in."*

Fred wrote on June 2: *"If I can catch a ride over from the farm to Anoka Thursday (a week), I shall pack my little hand box and climb into the 'auto' bound for Minneapolis.*

"I fear lest you would get lonesome if Miss E. left you Friday evening. Could I be company if I were able to get down on that day?

"I got to imagining yesterday so went over to Dr. Aldrich's and said that I wanted my throat, nose and lungs examined."

Fred continuously worried about his health.

"I am reminded of the men in 'Three Men in a Boat' who had everything but house maid's knee.

"Some doctors are more kind than others. Some will take all those diseases away from you by a process of logical exclusion from real symptoms of health. Others will give you some extra, or rare disease, especially if you have too much money. I did not have the money so had to lose all my ailments.

"I crave your sympathy!"

In Fred's letter of June 23, he discussed his last name. *"I suppose anyone who is 'ghostly' should take kindly to seances, table tipping and various other spirit manifestations. Perhaps we shall be ghostly authorities someday. How can you take kindly to such a 'spooky' name?*

"I shall expect you to own me even if I am tanned to 'sole leather.' Can you begin to imagine what will be expected of you? And do you begin to regret that you spoke out of your heart, instead of from cold reason?"

Mary wrote to Fred the same day. *"Yes, I know I'm horrid. I've just been thinking that perhaps you and I would both be happier if we had never met. Are you shocked? Well, I honestly think it when you are away. I'm truly sorry if I have hurt your feelings."*

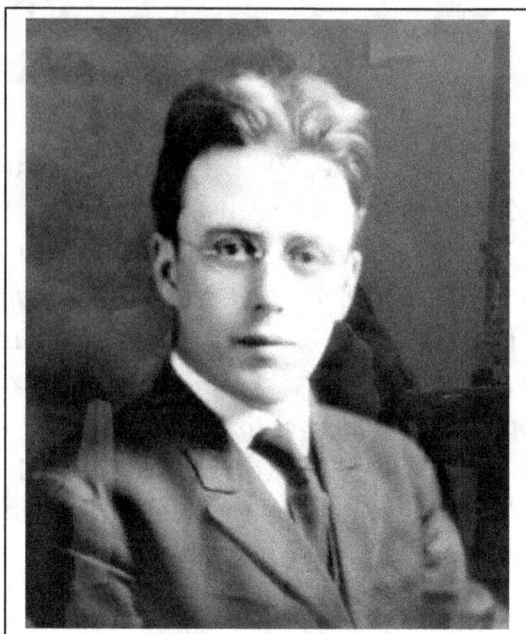

Fred Ghostley
Erin Barthel collection

Fred wrote a second letter to Mary on the same day. *"Mary, I have a plan to propose to you (you didn't think I could propose twice to you). There is a N.P. train which leaves Mpls. For Anoka 8:30 P.M. July 3rd. If you had to work Friday it would go back Friday 6 Klock [sic] A.M. I should like to have you spend July 4th in Anoka with me. My 'Ma' said she would like to have you come up. Now, won't you come, 'Little Girl?'"*

Mary, too, wrote a second letter. *"I wonder if you'll ever forgive me for writing you such a horrid, horrid letter as was my last one. I was sick and had the 'blues'—that isn't any excuse I know …guess the only thing for me is to learn to control my villainous temper.*

"Now about your proposition. I'd 'just love' to go. I wonder if your mother would think it presumptuous, do you suppose? If I went, wouldn't it be better to go on the morning train? I'm sure it would inconvenience if not annoy her to have a stranger there so long."

Mary teased Fred in her letter of June 26. *"Oh, by the way, Mrs. Cowie's folks are at the lake (Minnetonka) and Lew asked yours truly to go there to spend the 'Glorious 4th' with them. I really think I shall go."*

Fred wrote on June 27, *"I received both of your letters last night after I got home. It was the next best thing to getting home and finding you. I want you to always write me* just the way you feel. If you cannot write me 'clouds' as well as 'sunshine' when you feel lonely and sick, I do not justify the trust and affection which you have placed upon me. Mary, I always want you to write me anything you want to. If I were with you, I would talk, laugh, and love you out of those 'blues.'

"A big strong girl like you, partly educated in professional medicine, and 'with a feller' getting a slight attack of hypochondriasis. I shall have to come down if you have them again. This is not a nice way to write either, for you were sick. I am very sorry, for I do love you 'little girl.'

"It is best for you to come up evening of July 3rd. It will not be presumptuous. My 'ma' knows that we intend to practice together some day. There will be no inconvenience."

On June 30, Fred had been reading *The Rubaiyat* from his hammock. "I take the liberty to repeat a few lines," he wrote. Then, he proceeded to fill the letter with those "few" lines.

Mary wrote on July 1, "I have decided to go to Anoka the morning of the Fourth. You may pooh-pooh the conventionalities as much as you please; but I think you will agree with me that my decision is sensible. I would personally prefer the other plan; but under the circumstances I think it wiser to be guided by reason.

"Miss Evarts and I packed a grip with pillows, book, lunch and writing materials and I came out here to the end of the 'Eighth and Central' to have a quiet day. Under the trees a bit back were two wee lassies with a pitcher of really truly milk and a jar of lemonade. We stopped and had a drink. It was very good and quite cold too. Now don't say 'bugs.' They washed their glasses carefully and were as clean and neat as could be and kept their wares carefully covered in a big pan with a chunk of ice."

In Fred's letter of July 2, he expressed: "Was disappointed to learn that you were not coming up until July 4th morning.

"Am feeling very well. Expect to have two teeth filled this afternoon. It means an hour of unpleasantness. A good deal worse than pulling teeth!"

Mary visited Fred in Anoka for the Fourth, and he and his mother talked her into spending the night. On July 7, Fred's mother included a letter to Mary in Fred's envelope:

"My dear Miss Chapman,

"I must write to apologize for giving you an old night-gown. I was so astonished when I went upstairs and saw I had given you that old thing. I had forgotten it was in the drawer with the others and took it by mistake. I will try and give you a better one next time.

"I hope your cold is better.

"Lovingly yours, Catherine Ghostley"

Mary wrote Fred on July 8, "*I thoroughly enjoyed being there, more I'm afraid, than your people did having me there. I should not have staid [sic] over if your mother had not said 'Fred tells me you are to be my daughter some day; and I want you to stay so that we can get acquainted.' Then she wished me happiness and kissed me. Bless the dear little mothers! We don't half appreciate them, dear.*

"Evarts got really brilliant the other day when I was telling her how dead Anoka was and remarked that it was an appropriate place for Ghostley people to live in there. I think I will take Chapman for our name. What do you say?"

The same day, Fred wrote to Mary and asked if she enjoyed seeing the reproduction of 'Joan of Arc.' "*Did it call up a desire in you to do things ... the feeling which some women have misinterpreted as a desire for so-called 'Woman's Rights?' Of course you and I know that a man and woman have separate works to do; that it is just as great to be a woman as to be a man; that manhood and womanhood are equally good; and that one is the complement of the other.*"

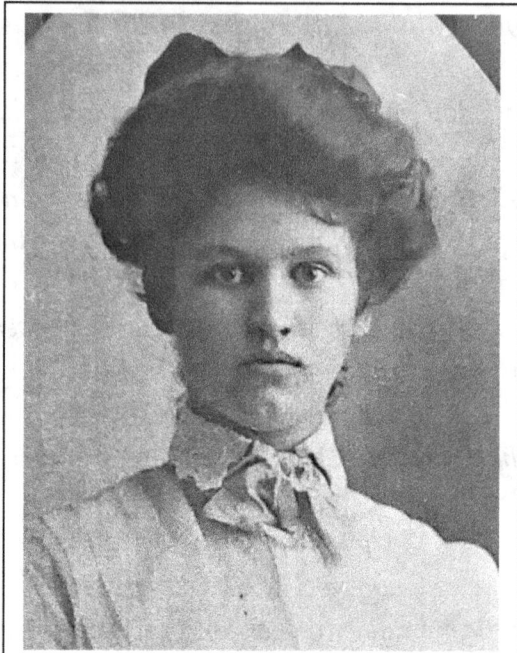

Mary Madison Chapman
James Ghostley collection

On the 10th, Fred wrote, "*I expect to drive back with horse and buggy to fetch mother over to the farm. She is going over to pick raspberries.*"

Mary wrote on July 11, "*I'm so glad you are coming down next week. Certainly, you'll take the board. And you'll pass too. You know that.*"

But on July 12, Fred wrote, "*I shall be down Wednesday. I do not know whether or not I shall take the pharmacy exam. It will only be for assistant anyway for I have only worked about 2 years.*"

Mary wrote on July 15, "*Let me tell you how indolent (that is more euphonious than lazy) I was this morning. I never got up until one o'clock. There! The only thing I regret is I have been cheated out of one meal.*

"By the way, there was only an eight cent fine on those books of yours. I bot [sic] fire crackers with the remaining seven cents and celebrated the 'Fourth' properly. Anoka was altogether too sane for me."

Two days later, Fred wrote, "Last Saturday morning it was raining, so I went fishing. I caught two pickerel and 8 or 9 bass. There was a small creek flowing into the river directly across from where we were fishing. We thought that there would certainly be fish at the mouth of it, so we took our fish poles and swam the river (across). We did not catch any fish there, but I caught a very bad sore throat. Looks like little canker sores all over my tonsils. Dr. Aldrich cleans them off every day and I touch them up every 4 or 5 hours."

Mary scolded him in her letter of July 18. "Really, when you know how susceptible you are to attacks of that nature, I think you might be more careful. I—even I—would not run such a chance of taking cold as you did.

"The drs. Monahan are in town. As yet they have been, as Bob expresses it, 'Out to pasture.' They came to get their 'outfit.'

"I talked with Rob for a while and he told me Prof. Dunn said I had done very well. I have been trying to interpret that to mean, 'She passed Anatomy.' There were twelve who failed, however. I'm afraid you were one."

The next day, Fred wrote that his throat continued to be very sore.

In his letter of July 20, he told of the heat bothering him. He left large spaces between the lines of his writing. "It is so hot, I thot [sic] I would leave plenty of room for the small breeze to blow between the lines.

"The doctor said my throat would probably be well by Sunday or Monday. It looks a great deal better, but feels about the same," he wrote.

On July 22, Mary wrote, "Oh, Honey, I've a beautiful compliment for you. Mrs. Dr. M (Monahan) *thinks you are handsome!* I hate to miss the look of scorn which will sweep over your expressive, handsome countenance when you read that.

"You asked me to raise my estimate of your judgement in regard to me. If you had acted more discretely on several occasions, particularly one memorable one, mentioned casually in your last epistle, I could truthfully say you were a man of sound judgement, but as it is, you know the adage which says, 'If you can say nothing good of a man—say nothing at all.' Therefore, I remain silent."

Fred wanted to see Mary, but he wrote on July 23, "It is best for you to go home and rest up for the remainder 1½ months before your winter work commences.

"My throat is nearly well. Just three ulcers left."

Two days later, Mary wrote, "My little brother came Monday. He has been having pleurisy and is not very strong so they sent him a day earlier to prevent his getting into the excursion crowd which came down today. We shall probably go home Saturday eve, however if we stay over Sunday we will be in St. Paul. I could not think of going home without seeing you if it is not absolutely necessary. Can you come down Friday?"

The next day, Fred replied that he would be down Friday to see Mary.

He did return to Minneapolis but had about 100 specimens to mount, so he wrote a quick letter to Mary rather than visiting. He also told her he had bought a stethoscope for their future medical practice.

Fred stayed for a few days, then left for his aunt's. Mary wrote, "*By this time you are in Grey Eagle. What if you commit indiscretions in matters of diet there? Were I your mother, I'd be afraid to let you go from home for a single night, without the usual maternal injunction to all small boys about buttons and ears ... peas and noses, green apples, etc.*"

Fred lovingly filled an envelope again with flowers for Mary, but her response wasn't what he expected. "*Thank you for the goldenrod and sunflowers. Why, may I ask, didn't you permit the beautiful blossoms to remain? They only withered and you robbed someone else of the pleasure of seeing them grow. I think it is sort of a spirit of vandalism which prompts people to pick flowers.*" However, nearly 115 years later, the dried flowers remain in the envelope they were mailed in, alongside the many other letters Fred and Mary exchanged before they married.

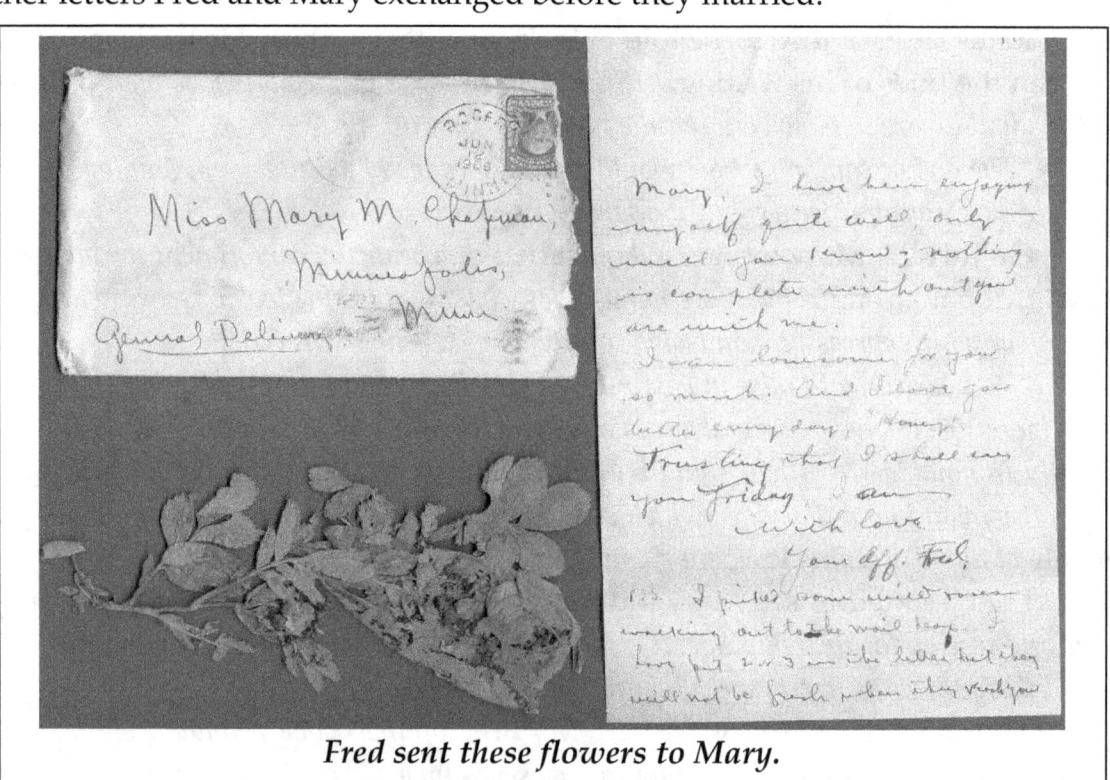

Fred sent these flowers to Mary.
James Ghostley collection
Pat Nelson photo

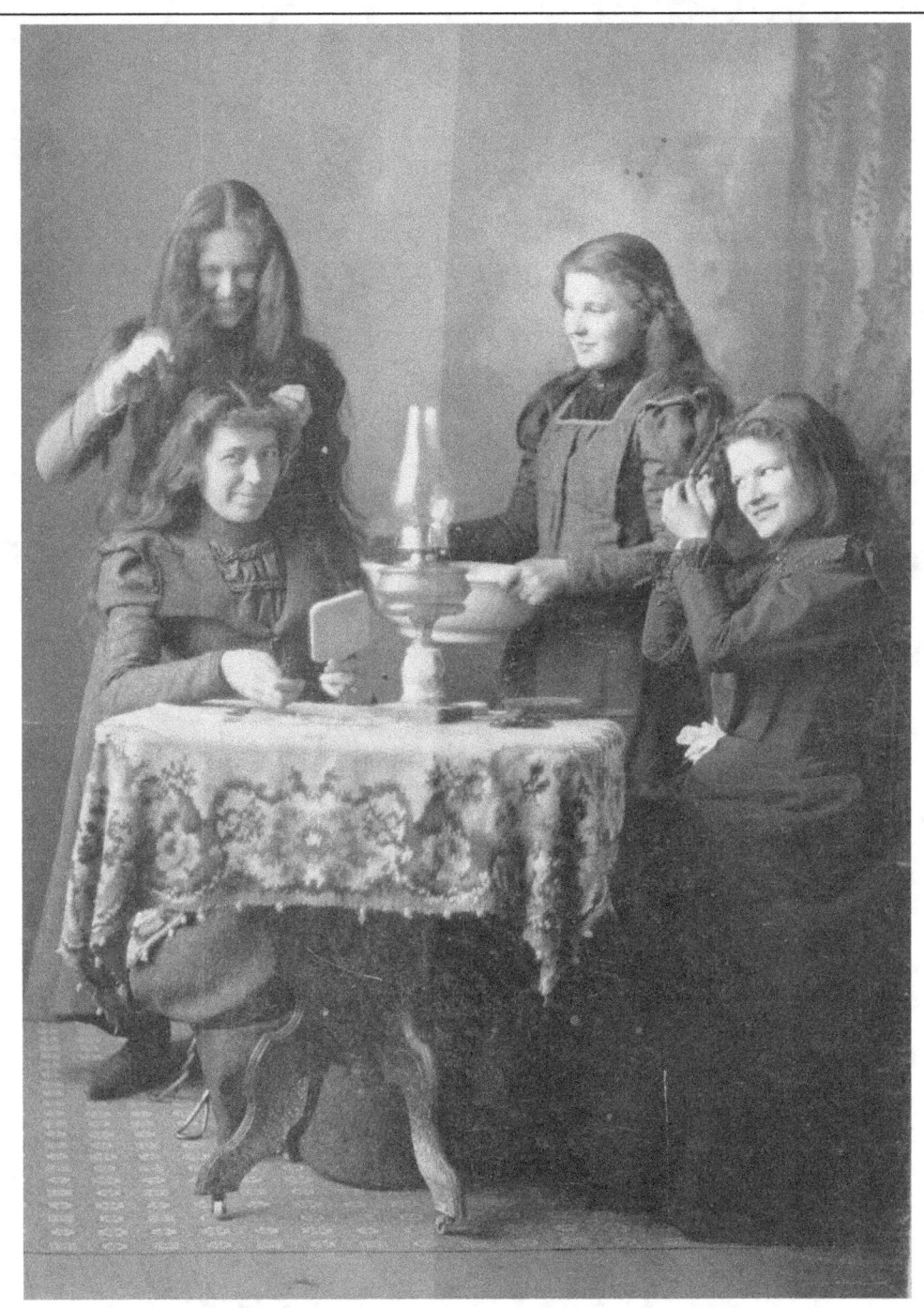

Mary Chapman combs her mother's hair.
Sisters Margaret, center, and Anna, right
James Ghostley collection

Chapter 12
Mary Takes a Break with Family

"Mother went to Milbank yesterday," Mary wrote, "and I'm the head of the family. Baked bread today ... washed yesterday and cook horrid stuff to eat all the time. I just despise housework. Learn all you can, my dear, while at your aunt's."

Fred wrote on July 8, "Still tired of my cucumber which I ate Saturday. Have some abdominal pain. Getting lots better tho."

"Let me see," Mary wrote on July 10, "you said several things which I feel called upon to speak about. Firstly, that some day you would ... or might ... say that the property of the firm belonged to the junior partner. My child ... the proposition is absurd. The senior member has the most rights in company matters. Then too please remember, 'What's yours is mine—what's mine ... is my own!

"Secondly. Please do not forget that I shall insist upon my right to direct our affairs.

"Thirdly, you resented Margaret's criticism of your chirography. I have assured you, times without number, that when you chose, you wrote very well indeed. But ordinarily your writing is not pretty and sometimes scarcely legible and you know this, don't you?

"It behooves each one of us to do his level best (Ahem!). After this I can see the straight little lines come between your eyebrows, and your brown eyes grow dark, and you launch into a lengthy, complicated argument to prove me wrong. I don't care. I'm right because!

"It is delightfully quiet and restful here in the country; but you don't know (not being a silly, fussy woman who is affected by such trifles) how annoying it is to be where everyone is so deeply concerned about everyone else's affairs. We go to church in the afternoon and come home to pull the poor, dear preacher's sermon to pieces and say uncomplimentary things about everyone else. As you have probably observed, my 'besetting sin' is a love for poking fun at people."

Fred wrote on August 5 that he believed he had obtained a crude idea of carcinoma, sarcoma, acute and chronic nephritis, cirrhosis of the liver, etc. by looking at specimens.

He wrote again on August 8 to tease Mary about which one of them would oversee their professional partnership. "Have you forgotten that I am to direct the work of 'this company?'"

On August 11, Fred asked if he should write gossip. "Our cousin had a young man from N. Dakota staying at her house last week. Tuesday they drove out in the country to a lake all by their lonesome about 18 miles. She also has a young Anoka boy who lives in Montana on the string. Last holidays he lived in Champlain most of the time. And then there is our Cousin Harry. She keeps up quite a correspondence with all. Notwithstanding Nordan's statement that it is psychologically possible for an individual to love two or more of the opposite sex at the same time, we know and like those individuals who have enough integrity and sincerity of character to, at least, smother such other desires by auto-suggestion, etc. Personally, I do not accept Nordan's edict. Rather I think that we should regard such individuals who exhibit fickleness, insincerity, etc. as monstrosities or atavistic degenerates caused by heredity—prenatal conditions and later environment."

Mary commented on August 13, "I do not consider it impossible for a normal person to love more than one of the opposite sex almost equally well at the same time."

Mary teased, "It seems so pleasant not to be bothered with you, I never thot of you at all yesterday.

"We girls milked this morning. Margaret pointed out the cows which stood the stillest and were the easiest to milk. I 'bit' of course. Will do my own selecting next time.

"Only about five weeks and we will be back to work."

Fred wrote on August 18, "Went strolling last night. Saw our evening star; made me think of you, 'girlie.'"

He added, "Little Girl, you don't know how much I need you to talk with me; for you know that you and I can have 'heart to heart' talks only with each other.

"I swear, if you should die, that I shall never love or know any woman. I love you better than all else in the world."

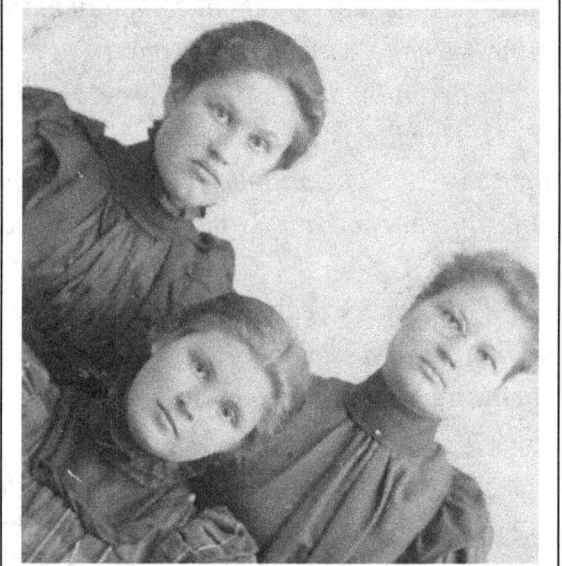

Mary Madison Chapman (left) and her sisters Margaret (center) and Anna (right) James Ghostley collection

Mary wrote on August 21, "We had callers yesterday. Some young folks who were married after I left last year. They used to be funny, jolly girls, 'good fellows' in any kind of fun, but all they can talk of now is 'my husband,' 'my baby,' and 'my house.' I think it makes people narrow to get married."

She wrote on August 26 of a new experience. "I was engaged for several hours in the interesting and new occupation of baby-tending. One of the neighbors went to town and left her four-month-old infant in our care. She's an exceptionally good baby and very *pretty (honest) so we don't mind her and she doesn't seem to mind us so we get on very well. "*

Fred had a toothache on August 30. *"It commenced about 12:00 last night so I read until four this morning. It is a tooth that I had filled about 2 months ago. Thot [sic] that I would settle it today, but found both of the respectable dental doctors off on vacation. They say that the remaining dentist here's unclean and careless and does not observe reasonable antiseptic and aseptic measures. I prefer the ache to possible 'blood poison' infection so shall wait and go to the city in the morning."*

Mary started her letter of September 1 with a complaint. *"To begin with, I think your name is the horridest one I ever tried to write ... Ghostley ... you just can't make such a combination of letters look civilized. How I dread to have always to put such a word at the close of my letters!*

"This has been a very <u>blue</u> day on the Prairie. Everyone has been shooting chickens. Our folks got only one; but yesterday, they got two. And we've been having a steady diet of duck lately.

"While I think of it, just permit me to disillusion you in regard to the shooting expeditions of Ghostley (me) and Ghostley (you). They <u>won't</u> occur on Sunday ... Never ... little boy."

Fred replied to Mary's comments on his name when he wrote on September 6, *"A name so suggestive of spiritualism should be ideal. Nearly all people hope for a life hereafter. 'Ghostly' people whom walk around, and who people can see perform the usual acts of life are convincing evidence of the existence of spirits."*

On September 12, Mary wrote: *"We had that model baby I told you of stay with us while her mother went to town yesterday. She never cried a bit. I think that child has had excellent advantages in the way of training and discipline."*

Mary and Fred could hardly wait to be together, and they decided to be married after Christmas. On December 4, she wrote to break the news to her mother, then wrote to Fred. *"She will be dreadfully surprised, but I knew she would prefer to know it now even if I would prefer to tell her when I got home. It wasn't so very hard to write it after all."*

Fred had been ill again, and on December 5, he wrote, *"I feel a great deal better this morning ... in fact, all well again except for a little bit of 'unsettledness' in my stomach and a little 'tinnitus aurism.'*

"I slept in your bedroom last night. The walls and every thing told me of you. And I heard the all and I liked it. Your soft arms, loving cheek and womanly spirit ... you know Mary, I want you.

"If our time of probation was more than two weeks, I do not believe that we could wait for it to pass."

Mary's study partner at school was Fred's roommate, Mr. Beardsley. Mary wrote on December 6, "I hope you are recovering rapidly. I miss you very much and guess Beardsley does too. See, I'm just selfish ... want you to get well so you can come back ...but don't ... until you _are_ well.

"Beardsley and I finished the back and back of the neck today. All we have left now is the head, face and front of the neck. See where I burn some midnight oil to get ready for my final before Xmas.

"It was 40 degrees below in the amphitheatre this A.M. and a few degrees lower in the dissecting room this P.M. I know I've 'taken a cold.' That's one reason why you should hurry to get well and come back and another is a tall, dark, comely looking stranger appeared on the scene with Cramer this A.M. He is adorable."

Fred wrote on December 7 to request to see his "*Little Girl*" Sunday, but he wasn't sure he would be back at school. "If anything should possibly happen so that I cannot go down to school this week will you come up Saturday? Of course I expect to go down. I do want to see you, 'Big Woman.' Believe that I can almost start my dissecting exam when I get back.

"Seems as tho we shall finish our Mat. Medica before school is out. I do not believe I could finish this year out eating at the Restaurant. It is a good thing that we are going to keep house.

"I am going down to the P.O. now to mail your letter. I will send it to school for Monday morning. I got to the P.O. too late yesterday with your letter but he promised to unlock the mail and put it in.

"Dear Girlie, I can hardly wait for three weeks until we shall be living together. It will be the greatest happiness that is possible to be, Mary."

The same day, he wrote, "You have heard the story about the woman who made a white chalk mark on the stovepipe every time her 'man' John did something of which she approved. This is the second letter that I have written you today, and I have phoned you once. I shall look for three white chalk marks on your stovepipe when I come down! I feel about all right tonight. My pulse is just a little rapid yet.

"I have another little donation for our family. Mother has a nice 'cobbler' bottom rocking chair that she said she did not need and offered it to us. I assure you that it was entirely voluntary. I was not even talking about furnishing our house."

He continued the letter the next day. "I am going to stay home alone (with you). I shall take two potatoes, fry a piece of beefsteak and make some cocoa. There will be a plate and cup and saucer for you beside me. I shall have supper ready for us at six o'clock. Mary, *so you know how much I want you all the time? When ever I am out in the kitchen wiping dishes, etc. I do want you here so much, Little Girl."*

Fred didn't stay well for long. He wrote the 10th, *"My stomach 'kicked up' a little bit again Saturday night and Sunday morning. Am quite well again today."*

Fred and Mary were apart for Christmas, and he wrote: *"I shall wish you a very good and fair day. If wishes were equivalent of realities, we should wish ourselves together today. I am decidedly and markedly lost these few days!*

"Mother is going down with me Monday morning. Said she could help us all day, see us married, and come home at 11:05 P.M. Monday evening. Is your Mother and Father coming?"

Mary's parents did not attend, but Fred's mother was present when Mary Chapman and Fred Ghostley married on December 31, 1906. His mother returned to her home in Anoka after the ceremony.

Even though Mary teased Fred about his last name, she changed her name to his. She became Mary Chapman Ghostley, using her maiden name before her married name so that there would be no confusion with her school transcripts.[42]

༄༅

The letters showed Fred to be intelligent, well-read, and sensitive. Even though he loved books and the arts, he was also an outdoorsman who liked to hunt and watch baseball. He often teased and deliberately invited controversy to spark a lively conversation. Unfortunately, Fred was a sickly fellow who always seemed to come down with something during his courtship of Mary.

Mary's letters showed her to be honest and intelligent, but a bit of a tease who had a stubborn streak. She was fond of the theater but also liked spending time in the woods. She enjoyed a good discussion or arguing a point with Fred. She attended church but questioned religion. Although Mary enjoyed prose and verse, she wasn't as well-read as Fred.

---

[42] James Ghostley interview

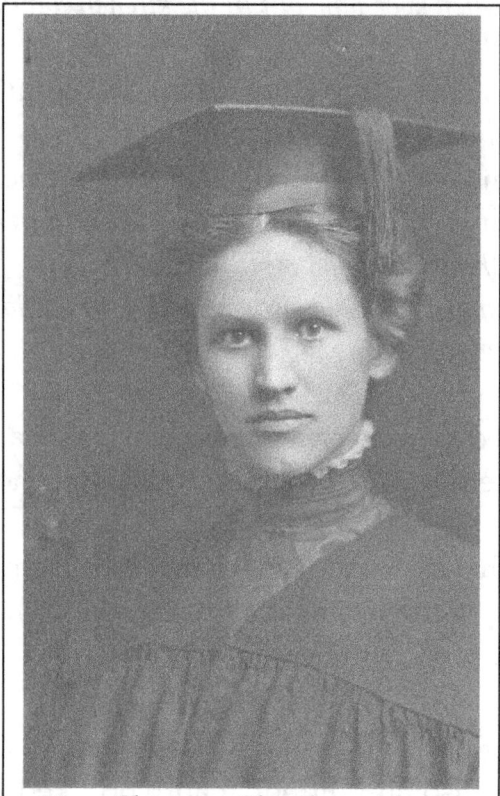

Mary Chapman Ghostley graduates from University of Minnesota Medical School in 1909
James Ghostley collection

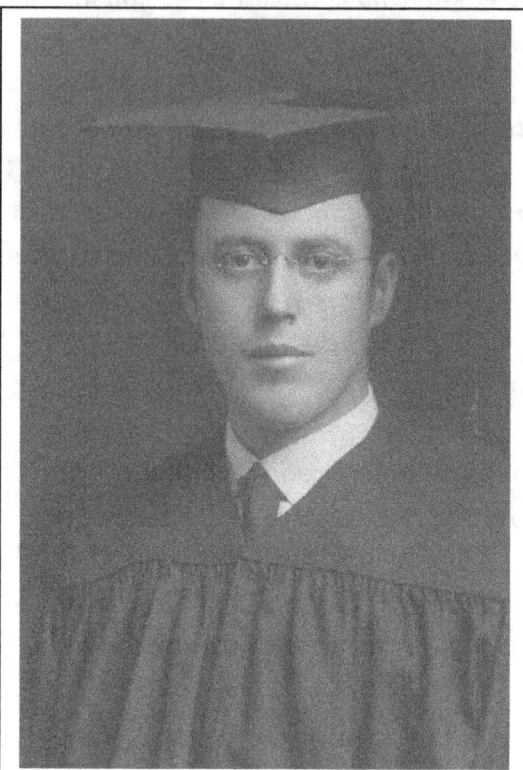

Fred Ghostley graduates from University of Minnesota Medical School in 1909
James Ghostley collection

In 1908, Hamline's medical school merged with the medical school of the University of Minnesota. Fred and Mary both graduated in 1909. As a part of their medical training, medical school taught them the fundamentals of diagnosis, treatment, and prevention of tuberculosis.[43] Before graduation, they made plans with former classmates Bob and Elizabeth Monahan of International Falls to practice medicine together.[44]

---

[43] *Invited and Conquered,* Minnesota Public Health Association, 1949
[44] James Ghostley interview

Chapter 13
Four Young Doctors

Robert Hugh Monahan was born in 1870 on a farm near St. Andrews, New Brunswick, Canada. He graduated from high school at age 17 and worked his way across Canada into California to meet an older brother, then traveled back through Montana. That is where Monahan became an American citizen. He then went to Minnesota, where he enrolled in Hamline University Medical School.

Elizabeth Stevens was born in 1880 in Blue Earth County, Minnesota. She taught for three years, then decided to study medicine at Hamline. She enrolled in the same year as Robert, and they married in 1905, a year before their graduation. [45]Elizabeth was only three years ahead of Mary Chapman Ghostley in med school at a time when it was uncommon for a woman to study medicine, and it gave the two a strong bond.

The Monahan's first son, George William, was born in 1907 in Blackduck. Once the tracks extended to International Falls, the Monahans could not resist the new frontier, and the young family moved there.

An entrepreneur and timber baron named Edward Wellington Backus recognized the potential of water power to operate lumber mills. He opened the Minnesota and Ontario Paper Company along the Rainy River in International Falls in the early 1900s.

According to Hiram Drache in *Taming the Wilderness*, Backus was responsible for constructing the dam and power plant as well as the paper mill. He left it up to others to provide the medical services. In 1907, he contracted with Drs. Robert and Elizabeth Monahan and Bert F. Osburn to provide medical services through the M and O Hospital (Minnesota and Ontario). The hospital's first offices were at Blackduck and Kelliher.[46] Blackduck sits 24 miles northeast of Bemidji, and Kelliher is approximately 18 miles from Blackduck.

---

[45] Monahan family history
[46] *Taming the Wilderness*, Hiram Drache, 1992

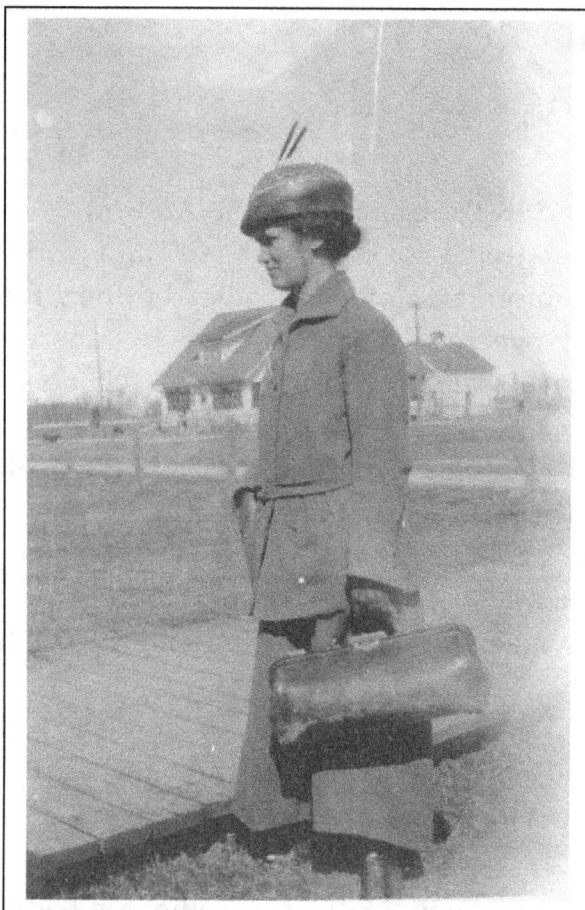

1909 on the boardwalk in Blackduck
James Ghostley collection

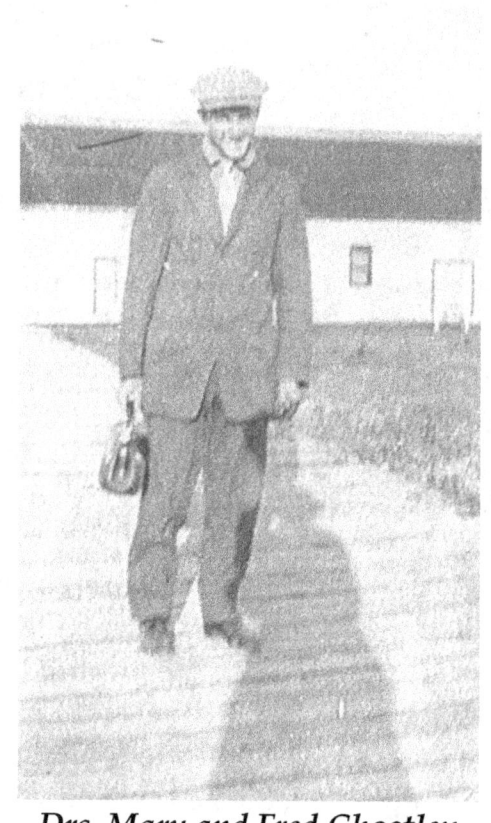

Drs. Mary and Fred Ghostley arrive in Blackduck in 1909 to practice medicine.
James Ghostley collection

Previously, the only doctors in International Falls had been M. E. Withrow and G. F. Swinnerton.[47]

The Monahans and Osburn were joined in 1909 by Fred and Mary Ghostley soon after their graduation from the University of Minnesota Medical School. In June 1909, the Monahan team began practicing in the Falls before the mill opened. The Ghostleys took over the Blackduck clinic as company doctors on the staff of the M and O Hospital Association.

On February 26, 1910, a meeting was held in Blackduck to organize the Northern Minnesota Hospital Association. The minutes listed Robert H. Monahan as president; Elizabeth Monahan, vice president; Bert F. Osburn, secretary; and

---

[47] *The Daily Journal*, International Falls, Minnesota, June 30, 2006

Mary C. Ghostley, treasurer. Directors were R. Monahan, B. Osburn, Frederick J. Ghostley, Clair C. Craig, and James Reid. The organization's purpose was to operate a general hospital, to construct more hospitals, and to buy and sell real estate and timber products. According to Drache, "Capital was $50,000, at $1 per share, of which $16,277 was paid at the time of the organization meeting."

The business was to commence on March 1, 1910. Physicians were to receive $150 per month as hospital heads, but lady members were to earn only $75. In no case was any physician to be paid more than $5,000 a year until the capital stock paid 10%, at which time he or she could draw up to $3,000 additional. When the stock paid 15%, the members could draw whatever was available. In no case was stock to be sold to anyone but the spouse of a stockholder.[48]

In the spring of 1910, some Blackduck residents started experiencing troubling symptoms such as fever, sweating, headaches, rash, diarrhea, abdominal pain, lethargy, muscle aches, and confusion. It was soon apparent that typhoid fever had Blackduck in its grips.[49]

The cause of typhoid fever remained elusive. People weren't yet willing to believe that inadequate sanitation compromised drinking water. As new frontiers developed, polluted water and typhoid outbreaks persisted.

Dr. Fred, exhausted after three days and nights of treating gravely ill patients, became ill himself on April 18. Mary knew how frail Fred had been in the past, so she insisted that they travel to his family in Anoka for a few days of rest. They planned to return to Blackduck and their practice as soon as he recuperated.

His physician in Anoka treated him beginning on April 22. His condition worsened, and after 17 days of illness, Fred died of typhoid fever on May 2, 1910, at 11 p.m. His new bride had quickly become a widow.

Fred was laid to rest at Forest Hill Cemetery in Anoka on May 5. Mary signed his death certificate, "Mrs. F. J. Ghostley," and she used his last name throughout the remainder of her long life.

Fred's obituary of May 6, 1910, read, *"To those who have known Dr. Ghostley in association with his esteemed wife, Dr. Mary Ghostley, this companionship both in*

---

[48] *Taming the Wilderness*, Hiram Drache, 1992
[49] *The Daily Journal*, International Falls, Minnesota, June 30, 2006

private and public life was ever the closest and most harmonious, and this fact causes us to feel so much more deeply in sympathy with her in her hour of deepest sorrow."[50]

The *Blackduck American* reported that in the short time Dr. Fred Ghostley had been there, he had established a reputation as a physician of more than ordinary ability as both a student and practitioner of his art, saying he was probably one of the most widely read and best practical medical men in Northern Minnesota. *"Many can attest to his absolute moral integrity and conscientiousness and his kindness and gentleness in the everyday care of the sick."*

Among those attending the funeral were F. Osburn, James M. Smith, E.N. French, Dr. C. C. Craig, and Dr. Mary's friend and business partner, Elizabeth Monahan.[51]

---

[50] *Blackduck American,* May 4, 1910
[51] *Blackduck American,* May 11, 1910

Chapter 14
Dr. Mary Relocates

When Mary returned to Blackduck, she was a brand-new doctor away from friends and family, and she felt alone in her grief. Tragedy seemed to engulf Mary in the small village. The town of Blackduck had problems, too. Just two days after Fred was laid to rest, the big old Teepeetonka Hotel in Blackduck, once a famous landmark because of its four-story construction from Norway pine, caught fire and was reduced to ashes. It had been empty for many years and had attracted vagrants, who may have started the fire.[52] Then, a few days later, Blackduck was hemmed in by forest fires. Farm homes narrowly escaped the flames.[53]

The partners decided to close the Blackduck clinic, and Mary moved to International Falls to practice with the Monahans. H. W. Froehich replaced Frederick Ghostley as part of the medical team. [54]

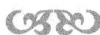

Elizabeth Monahan went to Crosby, nearly 170 miles south of International Falls, to start a new hospital facility. Besides her medical duties, Elizabeth assumed the work of the hired girl and the cook, who had both quit. She cooked for five staff members, three adult patients, and a baby—and that was before there were sewer and water connections. In December 1910, W. R. Beardsley joined the firm to operate the 10-bed hospital.[55]

The Minnesota and Ontario Hospital Association incorporated into the Northern Minnesota Hospital Association on March 1, 1911, to provide medical care and to train nurses. It had modern equipment and had grown from accommodating 25 patients to caring for 70.

---

[52] *Memory Lane,* Blackduck, MN March 11, 1987
[53] *Taming the Wilderness*, Hiram Drache, 1992
[54] *Blackduck American, May 1910*
[55] *Taming the Wilderness*, Hiram Drache, 1992

Even though it was unusual for a woman to practice medicine in those days, Dr. Mary didn't run into much trouble. People needed her, and she never lacked for patients. Residents were kind, and Dr. Elizabeth provided support.[56]

Dr. Mary encouraged women to enter the medical field, and she trained many for nursing careers. Her first nursing class graduated on June 4, 1913. The nursing school was one of the earliest such accredited schools in the state, and many of its graduating nurses went to work for the Mayo Clinic and other hospitals in the Twin Cities. Dr. Mary told groups of prospective nurses, "Anyone

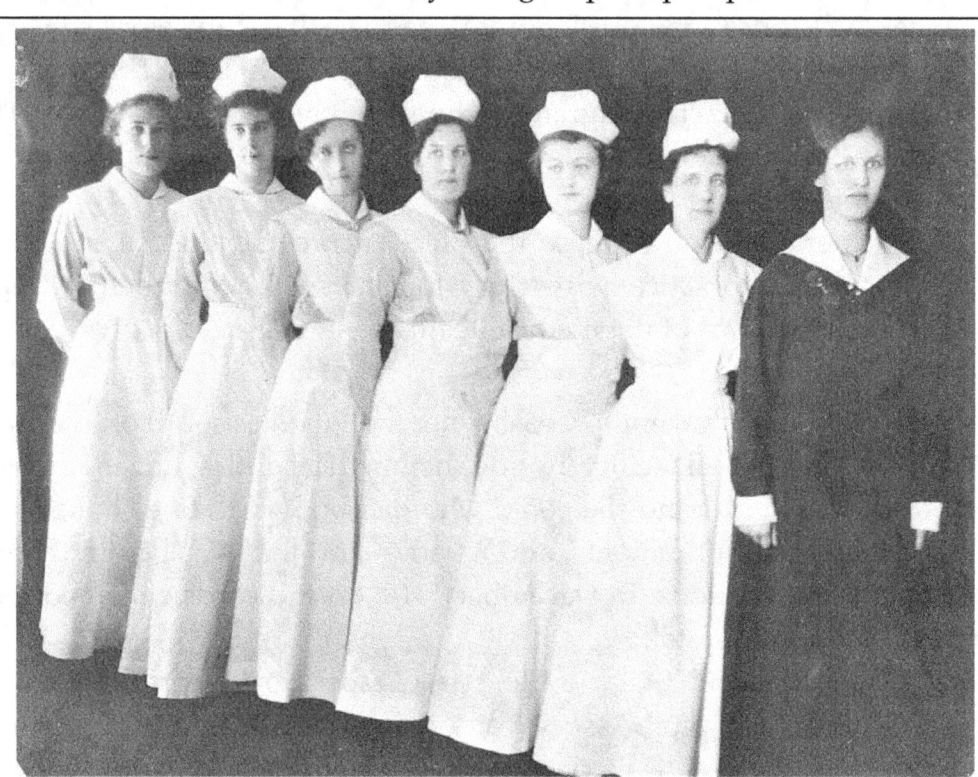

Dr. Mary's 1917 nursing-class graduates
Dr. Mary, far right
James Ghostley collection

---

[56] James Ghostley interview

interested in medicine should go ahead with their plans. There is a future in medicine for a woman, and funds are available to those who need help."[57]

The *International Falls Press and Border Budget* reported on July 2, 1914, "On Tuesday evening last, the third annual graduating exercises of the Northern Minnesota Hospital training school for nurses were held in the City Hall. Dr. Mary Ghostley presented diplomas."[58]

༄༅

The Monahans and Dr. Mary were active in civic and social life in the Falls. Doctors Elizabeth and Mary started a women's club called "Saturday Musicale" in 1915, Elizabeth as president and Mary as secretary. The group promoted music in Borderland—the area along the boundary between the U.S. and Canada.[59]

Mary was never afraid to support good causes. On June 22, 1916, she and Elizabeth Monahan were two of 20 women who wrote to thank Mayor Keyes for working toward a general and lasting cleanup, including his promise to remove curtains from pool halls and drink parlors and to ask undesirable folks to leave town before Saturday night.[60]

Women's rights, including the right to respect, meant a lot to Dr. Mary. When she heard that the local court provided entertainment for males by rude questioning of women charged with prostitution, Dr. Mary and Dr. Elizabeth Monahan appeared in court, and although remaining silent, their presence was influential. Soon, other women joined them, and that vulgar practice ended.[61]

Dr. Mary was active in the American Association of University Women. She helped local people get a college education, provided clothing for the needy, trained nurses and X-ray technicians, and allowed people to check out books from her library.[62]

༄༅

---

[57] *International Falls Press,* September 18, 1958
[58] *International Falls Press and Border Budget,* July 2, 1914
[59] *International Falls Daily Journal,* March 12, 2009
[60] *International Falls Press and Border Budget,* June 22, 1916
[61] James Ghostley interview
[62] *International Falls Press* and *Border Budget,* International Falls, Minnesota

While practicing in the Falls, Dr. Mary's brother Henry developed a glandular condition. She diagnosed it as cancer and sent him home to the Twin Cities. He returned to her with his doctor's warning: "Leave cancer detection to men in the profession." Her diagnosis had been correct, and her brother died of glandular cancer.[63]

Dr. Robert Monahan left the area during World War I and entered the Army as a captain in the medical corps. Dr. Elizabeth Monahan and Dr. Mary remained in general practice, and Dr. C. C. Craig joined them at the Northern Minnesota Hospital. In 1918, during the devastating worldwide flu epidemic, there were not enough doctors and nurses. Thank goodness Dr. Mary had learned to work long hours with only limited sleep, a practice she kept up throughout her career. She could shut her eyes for a few minutes and get the rest she needed, then continue her work.[64]

Dr. Craig and Dr. Mary were the only doctors in the area during the epidemic. They knocked on doors, each taking one side of the street, to check on the welfare of residents. The flu epidemic continued through that winter, but because of their diligence, the Falls death rate was lower than that of other neighboring communities.[65]

Robert Monahan returned from the war as a major in early 1919. During the war, he had served in a hospital in England under one of the world's foremost orthopedists, Dr. Robert Jones, and he decided to specialize in that field. In September 1919, he moved his family to Minneapolis, where he started his orthopedic practice. However, the family kept a cabin at Rainy Lake near International Falls. It served as their headquarters for more than 40 years.[66]

Dr. Elizabeth practiced eye care, and while back in the Falls in May 1920, she fit glasses at Dr. Ghostley's office for several days.[67]

---

[63] James Ghostley interview
[64] James Ghostley interview
[65] *International Falls Press,* October 4, 1956
[66] *Taming the Wilderness,* Hiram Drache, 1992
[67] *International Falls Press and Border Budget,* International Falls, Minnesota, April 29, 1920

In 1939, Robert Monahan returned to the Falls to go into general practice with Dr. C. C. Craig at the Northern Minnesota Hospital. He continued in this joint practice until his death in 1947.

Dr. Elizabeth remained in Minneapolis, where she was active in civic and social work until shortly before her death in 1951. She was in the first group to receive an award from the University of Minnesota for "Fifty Years in Medicine."

The Northern Minnesota Hospital building at Eighth Avenue and Second Street became an apartment house in 1948, then was razed in 1958 following a damaging fire. It had served its people well for nearly half a century.[68]

In those days, doctors often made house calls on foot because of poor road conditions. Horse-drawn buggies carried them to some homes, and in winter, sleighs often carried them across frozen lakes. Dr. Mary later traveled in her Hupmobile coupe with its California top. The roads were poor, and she often became stuck in mud or snow and had to walk anyway. When traveling by horse-drawn buggy, she sometimes dozed on the way home, so it was lucky the horse knew the way.[69]

Mary had made the hospital her home. When she moved into an apartment, it became the cultural center for the community, focusing on books and music. During the summers, her cultural gatherings of friends from both town and Rainy Lake at Ranier moved to her log house, "Rainbow's End," on the lakeshore at Birch Point.[70] People who might never have met did so through her get-togethers. She had a busy social life, and she started island-to-island swimming on Rainy Lake.[71]

People joked that wherever the stork went, Mary wasn't far behind. She delivered more than 2000 babies, and they were referred to with pride as "Dr. Mary babies." "When she went to a house to await a birth," Jim Ghostley said, "she kept busy cleaning and knitting socks or mittens for the older children in the

---

[68] *International Falls Press,* International Falls, Minnesota, May 14, 1958
[69] James Ghostley interview
[70] *The Daily Journal,* International Falls, Minnesota, June 30, 2006
[71] *The Daily Journal,* International Falls, Minnesota, March 15, 1994

family. Most people couldn't afford to pay. Instead, they would give her a chicken, a quart of cream, a promise, or just a thank you."

"Even in the ledger at her Rainy Lake cabin," granddaughter Barbara Fisher said, "family members found an entry where she noted that she had performed surgery in exchange for a chicken."

"To deliver babies," Jim Ghostley said, "she often had to travel over nearly impassable roads, in all kinds of weather, or over the treacherous frozen lakes."

ଔଃ

Dr. Mary bought a canoe that had belonged to a Catholic priest. It was a cargo canoe with no seats, and she had to kneel to paddle. Indians had paddled the large voyageur canoe when the priest rode in it.

An Indian named Wake em Up Old Man sometimes stopped by Dr. Mary's place. "Whenever he pulled up to her dock," recalled her son, Jim Ghostley, "she excitedly ran down to meet him."

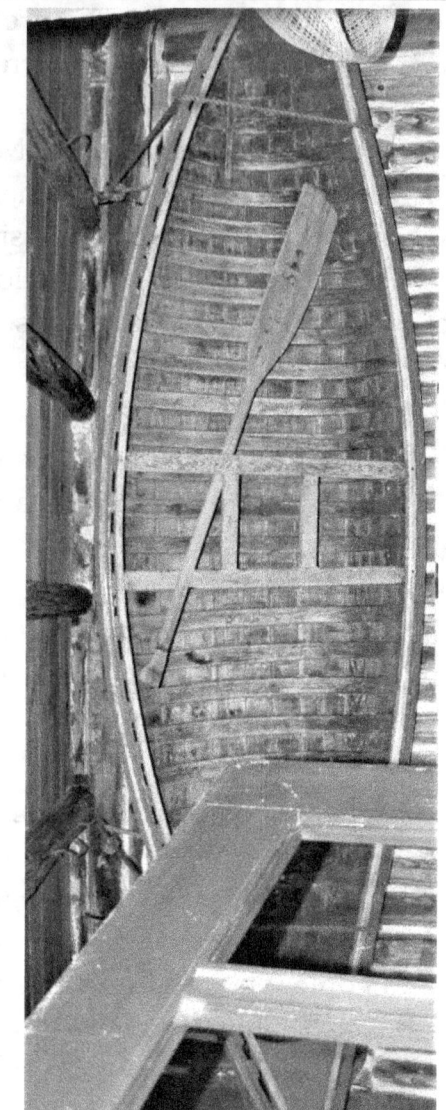

Dr. Mary's canoe
Pat Nelson photo

Dr. Mary was a women's rights activist and part of the suffragist movement to support women's right to vote.

She traveled by train on November 4, 1919, to St. Paul with a group of female delegates from International Falls. They demonstrated at the State Capitol in a nationwide campaign for women's suffrage.[72]

She also helped found the League of Women Voters in Bemidji.[73]

Her son, Jim Ghostley, remarked, "She didn't wait for legislation for women's rights; she just did what she felt was right, and nobody stopped her."

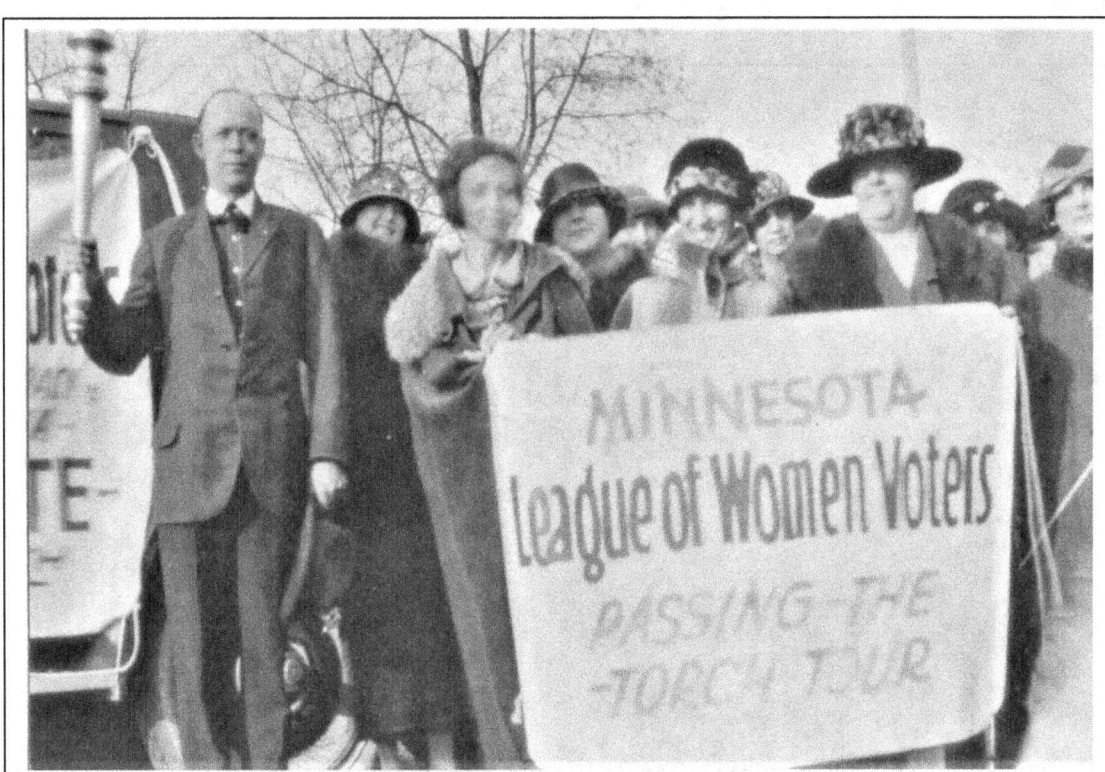

November 4, 1919, Mary Ghostley front row, center of sign. Delegates from International Falls travel to the State Capitol in a nationwide campaign for women's suffrage. James Ghostley collection.

---

[72] *The Daily Journal,* International Falls, Minnesota, February 20, 2002
[73] *The Bemidji Pioneer,* Bemidji, Minnesota, John Eggers, October 1, 2017

"My mother always stood up for her beliefs," Jim Ghostley said. "She had even fought people in the legislature."

☙❧

Dr. Mary had a keen interest in public health and administered the TB Mantoux test to thousands of Northern Minnesota schoolchildren. They lined up, and one by one, a small amount of tuberculin was injected by hypodermic needle into the layers of the skin of the arm. Forty-eight to 72 hours later, Dr. Mary checked their arms for reactions to the tuberculin. Most students tested negative, but if the result was positive, further testing was required to determine whether the student had active tuberculosis.[74]

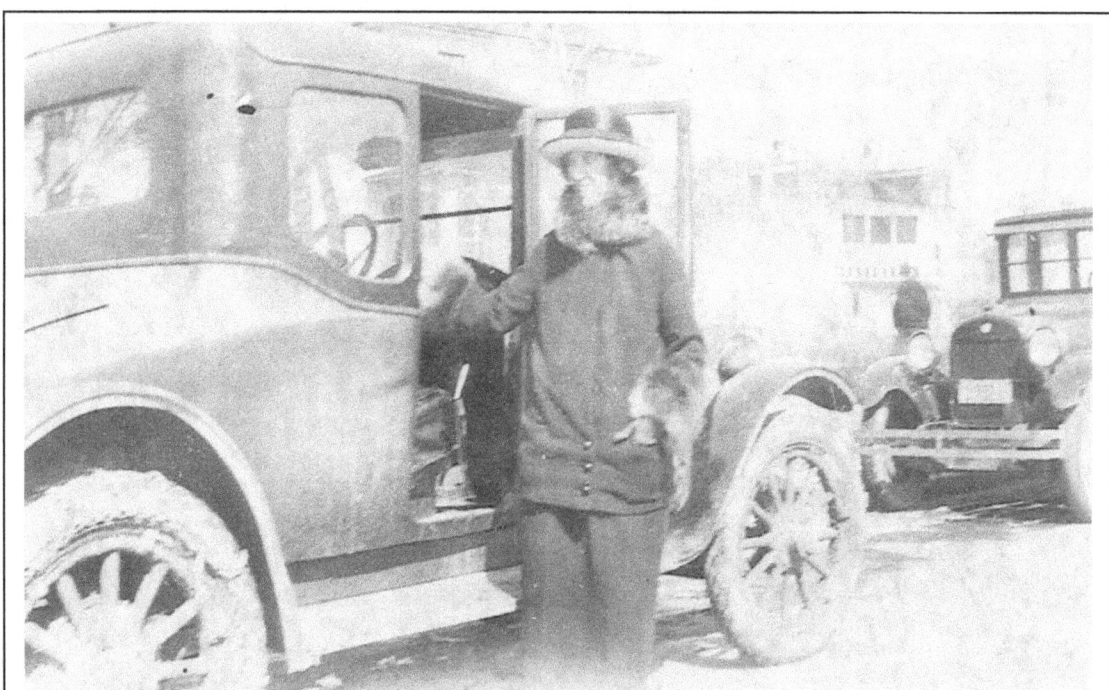

*Dr. Mary stands by one of her vehicles.
Notice the chains on the tires and the wooden spokes on the wheels.
James Ghostley collection*

---

[74] *Invited and Conquered*, Minnesota Public Health Association, 1949

Chapter 15
Dr. Mary's Bold Changes

On Monday evening, October 9, 1922, Dr. Mary married James Garnet Peterson, who went by the name Garnet. The ceremony was performed by Rev. A. W. McNeill at the home of Garnet's brother, Dr. Jack Peterson.[75]

Garnet was two years younger than Mary. He worked as an assistant cashier at First National Bank and had also sold life insurance. Both he and Mary were involved in civic affairs, and Garnet was on the local board for Koochiching County.

He had been married previously and had one daughter, Mary Jane.

Mary and Garnet had been friends for years and did many things together. However, many of their acquaintances were shocked to hear of the marriage. "Since the end of World War I," Jim Ghostley said, "Garnet had enjoyed the excitement of the Roaring 20s, and some friends weren't sure he was ready to settle down."

⁂

Just five years after her second marriage, Dr. Mary once again had a husband who was ill. On November 5, 1927, Garnet became a patient at the Lake Julia Tuberculosis Sanatorium,[76] where Mary had been a board member since 1925.[77] After a stay of just over three months, the disease appeared to be arrested, and the San released him. That wasn't the end of it, though, as the San readmitted Garnet in early June 1928. He was held one month for observation, and he was released because his TB was inactive.[78]

⁂

Two months earlier, Dr. Mary had become Health Officer in the Falls at a salary of $40 per month.[79] Around the same time, the San's board of directors,

---

[75] *International Falls Press and Border Budget,* International Falls, Minnesota, Oct. 12, 1922
[76] Minnesota History Center, Lake Julia Tuberculosis Sanatorium, Patient Register
[77] *Invited and Conquered,* Minnesota Public Health Association, 1949
[78] Minnesota History Center, Lake Julia Tuberculosis Sanatorium, Patient Register
[79] *International Falls Press,* International Falls, Minnesota, April 19, 1928

which included Dr. Mary, searched without luck for a doctor to take Dr. Laney's place near Puposky as superintendent of the Lake Julia Tuberculosis Sanatorium.

☙❧

In 1929, a young, unwed woman contacted Dr. Mary after she became pregnant. She had known the father only a short time, and she did not know what to do. She did know that she could not raise a baby by herself. In May 1929, Dr. Mary delivered the baby girl.

At age 48, Mary regretted that she did not have children of her own. She became the foster mother to Katherine, the baby who had looked into her eyes first when she entered the world. Dr. Mary nicknamed her Cathie and started the adoption paperwork. She wrote to friend Rosa Oberholtzer, "I have a baby girl."[80] She didn't say "we," so perhaps it was all her idea.

Even as Mary adjusted to motherhood, the other board members begged her to fill the position of superintendent at the San. There was a lot to consider. Where would Garnet work? He had a job at the bank in the Falls. There were few jobs in Puposky except at the San. How would she protect her new daughter from tuberculosis? How could she afford to hire someone to help with the child while she went to work at all hours?

Shortly before the end of the year, Dr. Laney was ready to leave, but no one would take his place. The board agreed to pay Dr. Mary the same rate that Dr. Laney earned, $400 per month[81]. That was a grand wage for a woman, and it would allow her to hire a caretaker for Cathie. The family would have a nearly new log cottage to live in near the San so that Mary could be close to the baby. And if Garnet's tuberculosis again became active, he would be at the San where he could get care. Those benefits, along with a sense of duty, compelled Mary to accept the position.

Before Dr. Mary left for Lake Julia to assume her new responsibilities, members of the Falls medical profession honored her at the home of Dr. and Mrs. C. C. Craig.[82]

Mary, Garnet, and baby Cathie moved to Puposky, where they became the second residents of the San's log house.

---

[80] Minnesota History Center, Dr. Mary Ghostley correspondence
[81] Minnesota History Center, Lake Julia Tuberculosis Sanatorium, Expense Report
[82] *International Falls Press,* International Falls, Minnesota, January 10, 1930

Garnet became the bookkeeper, and his wife became his boss. Accounting and bookkeeping methods were standardized for all of Minnesota's tuberculosis sanatoriums.[83] Garnet meticulously recorded income, expenses, and payroll, and he listed the infrequent voided checks as "spoiled," as he had done at the bank. He earned $70 per month, $330 per month less than his wife's salary.[84]

Census-takers in 1930 may have been confused about who wore the pants in the family. They first listed Mary as the head of household, then changed her title to "wife" and listed Garnet as "head."

☙❧

There was no doubt about Mary's deep love for the children, but when her nephew Percy (Peck) Brown and his mother, Anna Brown, visited Mary at Rainy Lake when Cathie was about a year old, Peck said, "I found it odd that Garnet didn't have much to do with either Cathie or his daughter Mary Jane."

Three months after Peck and his mother visited, Mary brought home a second baby, a boy named James, who she called Jim. His biological mother, Nelle Olson, had died of toxemia. Because his father, Melvin, could not care for his children, he placed the two oldest in foster care, and Dr. Mary adopted James. The baby was deathly ill for weeks. He might have died, but with her care, he became strong and healthy.

Jim's birth-siblings grew up on a farm, and they worked for room and board. "They were taken care of but had to work every day and help the farmer," Jim said. "My siblings and I got to know each other, and we became close friends."

Jim's daughter Carol Goplin stated, "I believe Dr. Mary not only saved my father's life as an infant, but she made his life through adoption."

---

[83] *Invited and Conquered*, Minnesota Public Health Association, 1949
[84] Minnesota History Center, Lake Julia Tuberculosis Sanatorium Expense Report

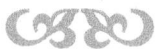

"Garnet liked to drive and to show off his latest cars," Jim Ghostley said, "and he was good friends with the Chrysler dealer. He was kind of flashy, kind of flamboyant in some ways. He had once owned a 1914 Stutz Bearcat, and many years later, I found an old Stutz Bearcat key fob on the mantle in Dr. Mary's cabin."

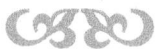

Many people were not surprised around 1935 when the marriage ended. Mary and Garnet divorced when James was five and Cathie was six.[85] Tres Lomen Hansen, a former nurse at the San,

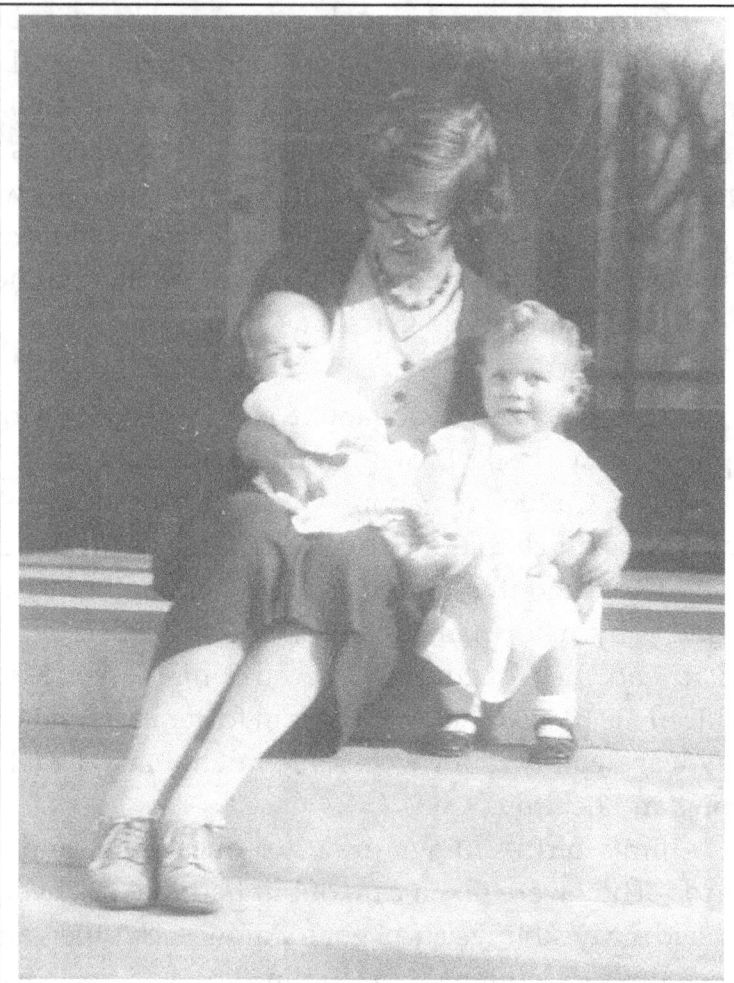

Dr. Mary holds her children, James and Cathie.
James Ghostley collection

recalled, "Dr. Mary and Garnet never seemed happy or like they had much in common."

"Mom and Garnet didn't get along very well because he liked to run and play," Jim said. "He and a friend would hunt and have drinking parties, and I remember plain as day that you couldn't go near them when they were partying; you would stay out of their way. I think one thing that was a real problem was that Mom was in charge. She made far more money than he did, and perhaps it

---

[85] James Ghostley interview

also bothered him that she hadn't taken his name because she had established her professional career as Dr. Mary Ghostley. It was a male-dominant time, and mother was ahead of her time in the decisions she made. I don't think Garnet took that well."

After the divorce, Dr. Mary had the last name of the children changed from Peterson to Ghostley. Cathie didn't like her middle name, so Dr. Mary changed Cathie's name from Katherine B. to Mary Catherine. Because Dr. Mary had never taken Garnet's last name but had continued to be Mary Chapman Gostley, mother and daughter then both had the initials, "MCG,"[86] and Jim, also, took the last name 'Ghostley.'"

Garnet moved to Hawaii, where he became a hospital administrator. Dr. Mary remained close to his brother, Dr. Jack Peterson, and his wife, Kitty. Dr. Peterson treated dental surgical problems at the San as needed, and he had a dental practice in the Falls.[87] Peck Brown remembered that Jack was always pleasant.[88]

"Garnet visited the family only once after the divorce," Jim said, "and that was to show off his Chrysler Air Flow, a flashy car. It was the strangest design. It set the whole auto world on its ear because it wasn't just straight up and down like a Model A, like the cars we were used to seeing."

"Life got better after he left," Jim said. "No question about it."

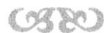

Jim Ghostley remembered that when he was little, both he and Cathie had identical teddy bears. "Oh, how I loved that bear," Jim said. "And Cathie didn't give a lick about hers. One day, my mother asked if she could have my bear; she couldn't find Cathie's. There was a little boy in the San who she said needed it more than I did. How I hated losing my bear.

"Mom brought home a photo of the little guy. He was cute as a button with big, dark eyes, and I could see that Mom had combed his hair just so, like she did mine, so that he looked neat as a pin. He didn't look sick, but I guess he was. I cried so hard that Cathie found her bear and gave it to me. I still have that lump of a bear. I looked in the records in later years and could find no admittance of a little child during that time. Chances are, he had lost his parents, and Mom just

---

[86] Ella Hedglin
[87] James Ghostley interview
[88] Percy (Peck) Brown interview

kept him there off the books until they found a home for him. I'm surprised she didn't bring home a brother for me. I thought once about writing a book. I was going to call it, '*My Mother Never Had Any Children.*' Well, she did, of course, but she had adopted us, and she was always delivering babies for other people."

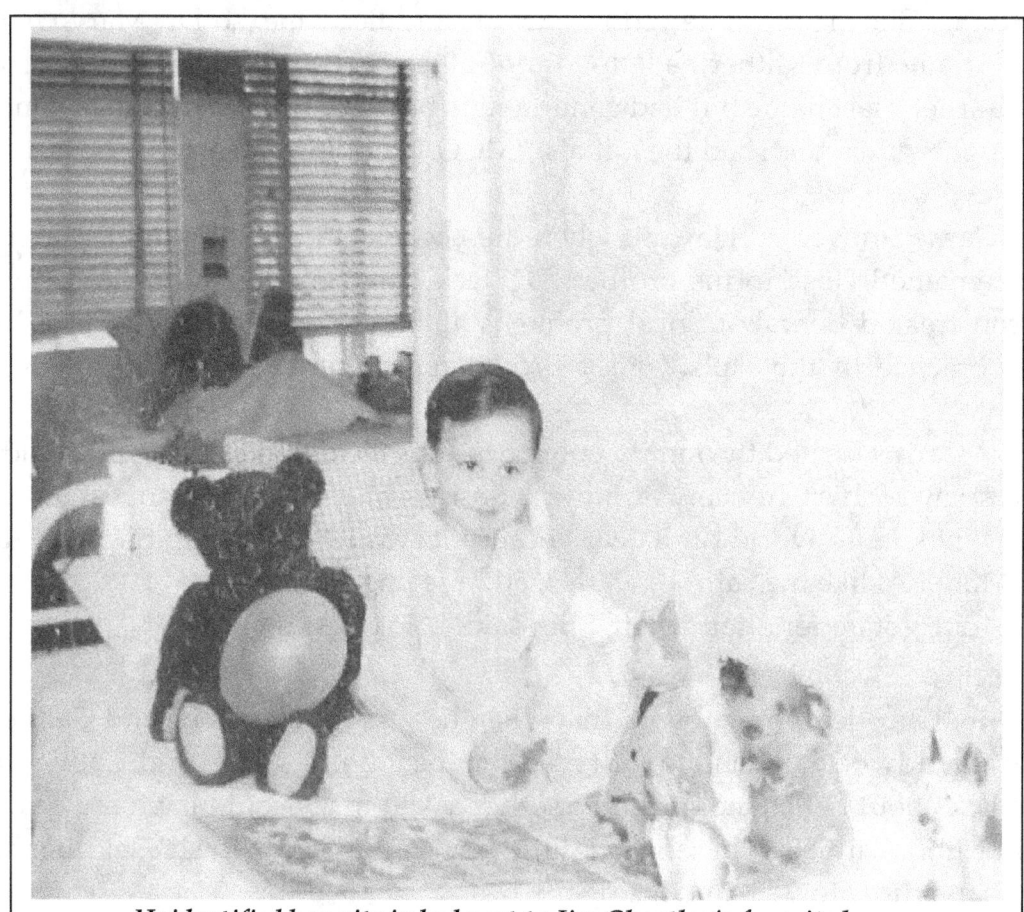

Unidentified boy sits in bed next to Jim Ghostley's favorite bear.
The child is in isolation.
A patient in the next room can be seen through the window.
James Ghostley collection

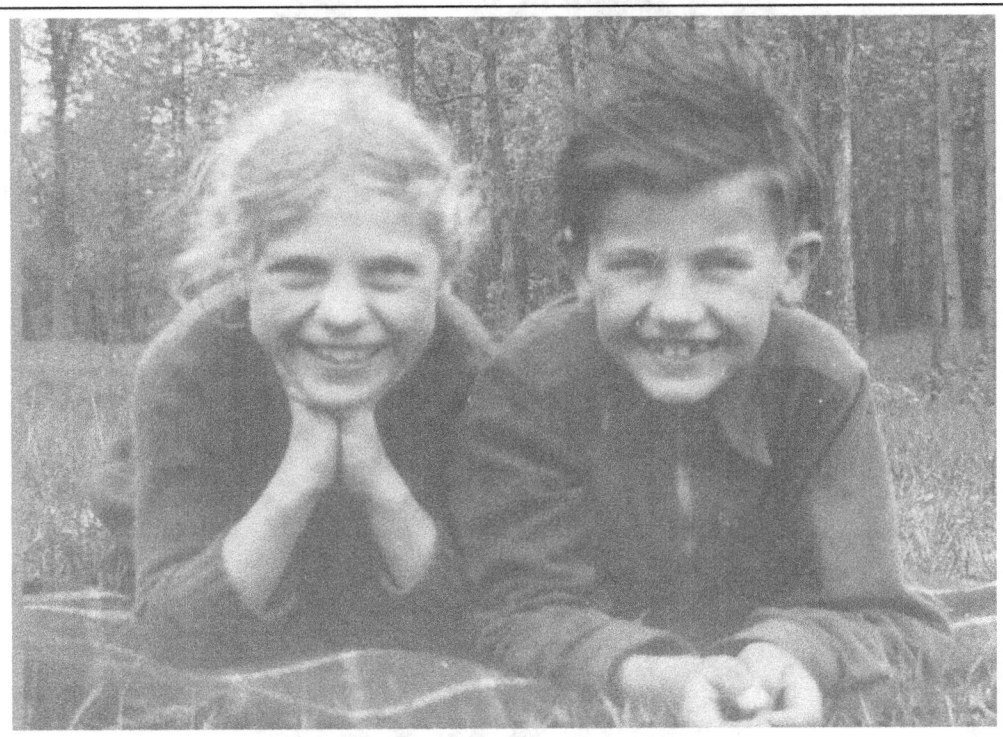

Cathie and Jim Ghostley
James Ghostley collection

Dr. Mary knew that if her children played outside at Lake Julia during the summer months, they would eventually encounter patients who had TB. "Summers, she sent us to our cabin at Birch Point in Ranier with our cousin, Wanda Brown, who had moved to Puposky from Washington State," Jim Ghostley said. "During the rest of the year, Wanda helped with office work and assisted with the kitchen, the gardening, and the crops at the San."

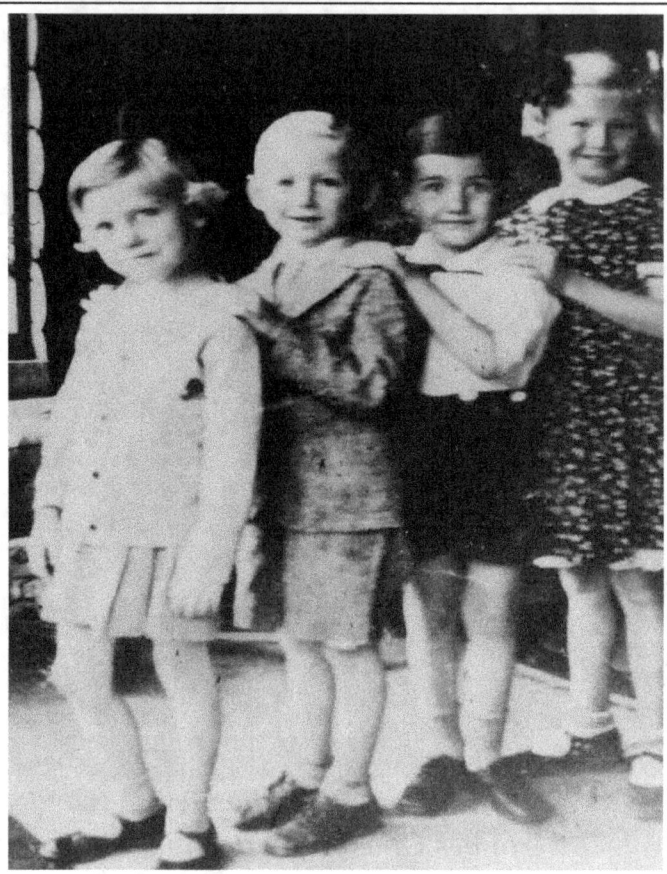

Cathie Ghostley, Fritz Becker, James Ghostley, and Ruth Becker
James Ghostley collection

Jim Ghostley proudly said this about his mother: "Her compassion and her attitude that 'it has to be done' helped her tackle the many challenges at the San.

"Dr. Mary oversaw everything: the hospital, the employees, the hay crops, the dairy herd, sheep, pigs, acreage, the greenhouse, the generating plant, the fruit trees, and the vegetable garden. She also canned vegetables and made kraut for the San. Cathie and I helped her collect maple sap for syrup and gathered mushrooms as a special treat for the patients."

Bob Maher lived on Lake Julia and had worked at the San as a steam engineer. He remembered Dr. Mary well and described her as a lovely woman and a good doctor. Because he lived near the San, he often went to find Dr. Mary when someone in the area was sick. His father, Harry Maher, had worked at the San for years and was good friends with Dr. Mary. When she told him what she needed, he made sure she got it.

Bob told of his father's ingenuity in constructing things for Dr. Mary. "There was a chain to raise the dumbwaiter. My father hooked up an electric motor in the attic, a knife with two blades, to make it into a powered dummy. The inspector saw it and put a stop to it because it could cause sparks. My father also made a reclining chair of metal pipe and a canvas sling, and he powered it with a generator."

After the divorce, some felt Dr. Mary got feisty with men. "Though most liked her," Bob Maher said, "some did not because if she had to, she could put her foot down. But with so much to manage, she sometimes had to be stern."

"My father used to argue with Dr. Mary," Patsy Maher Schwartz said, "and so did her secretary and longtime friend, Lucy Barrett, but they both loved her and couldn't get along without her."

Mary's nephew, Peck Brown, said, "Lucy was a nice lady. She was second in command at the San, even at the dinner table. She served coffee while Aunt Mary served the food. Aunt Mary held Lucy in high regard. Dr. Mary traveled a lot while working at the San, so Lucy looked out for things while she was away."

"Lucy Barrett had one speed," said Bob Maher. "She never got excited when Dr. Mary was upset, which might be why they got along so well."

Chapter 16
Dr. Mary's Friend Ober

Exposed rock formations add to the scenery in the border waters that separate International Falls and Ranier from Canada. Dr. Mary loved the rugged beauty, and she often participated in the varied recreation that the area provided: swimming, exploring, boating, and canoeing through interconnected waterways in the rugged northern wilderness. In 1916, Dr. Mary met Ernest Oberholtzer, who went by the name Ober. They both deeply loved the area, and they developed a close friendship.

○○○

Oberholtzer and an Ojibwe guide known as Billy Magee explored unmapped territory that had not been visited by white men since the 1700s. Ober had lived among the Ojibwe Indians in the territory north of, and tributary to, Rainy Lake, Ontario.

The Ojibwe people began calling him "Atisokan," legend or teller of legends. He learned to speak their language fluently, and he understood their way of life. The Ojibwe eventually accepted him as one of their own.[89]

○○○

Ober had heard of Dr. Mary before they met. In 1912, he learned that Dr. Mary, along with Dr. Robert Monahan, had tried unsuccessfully to save the life of E. Raymond Backus, son of lumber baron and industrialist Edward Backus. Raymond was accidentally shot while hunting on Dryweed Island just above Rainy Lake City, where the Backus houseboat was tied. His gun had accidentally discharged.[90]

People often called on Dr. Mary to provide emergency medical care. In early October of the same year, she was again summoned for a gunshot wound when a 13-year-old boy's pistol accidentally discharged, entering under his lower jaw, passing through his tongue, and lodging in his upper jaw. Then, another young

---

[89] *Keeper of the Wild,* Joe Paddock, Minnesota Historical Society Press, 2001

[90] *International Falls Press and Border Budget,* International Falls, Minnesota, October 10, 1912

man's 0.22 caliber rifle accidentally discharged while he tried to crawl under a fence, shooting off his right thumb and riddling his shoulder.[91]

Once they became friends, Ober quickly learned that Dr. Mary was always ready to go to someone's aid, and many of their visits had to end when someone needed her.

◈

In 1925, when Ober was 41, he learned that Edward Backus, whose paper mills were at that time the second-largest producers in the world, planned to build a series of seven dams to create four main water storage areas in the Rainy Lake watershed. Ober considered this an assault on the ecology and beauty of his beloved wilderness, so he organized a national effort to oppose the plan. He campaigned to halt the damming of area rivers for hydroelectric power. Oberholtzer, a strong advocate of conservation in Northern Minnesota, dedicated his life to preserving the border lakes wilderness. [92]

Dr. Mary corresponded with Ober several times in 1929 to assist him in battling what he considered as propaganda aimed at his efforts, and he was grateful for her assistance.[93]

◈

Dr. Mary's son, Jim, remembered Ober fondly. "He was a tiny little guy. He had an Indian drum tied to his ceiling, and he was proud to be able to kick it. He was very agile. He could fold his legs and walk on his knees, all folded up. Quite a crowd was gathered at his island once when he did that. He got cramps and was in severe pain. Mom got everybody out of there and got him untangled. Those of us waiting out of sight could hear his screams."

Ober's love of music and books, his passion for the borderlands, his sense of adventure, and his never-ending supply of stories were among the things that cemented his friendship with Dr. Mary.

---

[91] *International Falls Press and Border Budget,* International Falls, Minnesota, October 10, 1912

[92] http://eober.org/pages/oberholtzer/o_timeline.html

[93] Minnesota History Center, Letter from Oberholtzer to Dr. Mary Ghostley, June 25, 1929

He died in 1977. Ober has been called "the original architect of the border wilderness,"[94] He helped found the Wilderness Society and served on its executive council for 30 years. [95] The outcome of his tireless efforts was the creation of the Boundary Waters Canoe Area Wilderness and Voyageurs National Park in Minnesota and Quetico Provincial Park in Ontario, Canada.[96] People continue to enjoy the wilderness he fought for, many never knowing that it was ever at risk.

---

[94] *Star Tribune* Minneapolis, Minnesota, September 6, 1993
[95] http://www.mnhs.org/library/findaids/00353.html
[96] *Star Tribune*, Minneapolis, Minnesota, September 6, 1993

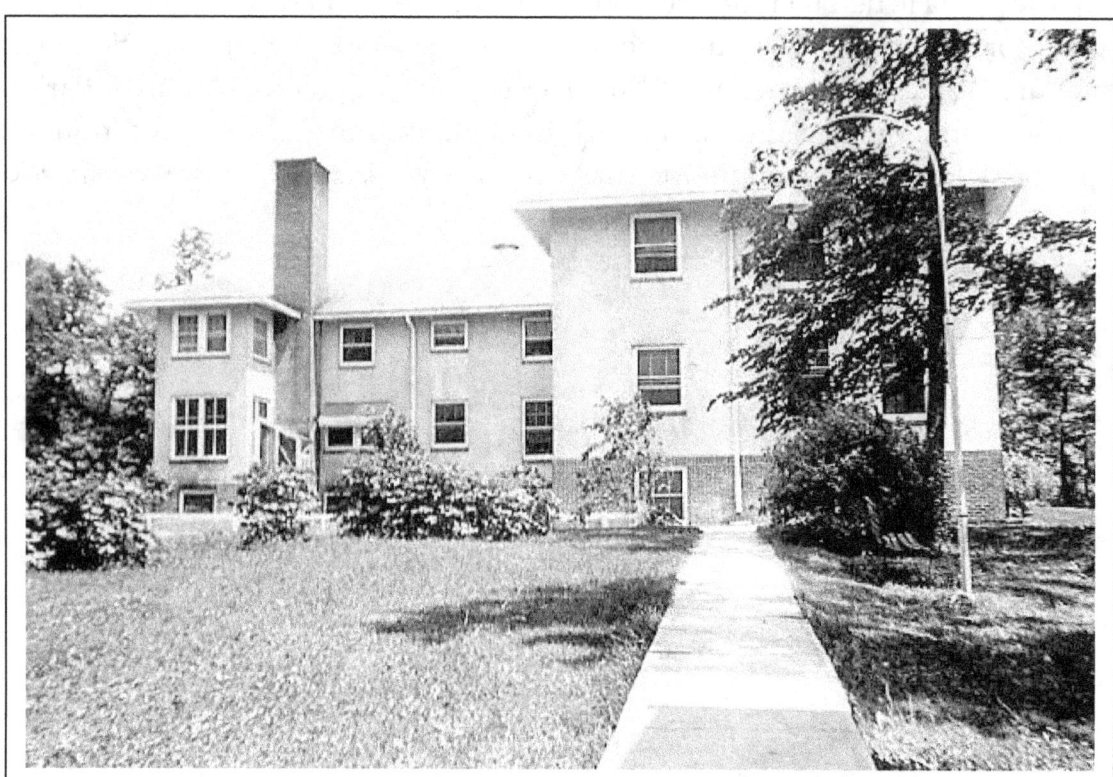

West Side of Lake Julia Tuberculosis Sanatorium
Walkway was referred to by some employees as "Lovers' Lane."
Art Holmstrom photo

Section Four: My Family

Chapter 17
My Mother's Path to the San

Ella Lillian Grande, my mother, was born on March 23, 1913, in Fergus Falls, Minnesota. Just over six years later, her family survived the Fergus Falls cyclone on June 22, 1919. Before she passed, she left extensive notes, especially about her childhood and young-adult life and her job at the San.

My grandfather, Johannes (John) Grande, owned an electric shop in Fergus Falls, which he sold in 1925. He traded their attractive, tidy house on Summit Avenue for 80 acres with a house near Wilton, plus $500. He liked the pines in Wilton because they reminded him of his childhood home in Norway.

My grandmother, Bertha, hadn't seen the place. The family drove to Bemidji, where the moving van was supposed to meet them at noon, but it didn't show up. They waited until midnight, and then Mom's father decided they should drive out to the place. The house turned out to be an old bootlegger's shack and a disappointment to my grandmother, who expected better. It was mid-October, and cold air pushed through the gaps between the logs of the house.

Mom's brother Clarence had moved with the family to Wilton. He wanted to earn some money but could not find a job, so in 1926 he tried selling Aladdin lamps and lanterns. One cold winter day, Clarence and his brother Russell walked 8 miles to Wilton to pick up the lights. Russell froze his feet, hands, and cheeks. The boys spent the night at a farmhouse where the owner had 15-year-old Russell soak his feet in kerosene to thaw them. Luckily, there were no ill effects. The young men felt uncertain about the kerosene treatment—because the man who suggested it had no feet himself! The next day, they got a ride home from a fellow with a team of horses and a sled full of hay.

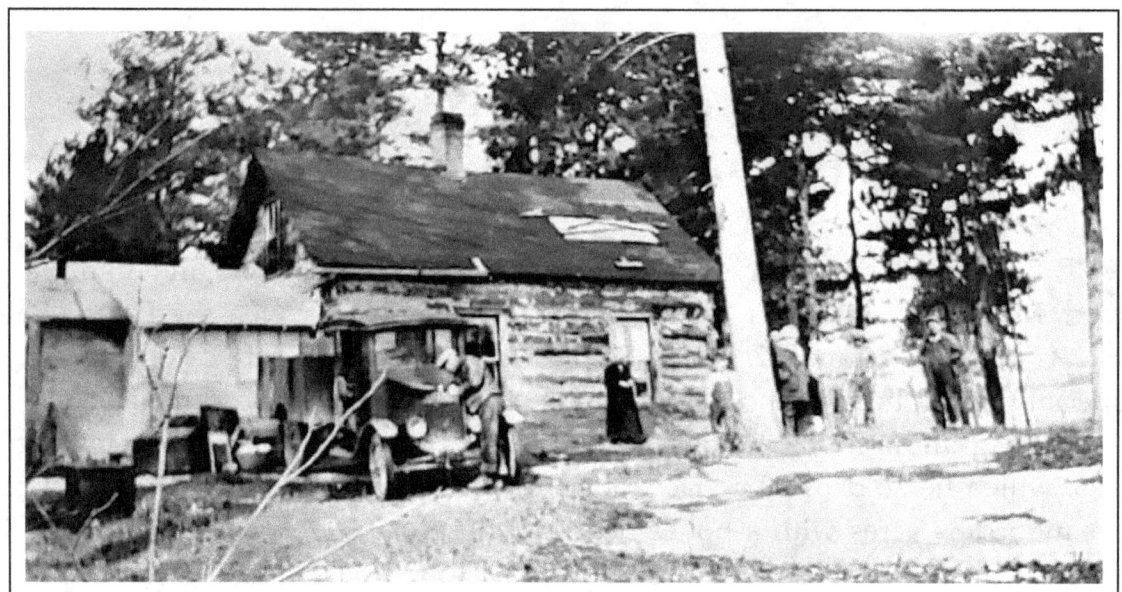

*My grandfather, John Grande, moved his family into
this old bootlegger's shack in the middle of the night.
My grandmother was unhappy about the condition of the house.
Ella Hedglin collection*

In the spring, Clarence still had not found work, so he decided to leave Wilton. The basement in their shack had a family of seven skunks. He needed travel money, so he trapped the skunks and got $1 for each. He hitched a ride in train boxcars from Wilton to Buffalo, New York. He jumped off before each town to wash dishes in restaurants in exchange for food.

My mother went to Pony Lake School and graduated from the eighth grade in 1927. She went on to high school in Pelican Rapids for a short time, but she had to quit because her family couldn't afford the tuition.

Like her brother Clarence, it was hard for my mother to find work. She left Wilton to find a job but eventually moved back home to help with her ailing grandmother, who had moved in with the family.

In July 1931, Mom's friend Eva Ihde started work at the Lake Julia Tuberculosis Sanatorium. She told my mother how much she liked pulling the chain to use the dumbwaiter (nicknamed *dummy*) that delivered the trays from upstairs back down to the kitchen, where there was a machine to wash the dishes. She expressed how helpful the employees were and how easy it was to make friends. "There's the most attractive, modern furniture in the dining room," she said, "and it's just a shame that so many patients have to eat in their rooms instead of enjoying it."

"Since grandmother passed on," Mom commented, "I need to find a job. I don't suppose the San has any openings."

Eva had taken the job at the San to earn money to buy a treadle sewing machine. One day when she went to work, she heard there would be a job opening for a maid. She had been doing summer relief work in the kitchen during vacations, and she needed a steady job. One of the maids, Violet Allen, had already packed for vacation, and Dr. Mary didn't have anyone to take her place.

Both Eva and her friend Emma Lovik considered the job. Eva didn't want to take the maid position because she was afraid to be in such close contact with the patients. After all, she already tested positive for tuberculosis, and she didn't want the disease to become active. Emma, too, was afraid of catching TB. Her parents were concerned about the risk. They told her that if she were to take the job, she needn't come home again.

Eva remembered that Mom was looking for a job, so she contacted her. My mother's need for a job must have been greater than her fear of tuberculosis because she started work the next morning.

Some of my mother's duties were to wash the patients' bedside tables and bed railings and to pass washbasins and towels before meals. Mom helped nurses pass out trays at mealtimes, too. She also cleaned patient bathrooms, washed door and window casings, and washed walls up as far as she, at 5 feet, could reach. It was then the janitor's responsibility to clean the higher places.

She was off work a few hours in the afternoon and returned in time to pass basins before the evening meal. After collecting trays, she was off work for the day, and she could return to her room in the nurses' home basement.

She was glad the job came with a warm place to call home and plenty of tasty, healthy food, and she liked making friends with the other employees.

After a couple of weeks, Eva left to work in Bemidji at the Birchmont Hotel, which paid a little more than the San position. Dr. Mary offered my mother a full-time job as a tray girl and dishwasher. Mom was happy to have kitchen work, and my grandmother was relieved to learn that she was no longer working in close contact with the patients.

When Violet Allen returned from vacation, she was Mom's roommate in the nurses' home. A maid had to be in close contact with the patients, and before long, Violet had contracted tuberculosis. She became a patient at the San at the beginning of 1933, at age 18, and was hospitalized until May 1934, then again from December 1934 to April 1937.[97]

On a visit home, Mom was excited to tell her mother all about her new job. "Others don't like the tray-girl job as there is so much to remember," she said, "but I like it. With 53 patients and many special orders, it is difficult to keep track of everything. That's part of the fun."

Each day, my mother set up trays with juices, butter, milk, etc., plus tea bags and other things at the last minute to be sure patients got what they had ordered. Then, she put six trays at a time on the dummy and pulled the rope, and the nurses on the second floor received them. Nurses on the first floor delivered the trays to their patients with the help of a maid. While patients ate, Mom served the up-patients—those who didn't have to remain confined to bed—in the dining room.

"I also serve three special tables in the dining room," she proudly told her mother. "One is for doctors and board members. Another is for nurses and employees. The third is for guests. I get to meet everyone!"

After people in the dining room finished eating, Mom helped clear tables. The empty trays from the wards went back to the kitchen. She ran the dishwasher, then scrubbed the sinks until they sparkled. Mom cleaned the whole area before setting up trays for the next meal. She toiled in steam, detergent, and bleach, doing her best to rid the plates, cups, and silverware of the deadly bacterium. It took about an hour to clear the dining room tables, clean trays, wash dishes, and clean the stainless-steel prep tables and floor, then to set up trays for the next meal. The workers had to be out of the kitchen by 1:00 for 'silent time.'

"I made up Jell-O® and some Norwegian buttermilk from a starter, and I had to have a little left to start a new batch," Mom told her mother on a visit home. She had never made buttermilk, and she was proud to talk about her new experience. "And on Saturdays, four of us girls cut and section grapefruit for Sunday mornings, enough for all of the patients and the help. That means there is no time off Sunday afternoons. And when the raspberries are ripe, we won't be off in the afternoons, either, because we'll have to pick berries. But toward the last of the berry season, Dr. Mary will let us pick a flat of berries to take home to our families. You'll like that, Mother!" she said.

---

[97] Minnesota History Center, Lake Julia Tuberculosis Sanatorium, Patient Register

About once a month, she bleached the dishes and polished the silverware. She put cutlery in a huge kettle on the stove to boil and added a disinfectant to the water.

The kitchen crew consisted of the chef and second cook, a relief girl (who took the place of other girls on their days off), a dining room girl, and a tray girl/dishwasher. The dining room girl and relief girl helped clear and set up trays.

There was also a rear dining room where employees, such as the truck driver, janitor, floor maids, nurses'-home maid, laundry girls, the two engineers who ran the heating plant, the teamster, and the extra men during haying ate their meals. They would ring a bell, and the waitresses would serve them. The dining room waitresses washed these dishes by hand in a separate sink, along with those of doctors, nurses, and guests. The girl who scraped the trays wore a gown and mask. Leftover food went over to the San Dairy to feed the pigs.

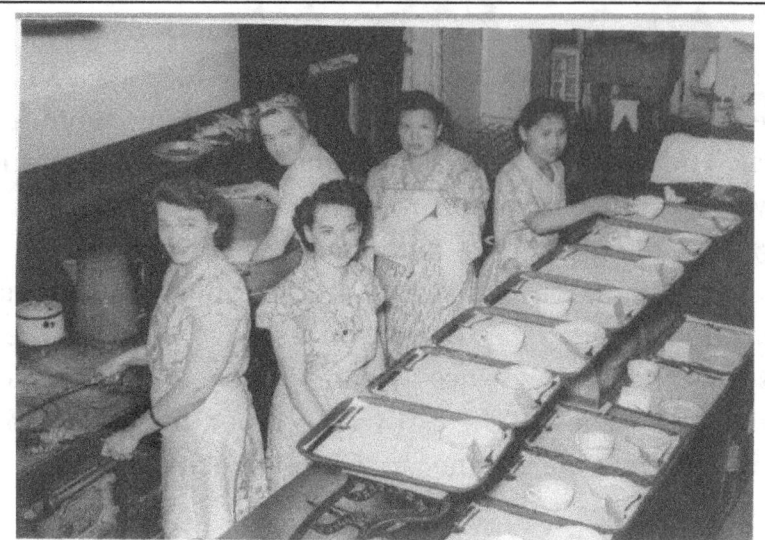

Kitchen Crew
James Ghostley collection

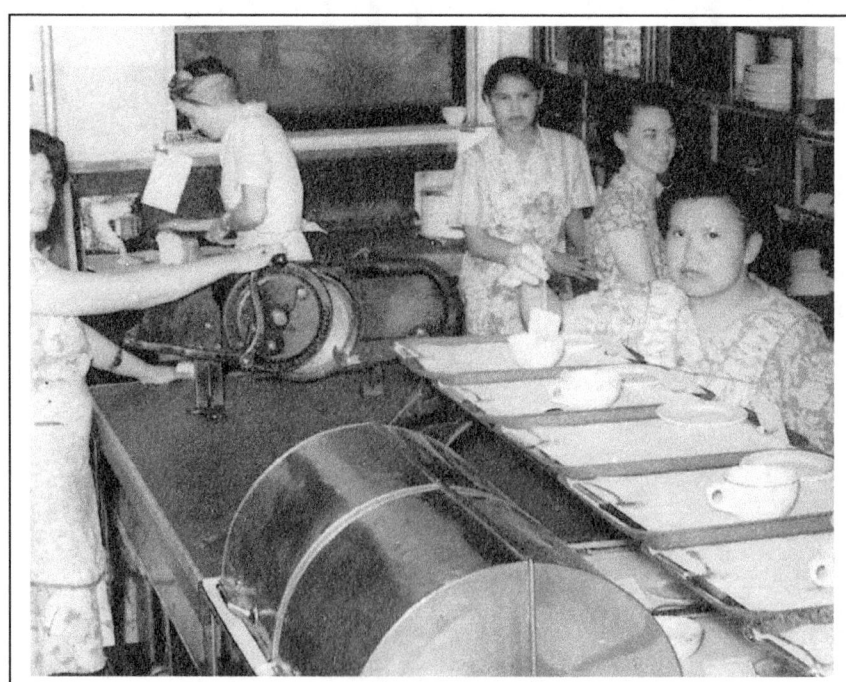

Kitchen Crew
James Ghostley collection

Chapter 18
My Father's Rocky Road

Lee Hedglin, my father, was delivered by his father, Edward, on October 20, 1908. The family lived in Maple Ridge Township, Minnesota, at Island Lake near Pleasant Valley School. The way Dad told it, there were "seven children in the first litter and six in the second." In the first family, there were Tom, Flo, Nell, Maude, Omer, William, and Luella Long, my father's half-siblings. In the second family, there was Harry, Dad, Ernest, Edward, Florence, and Opal Hedglin.

Dad's father abandoned his large family and ran off to live on the Red Lake Indian Reservation. His mother, Anna, was left penniless to raise the youngsters by herself on a mosquito-infested bog. With no money to buy shoes, she made moccasins for my dad and his siblings to wear to school.

Indians near my grandmother Anna's home befriended her and traded their wild rice for her cranberries. They sometimes borrowed her cast-iron skillets, then polished them with sand to a brilliant sheen before returning them. They stuck up for her when some in the area bullied her, and she valued their friendship.

Dad's paternal grandmother died before he was born, and his grandfather, George Webster Hedglin, died when he was 12. Just a few months later, on July 18, 1922, his mother died of appendicitis. There were so many children, but there were no grandparents to take care of them. When their mother died, the children went several directions because no one could afford to take in the whole family. Because there was no money, my father couldn't attend school again after he completed the seventh grade.

The San had many empty beds at that time, so Dr. Laney took in Dad's youngest sisters, Opal, 6, and Florence, 9, to stay at the San for a while because they appeared undernourished. Their names did not appear in the patient register because the San was only for tuberculosis patients, not for the poor, hungry, and orphaned.

The Hedglin boys stayed with their Uncle Charlie for a while. Later, some of them stayed for a short time with an older half-sister and her husband. Before long, Dad and his younger brother, Ed, who'd both had to grow up quickly, hopped freight trains and headed for Montana to look for work. They sometimes camped with Gypsies along the way, and other times they begged to sleep in jail cells for the night. The boys bought louse powder to sprinkle on the jail cots and down their shirts because they had heard lice were bad in jails. Newspapers covered the cots, and Dad and Ed could hear insects crawling across those papers all night.

Their sisters, Opal and Florence, who had been admitted off the record after their mother died, were officially patients at the San in 1927. Opal Hedglin became patient No. 577 on September 1, 1927, shortly before her 11th birthday, and Florence Hedglin Smith became patient No. 587 on October 30, 1927. Florence, at age 14, was already married.

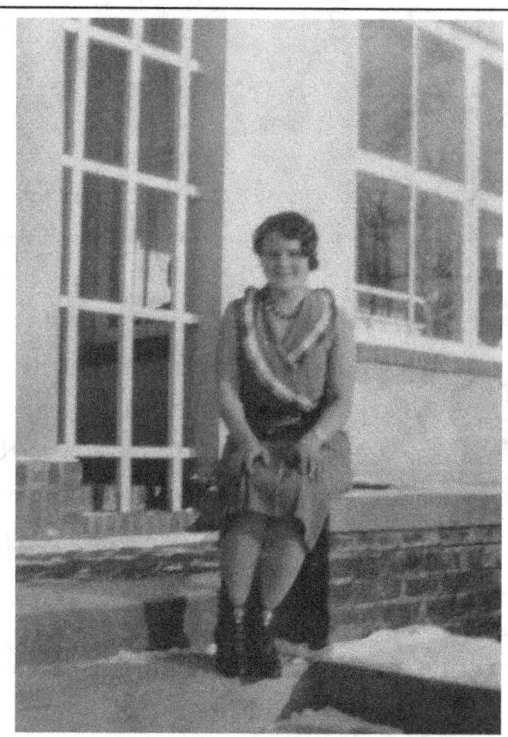

My aunt Opal Hedglin Smith on the San steps
Ella Hedglin collection

Florence's condition improved, and she left on January 22, 1928, after 85 days at the San. Opal, who had improved but was not yet considered well, left on the same day as Florence, but against doctor's advice. [98] Years later, Opal was back for a third time, this time as an employee.

☙❧

Dad finally found a steady job in October 1930 when he started working at the Lake Julia Tuberculosis Sanatorium as a janitor, earning $50 per month. His brother-in-law Dave Bruzelius, a former janitor at the San, helped him get the job. Bruzelius was married to Dad's half-sister Nell. He was her second husband. Her first husband, Hiram Flanders, had been admitted to the San in September 1920,

---

[98] Minnesota History Center, Lake Julia Tuberculosis Sanatorium, Patient Register

and 227 days later, he left against advice.[99] He eventually died of tuberculosis, as so many had.

Besides a job, my dad got a warm place to sleep each night. His little bed with its thin mattress felt like a luxury in the heated San basement, and he went to bed every night with a full belly. He got to know Bill Malterud, the yard man; Harry Maher, the engineer; Elmer Current, the night engineer; and others. Dad felt a sense of belonging and of being part of a family. He worked hard and took pride in doing a good job.

My father got to know the patients well because his cleaning responsibilities took him into their rooms. He had to learn to deal with being around illness and death. One day a patient, Elida Josephson of Pinewood, gave him a photo of herself. On the side, she wrote, "Lest you forget me." She died the day after Christmas in 1931. Dad never forgot her or others who died while he worked at the San. He kept Elida's photo throughout the rest of his life.

Dad and his brother Ed talked about going back to Montana, but then he met the new tray girl, Ella Grande, and he decided to stay.

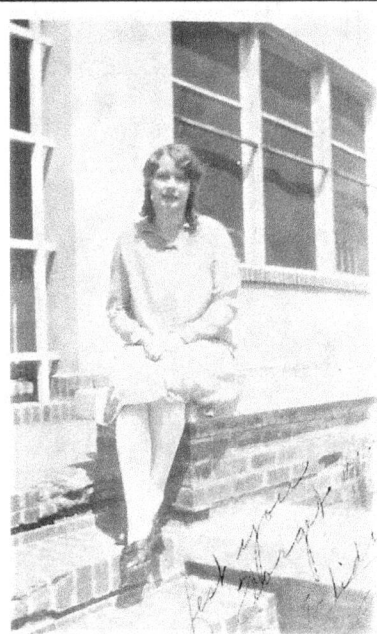

My father kept this photo that Elida Josephson gave to him. On it, she wrote, "Lest you forget me." She died at the San.
Ella Hedglin collection

---

[99] Minnesota History Center, Lake Julia Tuberculosis Sanatorium, Patient Register

Chapter 19
Marriage and Family

My parents' first date was to attend a church service together at the Puposky School. Soon, they made plans to be married.

Dad bought a suit from Everett McCarthy, a TB patient, to wear at their wedding. They were married on June 9, 1932, by the justice of the peace. My mother left these notes about the wedding: "I wore high heels. They hurt my feet, so I never wore them again. It wasn't a fancy wedding. I bought some flowered building paper for my parents' house to cover the mud-plastered logs. With my earnings from the San, I bought groceries for the celebration, and mother baked a cake. Our wedding party got together at my parents' house for supper. I didn't think about it at the time, but I suppose we could have found a better place for our wedding photo than in front of a barbed-wire fence!

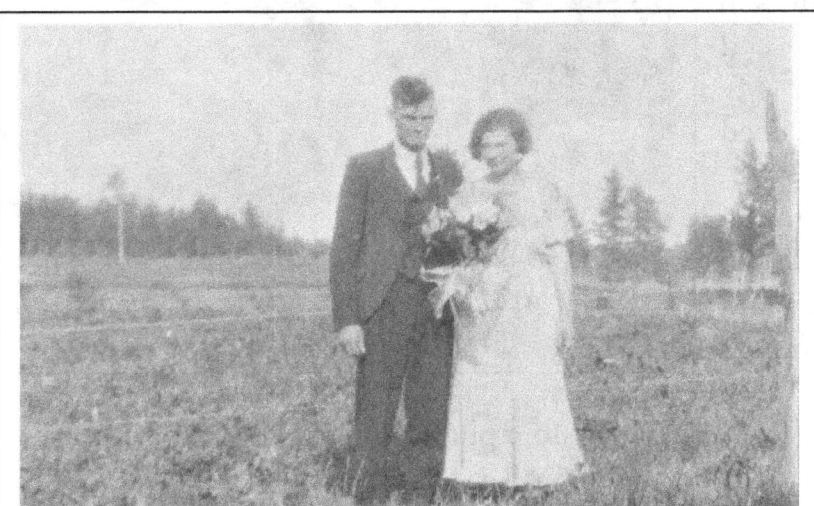

My parents' wedding photo
Lee Hedglin and Ella Grande
Ella Hedglin collection

"We borrowed a car for our honeymoon, and a friend offered us a place to stay. It rained hard that night, right through the roof of our wedding-night lodging, so we had to move the bed from place to place to find a dry place to sleep."

After marrying, they moved out of their separate San accommodations into Dad's brother-in-law Dave Bruzelius's place in Puposky. They rented their first home for $5 per month.

The house had broken plaster on the walls and unvarnished floors. My mother told me she scrubbed floors with a brush every day. Because there were no shelves in the pantry, she used wooden apple and orange boxes to store dishes and supplies.

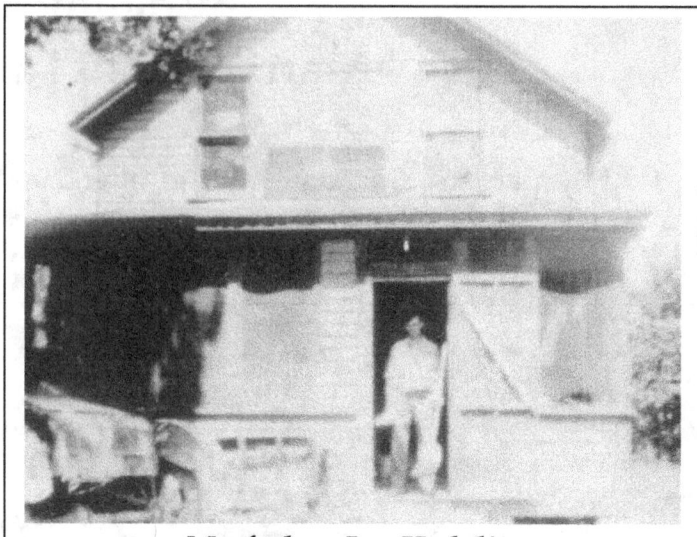
My father, Lee Hedglin, at the Bruzelius house, 1932
Ella Hedglin collection

Several neighbors shared a well. Mom put milk in a gallon pail with a cover, tied a rope to it, and let it down into the well to keep the milk cold.

Dad didn't want people to think he couldn't support his wife, so he didn't want Mom to continue to work. Once she left the job, she missed the work and the friendships, so Dad finally agreed that she could fill in during vacations.

My father slept at home but took baths and ate many of his meals at the San. My mother baked a lot of bread. Because Dad ate at the San and Mom baked, they were able to stretch their budget; still, half of Dad's monthly pay went to groceries, so they took in Clarissa Anderson, the schoolteacher, to room with them. That added $15 per month to their income.

My oldest brother, James Leroy Hedglin, was born on April 19, 1933. They called him Jimmie. Dr. Mary delivered him, and a Mrs. Luense was the midwife. Dr. Mary delivered babies free of charge for employees and others in the community who could not afford a doctor. Mom and Dad paid the midwife $15 for her services.

Dr. Mary expected new mothers to stay in bed for 10 days. One day, my mother complained of a headache, so the midwife let her sit up. The doctor stopped by to see how Mom felt, and she scolded her for sitting. Dr. Mary must not have been angry, though, because a few days later, she brought her children, Jim and Cathie, to visit the new baby.

When Jimmie was one year old, Dad transferred from his janitor position to be the dairyman for the San Dairy, the farm that supplied the San with milk and cream.

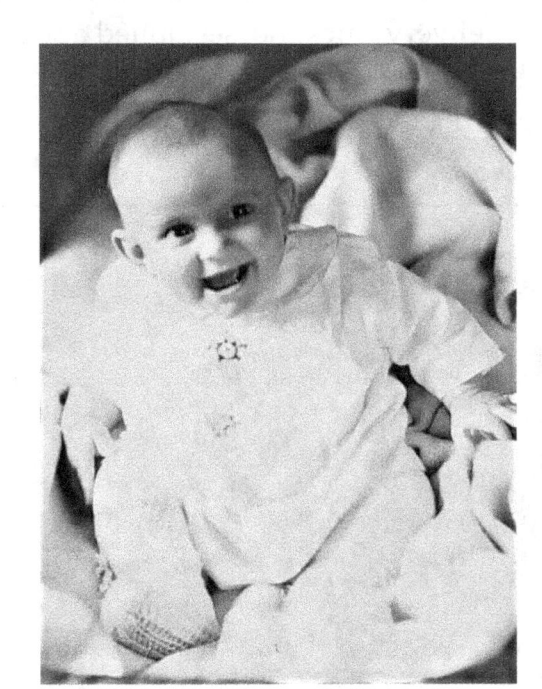

My oldest brother, Jimmie Hedglin, a " Dr. Mary Baby"
Ella Hedglin collection

The family moved into the house at the dairy, where they enjoyed running water and a bathroom in the basement. There were electric lights and all the milk the family wanted, even a little cream. Mom and Dad put up a small chicken coop for their 12 hens and a rooster, so there were plenty of eggs. On the San Dairy, milking started at 3 a.m.

The work was hard, but the pay and benefits made up for it.

∞

One day, Dr. Mary remarked, "Lee's barn floor is cleaner than the floors in most people's homes." The barn had a cement floor. Dad always hosed it down and kept it spotless.

The cows were milked with milking machines. Dad was proud of the way he cared for the animals, and he was happy to learn that one cow had topped production and butterfat for Holstein cows in Beltrami County.

My mother's job was to weigh the feed for each cow. She based the amount of feed on how much milk each one produced. She knew them all by name, even when they were in the pasture. All were black and white, but no two had the same spots.

My father weighed the milk at every milking, and he kept records. The county milk tester came by once a month, and he periodically tested the cows for TB and Bangs disease—an infectious bacterial disease of cattle that infects the genital organs and can cause spontaneous abortions.

After milking, Dad put the milk into cooling tanks, and in the morning, he separated it so there would be cream for the patients. In the evening, my parents worked together to bottle 200 half-pints of whole milk. Next, Dad thoroughly washed and sanitized the milking machine, separator, and other equipment, and he sanitized the milk-house floor.

In the morning, he delivered the bottled milk and cream and the milk for cooking to the San. He fed the remainder of the separated milk to the pigs. In the winter, when the snow was too deep for the delivery truck, horses pulled a wagon of milk to the San, and with each step the horses took, the loud, brassy, rhythmic sounds of leather and metal rang out through the cold air.

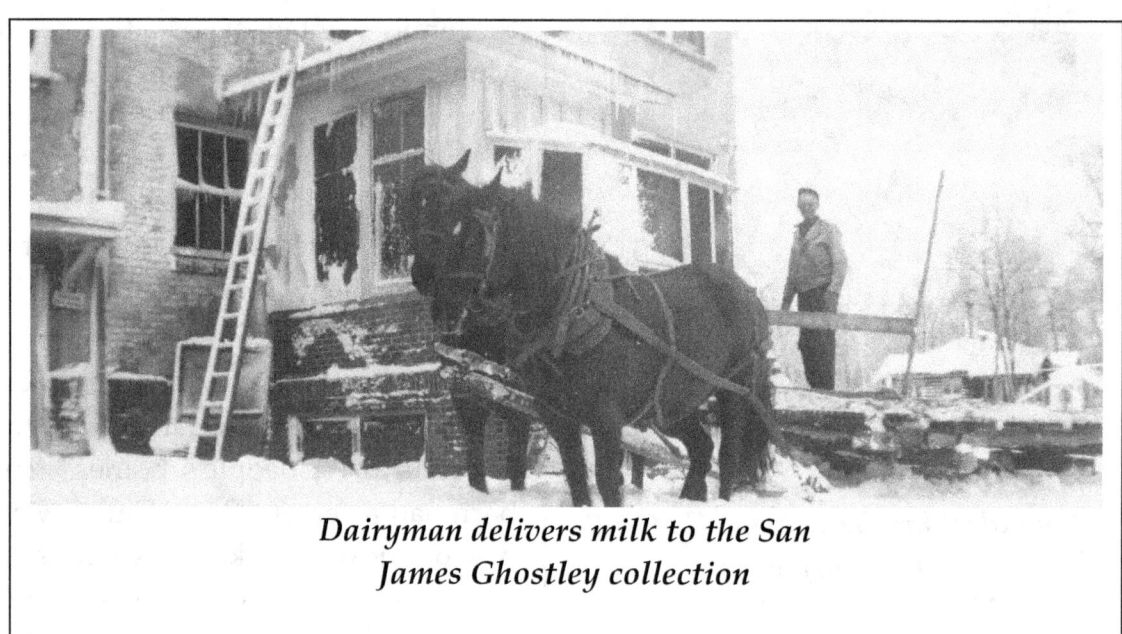

Dairyman delivers milk to the San
James Ghostley collection

Dad also raised pigs to butcher for the San. My parents usually got the heads, and Mom's brother Reuben helped make headcheese. They didn't waste anything that they could eat.

༺ཿ༻

There were many dangers for small children. Jimmie kept everyone on their toes. When he was a year old, he crawled over to Mom's brother while he read a book, and he bit Reuben's big toe. That should have warned Mom and Dad that Jimmie was going to be a feisty one. Jimmie used to crawl into the chicken pen through any hole he could find. One day my brother frightened a hen, and the Wyandotte rooster went after him. From then on, the rooster chased Jimmie every time he went outside. Soon, to protect the young boy, the rooster was butchered for dinner.

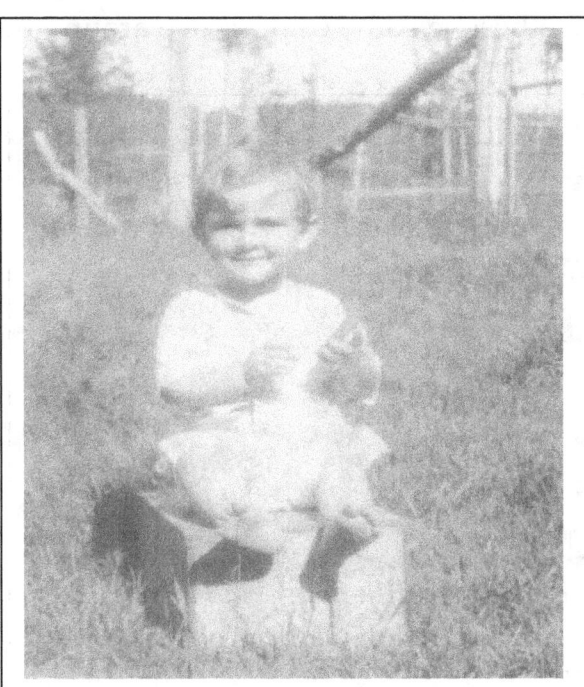
My oldest brother, Jimmie at the San Dairy
Ella Hedglin collection

There was one registered Holstein bull on the farm that was known to be mean. One day, Jimmie crawled under the gate and went into the L-shaped pen. When my mother saw him, he started to climb the 6-foot fence. She called for help as the bull approached and sniffed at her toddler. Jimmie slapped the beast on the nose. As he reached the top rail, Uncle Reuben grabbed him and lifted him away from the pen, just in time.

There was a big tank of kerosene on the property, and one day Jimmie opened the spout and soaked his shoes. After that, Dad put a lock on the container.

Another time, Jimmie climbed on top of a beehive and jumped on it. The bees must have been out because he wasn't stung.

Jimmie wouldn't nap, and it was hard to get him to sleep at night. The older he got, the more active he became. He was happy, but always on the go, and very quick to disappear.

In the morning, the truck driver usually left the keys in the truck when he parked in front of the milk house. One day, three-year-old Jimmie got in and started the vehicle. It went down the slope where it tore out the fence that was around the house. Jimmie, though, was OK. The truck driver and teamster laughed, which just encouraged Jimmie to be naughty.

Another time, Jimmie went behind the barn, and Mom found him in the truck with the motor running. He was proud, and he told her, "Me start car. Me start car."

Once when the truck was hooked up to the hay rope to pull hay into the hayloft, Jimmie had disappeared again. He was in the barn where he held the rope as the workers pulled in the hay. Someone heard his screams, so they stopped pulling. By then, the back of his hand was raw. Mom met them as they came from the barn. That's when she decided to tie a rope around Jimmie's waist whenever he went outside. She fastened it to the clothesline so he could move around but could not get to the barn.

Jimmie wasn't the only child who got hurt at the farm. My mother's nephew Clarence, 5 years old, tried to set the gopher trap and got his fingers caught.

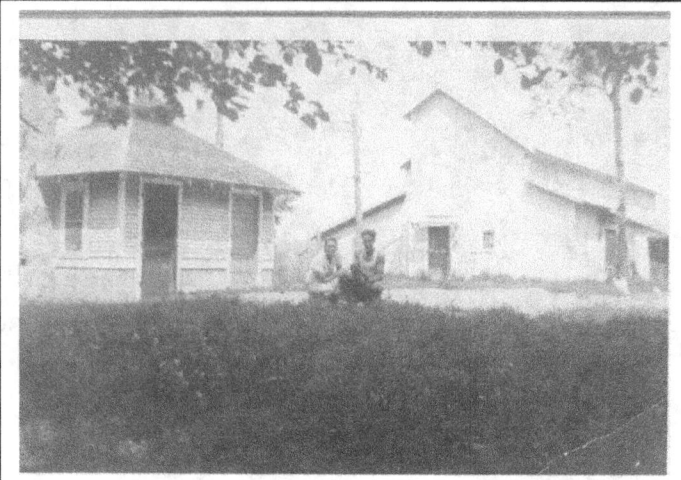
San Dairy milk house and barn
Ella Hedglin collection

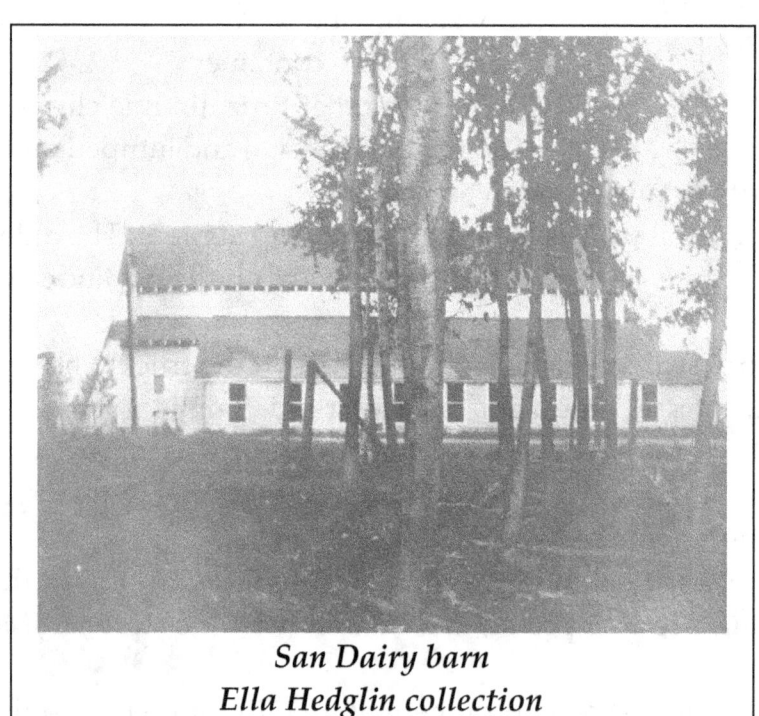
San Dairy barn
Ella Hedglin collection

Chapter 20
Leaving the Dairy—but not Forever

Jimmie kept getting hurt on the farm, so in 1935, Mom convinced Dad that they should move off the San Dairy. In hindsight, that might not have been the best thing to do during the Great Depression because, on the farm, they not only earned a wage but also had a warm place to live, a bathroom in the house, electricity, and food.

Their move began a long struggle to make ends meet. Those with jobs at the San had a different lifestyle than many during the Depression. Most Depression-era families could not find work, yet the San employed many.

My parents bought acreage south of Puposky. They stayed at Grandma Grande's house for a month while Dad built a small log house. There wasn't even an outhouse at first. No one had ever taught Dad construction, and there were big cracks in the floor. He built the house in the fall, and frost was already on the ground and crawling up between the floorboards. Mom wore wool socks and Dad's old felt shoes to try to keep warm. The temperature dropped to 35 degrees below zero. She was pregnant with my brother Lloyd at that time. She spent much of the morning in bed with Jimmie, trying to keep him warm.

My parents had to haul their drinking water from the neighbor's place in cream cans on a child's sled. Mom lugged snow in big tubs, melted it on the stove, and dumped the water into a big barrel in the corner of the kitchen to use for baths and for washing clothes and dishes. She couldn't afford the gas to operate her Maytag washer, so she washed clothes by hand using a scrub board. It took her all week to get enough snow melted to do laundry. She used bluing to scrub the floors with a scrub brush.

Dad cut wood for $2 a day in that bitterly cold weather. He sometimes worked for others at 25 cents per hour. At times, Dad worked as a teamster for the San, driving trucks. He farmed his land, painted walls at the San, and put up ice. One year, even though he had chickenpox, he stood in Lake Julia near the shoreline to cut two-foot square blocks of ice, then packed them in sawdust and sold them for 5 cents a block. He also sheared sheep with his uncle, Charlie Hedglin, and he found work wherever he could.

My brother Lloyd was born on April 23, 1936. By then, doctors had begun to complain that Dr. Mary took business from them by delivering so many babies, so Lloyd was delivered by Dr. Vandersluis. What the other doctors didn't know was that patients seldom paid Dr. Mary in cash. Instead, she often only received a chicken or a thank you and a promise for her services.

When Lloyd was five months old, the family moved out of the drafty little cabin and moved in with Dad's Uncle Charlie at Turtle Lake.

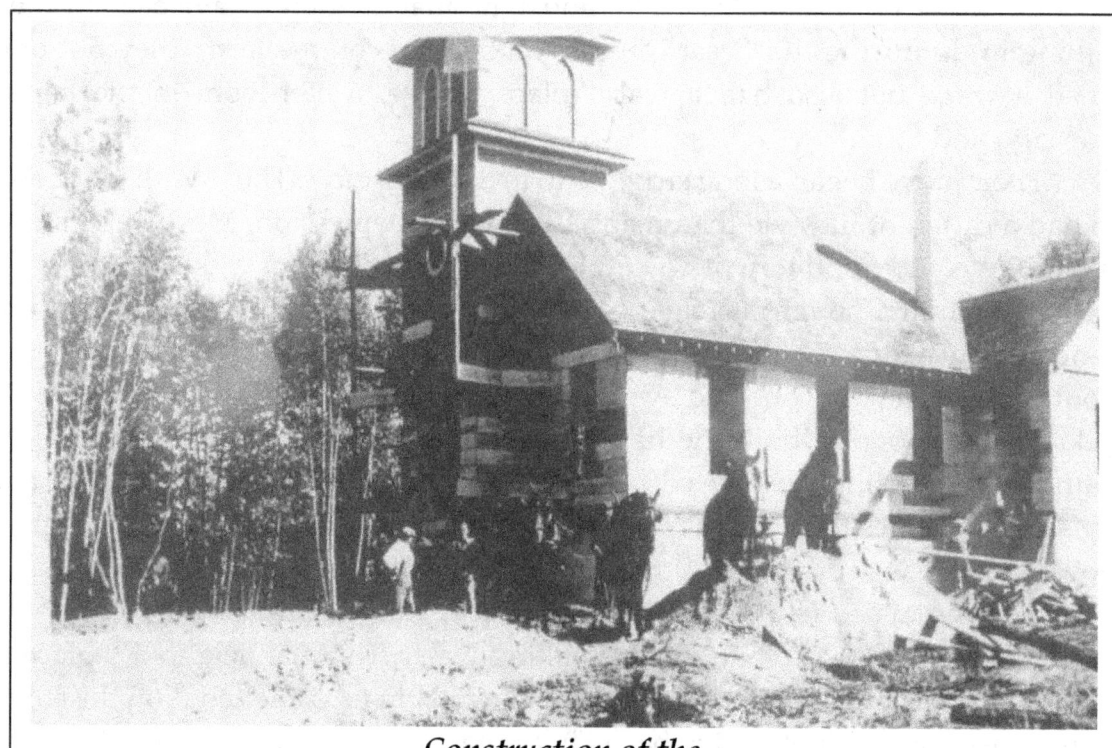

*Construction of the
Our Redeemer's Lutheran Church, Puposky
Ella Hedglin collection*

That year, Dad helped build the white Our Redeemer's Lutheran Church, where he and Mom were charter members.

The church was first under the direction of Rev. A. E. Hanson, who, beginning in 1931, agreed to be a temporary pastor. He came from Bemidji a couple of times a month to conduct church services in the schoolhouse or the town hall.

Rev. Jacob Stolee was in charge for seven years beginning in 1934. He and his wife, Alice, had moved to Puposky just before Christmas, where they lived in a small cottage on the San property.[100]

On September 5, 1935, a meeting was held to organize the Our Redeemer's Lutheran Congregation of Puposky. The congregation adopted a building program on February 2, 1936. Funds raised included a generous donation from Dr. Mary Ghostley. There were donations, pledges, and an $800 loan from the church extension fund.[101]

William Carlson donated stumpage on a tract of his land. The men of the congregation cut logs and exchanged them at Dickinson's Lumbermill for seasoned building material. The church structure was planned, complete with

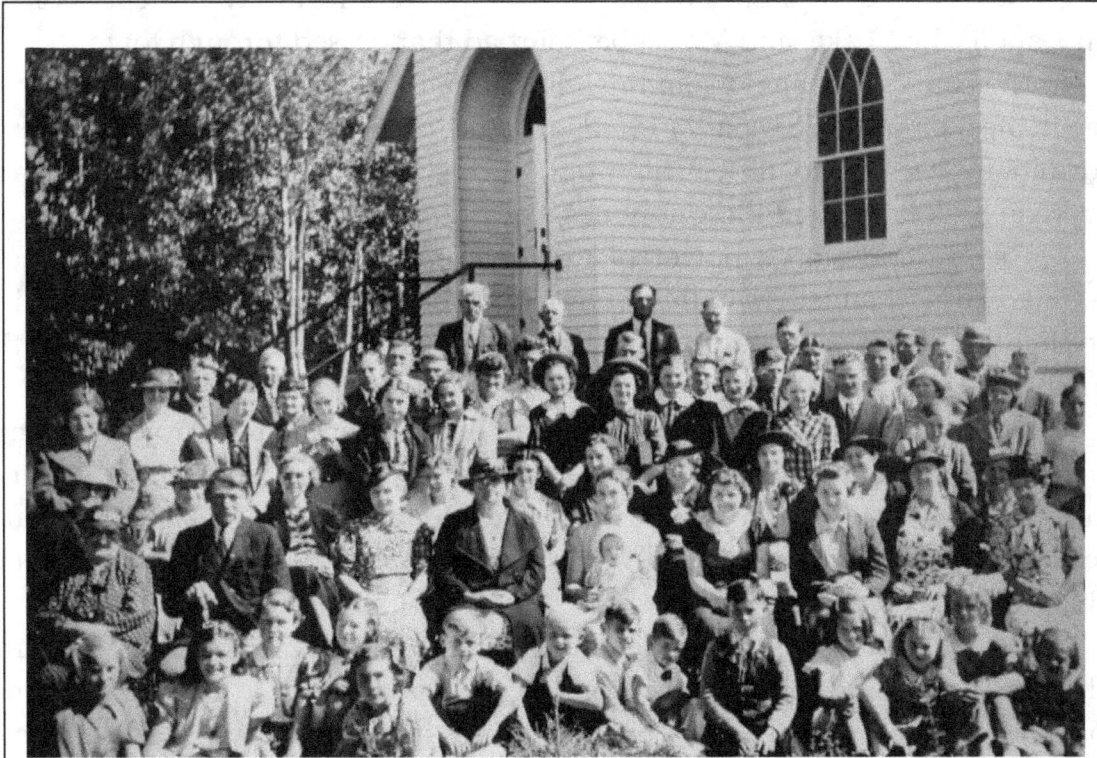

Congregation gathers at the Our Redeemer's Lutheran Church, Puposky
Ella Hedglin collection

---

[100] Ella Hedglin
[101] Puposky Centennial Booklet, 2005

sacristy, steeple, and basement. Mr. and Mrs. Carl Durand donated a site across from their store, which had first been owned and operated by Carl's father, Charles Durand.

Construction commenced in July 1936 and was nearly complete by Christmas. Charles Maher sawed wood into lumber. Other men cut firewood and hauled it to the church grounds. Before the congregation hired a janitor, Dad split firewood to keep the new church warm for Sunday services. It was a community affair.

The church was a frame structure of 28 feet by 40 feet with a full concrete basement,[102] a dining room, a kitchen with both a wood stove and a gas stove, and a church bell that came from a discarded locomotive. Windows were of gothic design with cathedral glass. Two rows of pews were formerly in depots of the Minneapolis, Red Lake, and Manitoba Railroad that passed through town.

The church had an outstanding altar and altar ring. The central spires had been in the old Luther Seminary in St. Paul before being removed and stored. They had initially been 12 to 14 feet high but were cut down to fit the new church. Reverend Stolee acquired these antiques, thanks to the influence of friends.

The Durand store's power plant provided electricity for lighting. There were two large chandeliers in the center, lights between the windows, and a big floodlight above the altar, plus a small sidelight on each side. Dedication of the church and laying of the cornerstone took place on June 6, 1937.

During the building of the church, Dad developed severe thyroid problems. An enlarged thyroid gland had caused massive swelling in his neck—a goiter—causing him to suffer from nervousness and palpitations. In those days, many people suffered from goiters; they were common until people started using iodized salt.

Just six months after he helped finish the church, on December 18, 1937, my father had a thyroidectomy. Following surgery, his doctor told him he could not work for three years. That wasn't the only illness in the family. While Dad was in the hospital, Mom and the two boys had whooping cough.

At that time, the family lived in an old shack that belonged to Dad's half-sister, Flo Mackaman. Some days, it took half a cord of wood to heat the place, and luckily, Mom's brother Reuben cut the wood for them. Dad had frequent doctor's

---

[102] Puposky Centennial Booklet, 2005

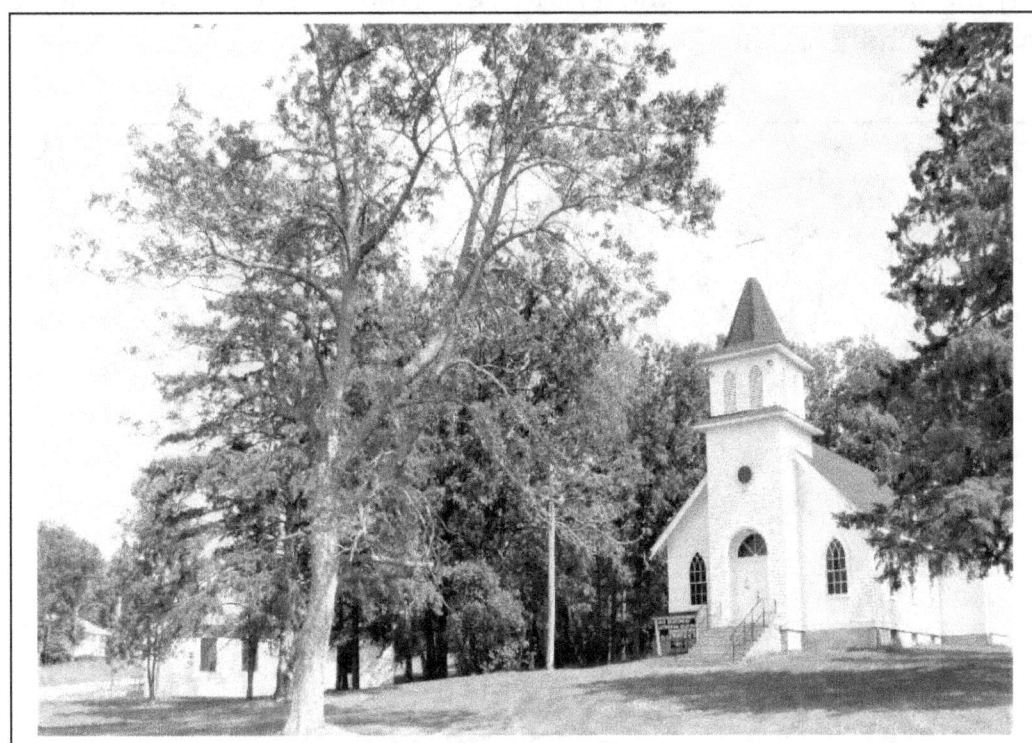
Our Redeemer's Lutheran Church, Puposky
Pat Nelson photo

appointments in Bemidji. Miss Kjome from the relief office said the place wasn't fit to live in, so one bitterly cold day, Mom hitchhiked to town to talk to the men at the relief office about getting a place in Bemidji to live while Dad recuperated. They refused to help until Miss Kjome overheard from her office and stepped in.

Soon the family moved to a two-room apartment on Eighth Street. Things were quiet at first while the landlady's husband was away, but once he returned, he was loud and disruptive to his neighbors.

My mother heard the rumor that he pawned anything he could, including his wife's iron and his clothing, to buy Heet to drink for the effects of its primary ingredient, methanol. She was afraid to stay there and started looking for another place to live. She asked Dr. Mary for advice.

Luckily, a little house was vacant on the San property where the cook and baker, Adolf Becker, had lived. She offered the house to my parents at $5 per month.

The Becker family—Adolf, his wife, Johanna, and their children Ruthie, Fritz, and Rolf—had recently returned to Germany. Dr. Mary had cried when they left. My mother was sad to see them go too, even though she was happy to be able to move her family back to the San property.

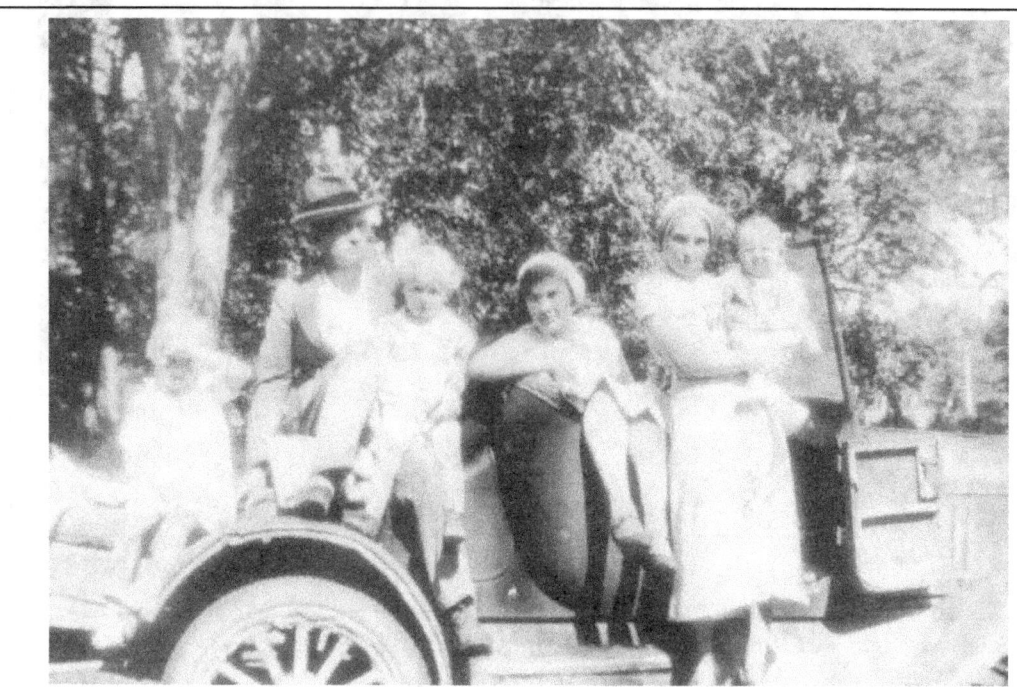

Adolf Becker family, 1932
My mother, Ella, seated in automobile
Ella Hedglin collection

During the Great Depression, the Works Project Administration (WPA) was one of the programs instituted by President Franklin D. Roosevelt to restore prosperity to Americans. Unemployed women like my mother found work in sewing rooms where they could earn money by making clothing for other low-income Americans. By the end of 1941, nearly 137,000 Minnesota residents received federal aid, close to 30,000 of them through the WPA, and close to 3,500 in Civilian Conservation Corps camps.[103]

Mom needed to work to provide for the family, but there were no openings at the San—no one wanted to give up a job during the Depression. For the next six months, she lived in Bemidji during the week while working for the WPA Sewing Project. She returned home on weekends.

---

[103] *Minneapolis Tribune*, Minneapolis, Minnesota, October 21, 1979

Even though my father wasn't supposed to work, he had to take care of my brothers, which was often more strenuous than having a job. Luckily, Grandma Grande helped with the boys.

After completing the maximum allowed months of work at the Sewing Project, Mom worked as a cook at the Puposky School for nine months, also under the WPA program. Then, she returned to the Sewing Project for another three months. In 1938, she took an opening at the San to fill in during vacations and soon got her old job back as a tray girl and dishwasher at $35 per month. When Dad was released to work, he went back to the San as a teamster making $30 per month.

Each fall, the boys and Dad cut Christmas trees. They got 25 cents each for the small ones and 50 cents each for six-foot trees. Dad cut the trees, and the three of them carried them out of the forest.

Clarissa Anderson again wanted to board with my parents when she was Jimmie's fifth-grade teacher, but by then, there wasn't room for her to stay long because Mom and Dad had a foster child, 11-year-old Joyce Seado, living with them. When Joyce's mother died, Joyce moved into a foster home because there were only her father and three brothers at home. Her sister, Pearl, a nurse at the San, asked Mom to care for Joyce. Pearl had been a patient at the San at age 14, going in once in 1923 for 144 days and again nine months later, in 1924, for a much longer stay. [104]

Welfare paid Mom $5 month, and Pearl matched that amount. My mother didn't know that welfare paid a month in advance, so she didn't claim her first payment and never received it. "Money was tight," she wrote in her notes, "and we had counted on that $5."

Jimmie still found ways to get hurt. When he was seven, he inserted his finger into an old cream separator and asked Lloyd to turn the crank. The separator ground his finger to a bloody pulp. Dad and his cousin took Jimmie to the San, and Dr. Mary advised them to take her car and drive Jimmie to Dr. Johnson in Bemidji to have the finger amputated. When the procedure was over, the nurse wrapped the damaged finger and the one next to it together. Jimmie, when he saw it, hollered, "You didn't need to cut them both off!"

---

[104] Minnesota History Center, Lake Julia Tuberculosis Sanatorium, Patient Register

Dr. Mary and Miss Broomfield, the Irish head nurse, changed the bandages after school each day to save my father from having to make trips to town for the three months it took Jimmie's hand to heal.

◊

I was my parents' third child. I entered the world on September 26, 1947, in Bemidji. They named me Patricia Ann but called me Patty.

Dad returned to the janitor job at the San again in July 1948 at $100 per month. Nine months later, he was offered the position of dairyman, and my family moved back to the San Dairy. As I ran through the yard, my dog, Ring, and my pet lamb were never far behind. I spent hours playing on a uniquely designed swing that hung from a big tree near the house. I helped my mama gather eggs from the chicken coop, and I patted the cows on their warm bellies while I chattered to them. Sometimes I rode over to the San with my dad when he delivered milk. In the winter, my brother Lloyd helped me build snowmen. The San Dairy was a fine place to live.

◊

In 1951, Dad asked Dr. Mary for a raise but didn't get one. He didn't know that she had already seen the writing on the wall. Perhaps she suspected that tuberculosis sanatoriums would soon be a thing of the past and, rather than keeping Dad there until the end, believed it would be better if he could move on to a more-promising job. My father quit his job as the herdsman in September, then worked for the San as a farmhand until November. That's when he moved our family 150 miles south to Sauk Centre, a town 100 miles northwest of Minneapolis and St. Paul. There, he operated a farm for Ann Voller at a higher wage than he had earned at the San.

Workdays on the Voller farm were long. Dad took care of beef cattle and pigs, and Mom took care of 200 chickens. She put out four or five large pails of fresh water for the chickens three times a day and cleaned the chicken coop. Mom also gathered eggs and gently wiped them with sandpaper before Dad delivered them to the store in Padua. My mother received a percentage of the egg money and could use all the eggs she needed for meals. She also cooked for the extra farm help for additional pay.

Soon, my father heard from relatives in the Pacific Northwest—in Longview, Washington— that Weyerhaeuser was hiring. The lumber company had been started by Frederick Weyerhaeuser of St. Paul, MN, who, by 1929 had built it into the world's largest sawmill.

The job sounded good, but Dad wanted to be sure the position would be permanent before moving our family. He quit his job on the Voller farm and moved us from the outskirts into the town of Sauk Centre. I started kindergarten in September, and Lloyd began his junior year of high school. Just over a month later, on October 9, 1952, Dad left for Washington. The rest of us followed in June 1953, three months before I turned six.

That was the beginning of a 21-year career at Weyerhaeuser in Longview, Washington, for my father. Unfortunately, his vision deteriorated over the years. When he was declared legally blind, he was forced to retire.

Though his doctor never knew for sure what had caused his progressive eye disease, he said it could have been tuberculosis of the eye. Tuberculosis can strike many parts of the body, not just the lungs.

Most who worked at the San tested positive, even if the disease had never become active. Once a person tested positive, he would always remain positive, so there was no longer a reason to perform the Mantoux test. Instead, technicians periodically took chest X-rays. Those who worked for the San received chest X-rays every six months, but the tests only revealed tuberculosis in the lungs, not in other parts of the body.

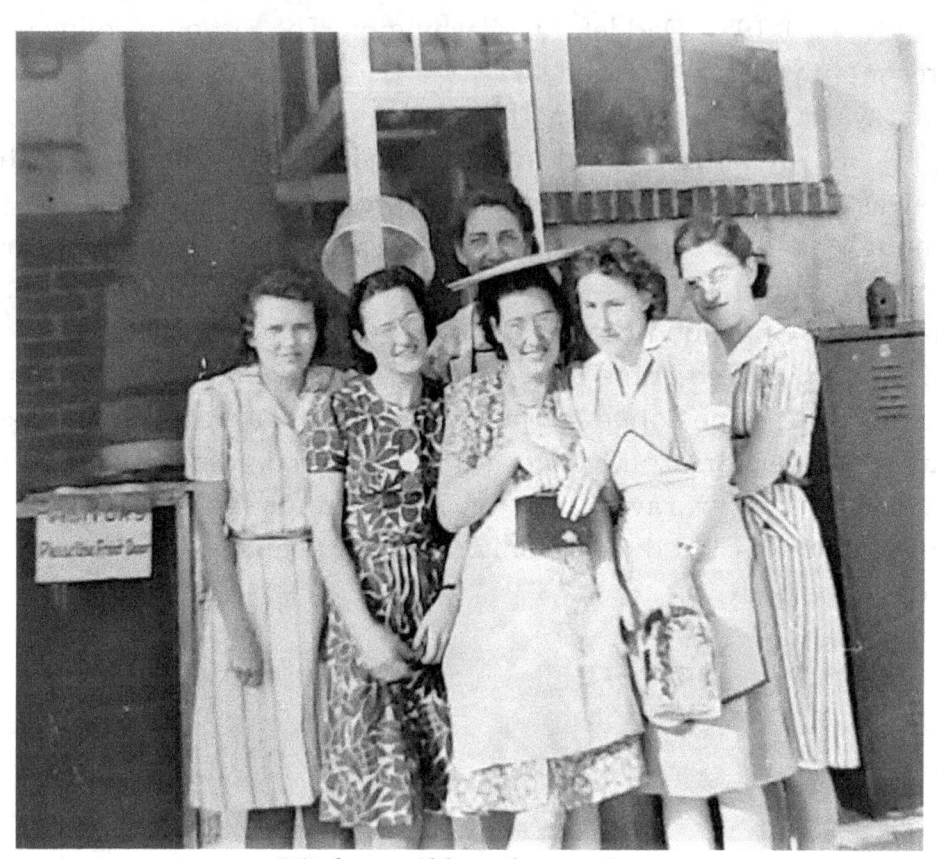
Kitchen and laundry workers
Ruth Hayes, Fran Vick, Mabel Wilcox, Millie Johnson, Bernice Bakke
Ida (Mac) McDonald in back row
Ella Hedglin collection

Chapter 21
Bernice Bakke, Laundress

Bernice Bakke married my uncle, Norman Grande.
She accompanied me on my trip to visit the San in 1985.

Bernice remembered well what had brought her family to Puposky. Life in South Dakota had been tough during the "Dirty Thirties." Drought had caused dust storms that blocked out the sun and drifted like snow. Some friends and relatives of the family had moved to Puposky, Minnesota, and they encouraged Bernice's father, Elmer, to consider land that was for sale there. Elmer liked what he saw and purchased 40 acres. The family moved there with two cows and their dog, Shep.

Elmer's cousin, Ole Kalseter Olson, already lived on the property in a big tent with a double fly, so the whole family moved in with him. There were Elmer and his wife, Clara, and their four children, Bernice, Violet, Clayton, and Elwood.

"We dug a hole in the ground to keep the food cold," Bernice said, "and Mother cooked our meals over a campfire. The mosquitoes were terrible. We had to build a house before winter, so we weren't in the tent for long. First, we had to clear the trees, then we bought the lumber from the Bemidji Lumber Company to build our two-story, 16' x 16' house.

"Father worked for the WPA, and he also did some haying and general work, like hauling wood, for the San, so Dr. Mary knew the family. She asked if he knew anyone who would help pick potatoes. I heard the request and volunteered immediately."

The potatoes, once picked, were placed in sacks for storage, then stored in the root cellar at the San. "Jack Spicer drove the horses that pulled the potato digger," Bernice recalled. "I was the only gal amongst all the men picking, and they loved to tease me. Leo Rundell would throw the spuds back into my row. I remember having a good laugh one time when Jack got his pants caught in the digger. They ripped to shreds. Oh, how we all teased him. As Jack tried to hold his pants together, one of the men asked him, 'Don't you know there's a lady out here?'"

Dr. Mary noticed that Bernice was a hard worker, so when she needed to hire help for the laundry, she went over to the Bakke home and recruited her.

Bernice took the job and moved to the nurses' home at the San, where she shared a room in the basement with Ruth Hayes.

Patients were not allowed in the laundry. It was located a few steps down from the main floor of the San and a few steps up from the basement. The engine room, which provided heat for all the buildings on the San property, was next to the laundry room. One day, a flirtatious young man who had been in the Civilian Conservation Corps (CCC) camps, and who wore his CCC clothing, stood on the steps, just outside the laundry, and said to Bernice, "I could kiss you now; you've got your mask on." The CCC operated from 1933 to 1942 as a work-relief program for unemployed, unmarried men.

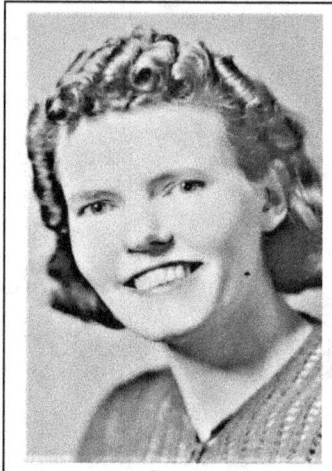

Ruth Hayes
Ella Hedglin collection

☙❧

Because it was her job to label clothing, Bernice got to know the names of all the patients. She did a lot of washing and also operated the mangle, a machine used to press flat items such as sheets, pillowcases, pajama bottoms, and straight pajama tops. Bernice also had the job of changing the linens in the basement for the men and cleaning their bathroom. She used acid to clean the toilets, and it burned her hands.

☙❧

In the laundry, the big electric washer that Bernice used was about 4 feet long with a cover that raised and an agitator. Bernice filled it from a hot-water hose that hung on the wall next to it. "One time, there was so much pressure in it," Bernice said, "that when I barely touched the hose, it exploded and burned me with scalding water. The pain was awful."

Dr. Mary applied salve and bandaged Bernice's blistered legs. She wouldn't allow Bernice to return to work until the injuries healed.

"I got so hot under my mask, but it was important to wear it so that I wouldn't get TB from handling the laundry," she pointed out. "We didn't wear gloves, but we sure washed our hands a lot." Bandages had to go through a sanitizer, but Bernice didn't handle those. The nurses had that duty.

Another time, Bernice got overheated and shook uncontrollably. The doctor who was filling in during Dr. Mary's vacation was on the lake in the rowboat. Someone took Bernice to the nurses' home, and Eva Yerbich, who was a part-time laundry employee, ran to the lake, waving a towel to summon the doctor. The head nurse, Miss Anderson, rushed to the attic for the rhubarb wine, hoping to calm Bernice. The doctor arrived and treated her. It took a week for Bernice to recover. It's not known whether it was the professional care or the rhubarb wine that did the trick.

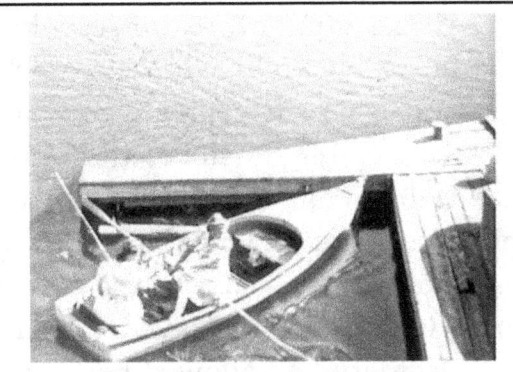

Rowboat on Lake Julia
James Ghostley collection

"Ruth Hayes took care of the nurses' uniforms because she was the best at getting them just right," Bernice said. She also did any darning that was needed to repair socks and holes in garments. Some patients had stylish clothing that required special care and ironing, and Ruth was in charge of that. There were laundry tubs for washing by hand and two more cement laundry tubs for hot and cold water. The San ordered soap in large quantities.

"Once while I worked there, a fellow named Kenny Haffner got his arm shot off while duck hunting on Lake Julia. Dr. Mary served as the 'emergency room,' and we in the laundry had the unpleasant job of washing the bloody sheets.

"We used an extractor to get most of the water out of the clothing for faster drying," Bernice explained. "Before ironing and starching the uniforms, they had to be damped. Ruth usually mixed up the starch and took care of the uniforms because the nurses wanted different amounts of stiffness. There were about 32 white nurses' uniforms and two ironing boards. Some patient dresses, too, required ironing. If Ruth had too much work to do, I helped. We sent all the folded clothing out on carts."

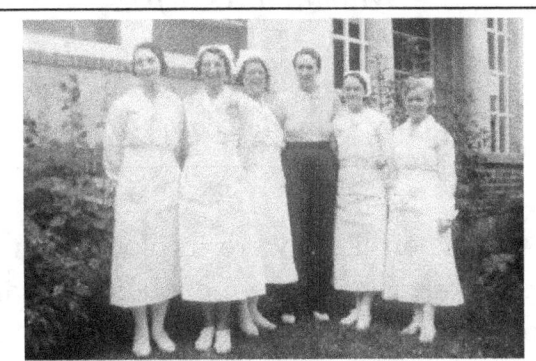

Wilma Watts, far left.
Ivy Budd, fourth from left
Olga Christianson, second from right
Ella Hedglin collection

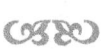

All the nurses wore dresses when Jim Ghostley was a child except for one county nurse, Ivy Budd, who wore slacks. Jim remembered thinking it looked odd to see a nurse in pants. Times were changing.

He fondly remembered a nurse named Wilma Watts. "She was really part of the place," he said. Once when Jim was at his mother's Rainy Lake cabin, Wilma stopped by because she loved the place where Dr. Mary had allowed her to visit for vacations. She later moved to Montana.

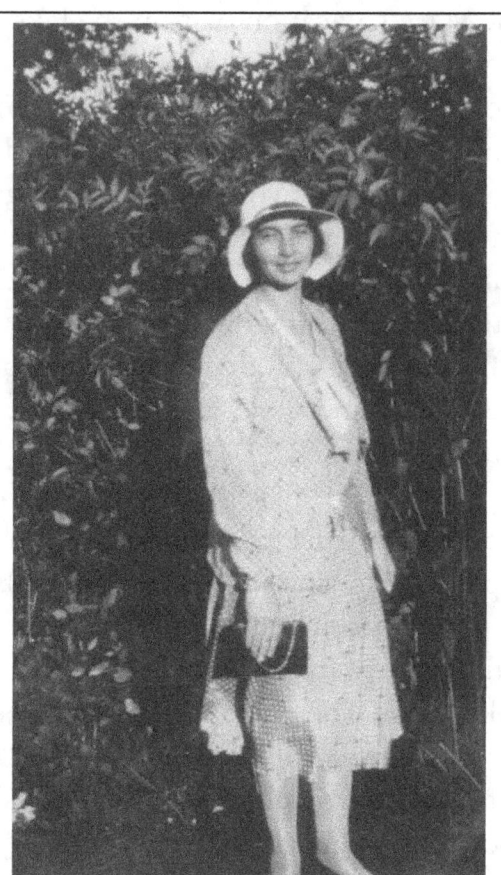

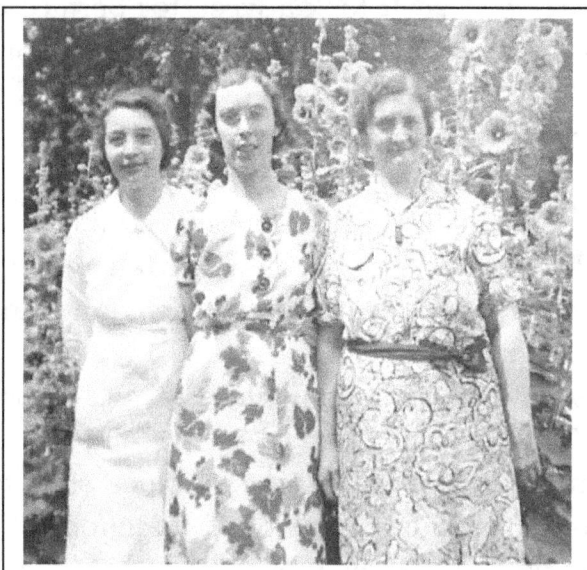

Wilma Watts (left)
Gladys Maki (center)
Vivian Moe (right)
James Ghostley collection

Wilma Watts
From her San photo album
which will be donated to the
Beltrami History Center.
Beth Watts collection

"When lilacs were in bloom, employees placed the fragrant blossoms in tubs of water in the basement before arranging them in jars and distributing them throughout the San," Bernice recalled.

She remembered that some of the patients played croquet. Dr. Mary had added a croquet court, and she had benches placed throughout the yard so the patients could rest while exercising outdoors. Charles Thoraldson was good at the game. He was a patient at the San three times beginning in August 1936 at age 17, and he later was a San employee. He also picked mushrooms, and the kitchen used them in dishes for the patients.

One of the laundry employees was Ida (Mac) McDonald, a tall woman whose first husband had been close to 7 feet. She had admitted him to the San, then got a job there to be close to him. Mac wasn't the only one who got a job at the San to be near her patient-husband. So did Agnes Lessard and several others.

Mac's husband died, and orderlies took his body to a little room by the laundry where the San stored the sack-salt used to melt ice. Then Mac, whose father was an undertaker, embalmed her husband herself before his burial at the Oakhill Cemetery.

The property was sometimes called the Poor-Man's Cemetery. There were Indian burial mounds in the area. A Peterson family owned the land, and they had buried a baby there. Later they began to lay other family members to rest on the three-acre site. Eventually, anyone who couldn't afford a spot could use it.

On one of my trips to the San with cousins Paul Grande and Barbara Madsen, we inquired about the San at the courthouse. An employee told us we should take a look at the old Oakhill Cemetery where some patients were buried, and that the county was working in the area. We drove out near the cemetery, on the north side of County Road 26, across the road from the San Dairy, where I had lived as a child. We parked the car and told the construction workers why we were there.

"Follow me," one worker directed. "I'll doze you a road." And he did. Grave markers sat askew or were on their backs or sides. Some graves had been torn into by animals, exposing casket handles and bones. The cemetery committee had plans to dig, sift, and rebury any unearthed items. Some graves had become unmarked. Names and dates I read on headstones were:

- Addie McKnight November 28, 1849-November 11, 1913
- Grandmother Carrie Peterson 1839-1923
- Mackaman Baby
- Archie H. Watson 1862-1924
- Cordelia G. Watson 1824-1911
- Bish (Rella), who died at the Lake Julia Tuberculosis Sanatorium on November 24, 1916[105]

---

[105] Minnesota History Center, Lake Julia Tuberculosis Sanatorium, Patient Register

- Carie C. Krantz 1888-1/1889

The railroad that ran from Bemidji to Red Lake was near the cemetery. According to Patsy Maher Schwartz, her father, Harry Maher, had at one time owned that piece of property. In summer, Patsy said, he would take the calves and sheep up there to keep all the brush eaten down, but some people didn't like the animals being there.

"I remember going to a funeral there when I was five or six," Patsy said. She also recalled that her father took people to the "Poor-Man's Cemetery" for burial while he worked at the San and that the janitor sometimes had to build the box for a coffin and dig the hole.[106]

Bernice felt nervous about going into that little storage room where Mac had embalmed her husband. She could see into it from the laundry when the undertaker came with stretchers to take the bodies away. Bernice didn't believe in ghosts, but sometimes when she was working, she could see movement through the window when no one was there.

While Mac worked in the laundry, she eventually met Charles Thoraldson. He had TB of the throat and had a long scar on his neck. The laundry workers frequently saw Charles when he brought the laundry part way to the room. His sister Margaret worked there too, and sometimes she got to talk with him when he dropped off the laundry at the top of the stairs. That's how Margaret had the opportunity to introduce him to her co-worker, Mac McDonald.

Later, when Charles had recovered and after they had married, Charles and Mac would take off from the San part of the year and follow the carnivals and circuses from the Southern U.S. northward and back south from April to October. They carried a freezer. When they reached a town holding an event, they would contact suppliers, order ice cream, and cut it into bricks, then put it between graham crackers or chocolate crackers. They sold these as ice cream sandwiches.

---

[106] Patsy Maher Schwartz interview

Section Five: The Holmstrom Family

Chapter 22
Family History

TB struck Art Holmstrom while he looked forward to graduating as valedictorian of his high school's senior class. These are the stories Art told me about his family, the illness that changed his life, and the lady doctor who cared for him.

"**O**h my, yes!" was 19-year-old Elizabeth Eleanora Goransson's enthusiastic reply in 1912 when her beau of two years, Carl Gustaf (Gust) Holmstrom, traveled from Minnesota to Seattle, Washington, to ask her to be his wife. The Swedish couple had met on the *SS Mauritanis* while Elizabeth voyaged from Sweden to Seattle with her uncle. Upon the ship's arrival in Seattle, Gust departed for Minnesota, the home he had left eight years earlier at age 20.

It didn't bother Lissie—Gust seldom called her Elizabeth—that Gust was more than nine years older than she. He was great with numbers and had already proven that he could make a good living for a family, having worked construction, laid railroad, farmed, and logged. He'd even gone to business college. Lissie couldn't believe her good fortune.

During their engagement, Lissie stitched a quilt for her hope chest and imagined sleeping beneath it with her beloved in their future home. *We'll entertain guests at a grand table covered with the lace tablecloth I carried in my trunk from Sweden*, she thought, *and a big bouquet of bright flowers from my garden will sit in the center.*

She dreamed of how she would make Gust's home the perfect place for him to return to after work, with freshly baked bread and pies coming from the oven as he stepped through the door. The pair would have beautiful, healthy, yellow-haired babies who would grow up to be tall, smart, strong Swedes like their father, and life would be perfect.

When Gust arrived in Seattle to propose, and soon after, when they moved to Minnesota, it was a dream-come-true for Lissie. That dream was right on track in September 1913 when their first child, Ruth Elizabeth, was born in Minnesota. But the baby was frail and sickly from the start, and poor Ruthie lived only 18 months. She died in March 1915, just as Lissie suspected another child grew in her belly.

Before Christmas, a second girl, Elsie Ruth, was born in Duluth. Lissie felt relieved that their new daughter appeared to be strong and healthy.

A few months later, Gust came home from the shingle mill with unexpected news. He popped through the door with excitement in his voice. "Lissie, pack the bags. I got a job out at Remer, and I start next week."

"Will we have a house?" Lissie asked. "A nice big house for Elsie, with room for more babies?"

"When the time is right," replied Gust. "For now, the boss from Montreal said he'll provide a little place for us to live, and I'll make more money, too! We can save up for a place of our own."

"Can't we go out and take a peek first? To make sure it's a suitable place to raise children?"

"I can't pass up this opportunity, Lissie. I already told him, 'yes.'"

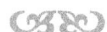

When the Gust Holmstrom family arrived at Shovel Lake near Remer, Lissie realized "home" was just a small, dank shack in a logging camp. There were no other women, just lumberjacks with crude mouths. Gust worked long days, so Lissie and little Elsie were alone most of the time.

Lissie did her best to make the shack a home, but it wasn't easy adding a woman's homey touch to a man's world. She had never felt such loneliness. Most days, as Lissie held Elsie on her lap and pumped the treadle of her Singer sewing machine, tears boiled in her eyes. Every day, she taught Elsie and played with her, then cooked for Gust, but she was unhappy. What had happened to her dream? She longed to move to town into a real house, a place where she could hang lace curtains and invite guests to Sunday supper.

Life at the logging camp didn't agree with Elsie, either. She caught one cold after another and then had a frightening seizure, her little limbs stiffening while her blue eyes rolled back into her head. Lissie was alone and frantic. *Is Elsie dying? This dear baby can't die too*, she thought. Then, the child's limbs relaxed, and her eyes returned to normal. She played as though nothing had happened. Lissie released a long breath.

Elsie repeated the frightening seizures a few more times. When Lissie told Gust she was again with child, he admitted the logging camp was no place for his growing family, but he was doing his best to be a good provider. In 1917, he rented a big white farmhouse near Remer, just a mile from the railroad tracks—a place Lissie was happy to call home while being close to a doctor for Elsie. In their new home, Lissie's Singer sewing machine sang as she made curtains for the house and dresses for Elsie, and she hummed along with the tune of its pumping treadle. *Living here is more like my dream*, she thought.

◦✿◦

Just after the midwife arrived on June 12, 1918, for the birth of the couple's third child, there was an awful ruckus. A big storm came up while Lissie was in labor. As she screamed out in pain, the wind grabbed shingles and tore them from the big white house. Just as baby Joseph entered the world, the roof sprang a big leak right over Lissie's sewing machine, and she belted out an even louder cry, long and agonizing. The train whistle blared, and more water, seemingly on cue, cascaded in through the roof, leaving soggy strips of tarpaper dripping onto Lissie's beloved Singer. That's when lightning struck the shingle mill at Shovel Lake and burned it to the ground. Amongst the chaos, Joseph Holmstrom entered the world, red-faced and crying, to face his own storms.

Chapter 23
Getting Down to Business

The storm quieted, and so did Lissie and their new son. But although the skies had calmed, the family soon learned that the turbulence in their life was not over. The owner of the shingle mill had struggled to make a profit. When the mill burned, he counted his blessings, took the insurance money, and left the area. Just as Gust's family had grown again, his means of supporting it had vanished. He could not find work.

"Lissie," Gust mentioned one day, "I have an idea."

"We need one," Lissie replied. She wondered how much longer they could afford to stay in the big white house.

"I know two other good men who are looking for work. We'll start a mill ourselves."

"You're good at organizing crews, and you have plenty of experience with numbers." Lissie's eyes brightened with renewed hope.

"Yes, I think I would prefer to run the crews. One man could operate the sawmill, and the other has bookkeeping experience. All three of us can make a good living."

The two other men were excited about the idea. Soon, Gust and his partners had become successful business owners.

Things went well, and a few months later, Gust commented contentedly at supper, "I like owning my own business. The mill is doing fine. I should have done this years ago."

"You're a resourceful man, Gust Holmstrom," Lissie replied proudly. "I didn't know how we would get by, but you figured it out, just like you always do."

But their days of doing well ended abruptly when the bookkeeper liquidated everything and ran off with all the money. Gust and his other partner had not just lost their jobs this time; they had lost their investment, too.

Chapter 24
The Job Search

Gustaf found another job, but it didn't last. He searched for work every day and returned home wearing discouragement like a heavy coat on his slumping shoulders. He had inquired all over International Falls and the surrounding areas without luck. In 1919, he was offered a lead on a job as manager of a logging operation in Washington State, and he acted quickly.

"But I don't want to leave," cried Lissie. "This is the first place we've lived that feels like home."

"We'll have to leave here anyway if I don't find work," Gust replied. Lissie didn't seem to understand that he was doing the best he could.

With baggage and babies, they moved to Spokane, Washington, where they again rented a house. They didn't stay long. They moved once more in 1920, this time to Kalispell, Montana.

Gust's job was steady, but Kalispell didn't feel like home to him. He didn't consider the move a permanent one. The next year, when Gust was 40, he heard that Backus and Brooks needed a camp and walking boss back near International Falls. He applied, anxious to return to Minnesota.

When Gust told Lissie about the Minnesota job opportunity, she put her foot down—flatly refused to go. She liked their home in Kalispell, and she was afraid the family would have to move back into a camp shack if they returned to Minnesota.

"I won't do it. I've moved enough," Lissie insisted sternly. "I won't leave Montana. It's my home now."

"But there's plenty of work now near the Falls. You can have a home there, maybe even a bigger house than the one we're in now."

"You came to Kalispell to work. You got exactly what you wished for, and you're a fool to want to leave."

Gust didn't like being called a fool. "Well, I've made up my mind, Elizabeth. I'm going, with you and the children or without you."

"And I've made up mine, Gustaf!" Lissie shouted at him. "We're staying here!"

In 1921, Gust left alone. In Minnesota, a severe cyclone had leveled a swath of trees around Thistledew Lake in NE Itasca County, laying them out on the ground like spilled toothpicks. It was Gust's job to salvage that timber. To do so, he had to build a railroad spur from Camp 29, near Craigville, eastward, and southward to Thistledew Lake.

Living at Camp 29 alone, Gust found that Lissie had been right. Minnesota didn't feel like home without his family. He missed Lissie and the children, and he always worried about Elsie and Joe, who both had grand mal epilepsy. He begged Lissie to bring the children to International Falls, where he would find a house so they could all be together. She stubbornly refused.

Things were difficult at work, too. His crew was tough to manage. The men cared more about the saloons and the ladies than about their jobs. On payday, they would spend their wages, not content until they had wasted every penny on booze and women. One time, when Gust tried to get them out of the saloons, some of his workers threatened to kill him. He had to have the police raid the saloons to get the men back to work, and they were even less fond of him after that.

Finally, in August 1923, Gust learned of an opportunity for the family to move back to the Falls into company housing.

"In the camps again?" Lissie asked.

"No, I know better than that," he declared. "The company wants to build a larger mill office, so they removed the old building. They hauled it away with horses and skids down a muddy quagmire of a street, the horses with mud to their bellies—you should have seen it—from Second Avenue to Sixth Avenue, where they located it in the 600 block of Sixth. There, they sawed it right down the middle into two identical apartment houses that contained four units in each half. They're called the Terrace Apartments, and they're quite nice."

At that time, Elsie was 10, and Joe was five. They were too strong for Lissie to handle when they had seizures. Besides that, they often cried for their father. Lissie needed her husband's support and physical strength.

Seizures were cruelly called "fits" in those days, and people discriminated against those with epilepsy in regards to both education and employment. Some people made cruel remarks about the children, as though having epilepsy meant they couldn't hear the hurtful comments or see the rude stares. Wherever they went, there were hateful looks and whispers. People pointed fingers at the children. The stigma attached to epilepsy isolated the Holmstrom family. It didn't help that their frequent moves had kept them from forming friendships.

One day Lissie wrote to Gust, "You're right. The children and I need to be with you. I can't deal with them alone anymore."

Soon, Lissie and the children joined their father. Gust worked to pay the bills, and Lissie busied herself with the many doctors' appointments for Elsie and Joe. Phenobarbital usually controlled Elsie's seizures, but she still sometimes had episodes, without even knowing what was happening. A cold or some other illness often brought them on, so Lissie became hypervigilant and watched the children for any signs of sickness or seizures.

Chapter 25
Another Son

In 1924, Lissie was relieved when her brother, George Goransson, came from Sweden to live with the family. Then, on January 25, 1926, Gust and Lissie's second son, Arthur Carl, was born. Arthur was the first of the Holmstrom babies to be delivered in a hospital, and mother and son received excellent care at the Northern Minnesota Hospital, just down the street from their apartment.

Lissie had longed for another baby, but at the same time, she was nervous. Arthur was her fourth child, and each of the previous three children had suffered from illness, with her firstborn dying. She fretted about the new baby's health, wanting to believe that life would spare him the pain the other three had endured. She knew from experience that not all dreams come true. The kind nurses at the hospital calmed her fears and assured her that little Art was a perfectly healthy baby boy.

The Terrace Apartments were noisy, and in 1928, when the Holmstroms had a chance to move out of the apartments and into a company house at 615 Fifth Street, they packed and moved again.

"At least we're just moving nearby," Lissie uttered, "and I've packed so many times that there's nothing to it."

⋄

Art lived his life with caution and only had a couple of seizures, both when he had a fever. Those two incidents were cruel warnings that his life, too, might be marred by illness. Lissie felt lucky to have a competent physician, Dr. Morrill E. Withrow, to watch over her children. As Art grew, Dr. Withrow told the family to be careful, not to let him play rough games or sports, because a head injury could bring on a seizure. Art generally exercised his mind more than his body.

He was an innovative thinker. As a child, he collected lead scrap metal to make toy soldiers and to form lead sinkers, which he sold for fishing. He turned wooden fruit lugs—boxes manufactured to carry fruit—into fish-shipping boxes.[107]

⋄

---

[107] Edith Holmstrom interview

Gust's job seemed secure, but he still had to be away from home a lot. He hated being away from his youngest son, Arthur. Gust had advanced from camp boss to supervisor of pulpwood production for the local Backus and Brooks paper mill. Because the job was in the woods, he was only home every few days, about once a week, until around 1930.

He'd planned to work for Backus and Brooks for the rest of his career. Then, at the start of the Depression, jobs were cut, and the company laid him off. Just two years later, Backus and Brooks went bankrupt, and the plant was taken over by the Minnesota and Ontario Paper Company.

When he lost the job at Backus and Brooks, Gust found work with Consolidated Water, Power, & Paper Co. in Wisconsin Rapids, Wisconsin. Again, Lissie refused to follow her husband.

When Wisconsin Paper Company had an opening in Canada, Gust moved his home base to Port Arthur, about 200 miles east. His work took him northward, then down toward Sioux St. Marie. Then it followed Lake Superior down to Duluth and down the south shore of Lake Superior and over to Ashland, Wisconsin. He managed the Minnesota and Ontario operations of pulpwood production to bring wood to Lake Superior. His crews formed log rafts, and tugs took them across Lake Superior to Ashland. In winter, they took the logs over the thick ice of the lake. The logs were then loaded onto flat cars and sent to Wisconsin Rapids for manufacture.

Lissie again was alone in dealing with the health issues of her children. She had no way to control Joe's seizures. He had attended the Alexander Baker School, but because of his epilepsy, he was placed in an ungraded room made up of first- to fourth-graders. Later, he was in an ungraded fourth-to-eighth-grade room. He was bright and a good reader, but when he reached 12, about the time his father took the job with Consolidated and left home again, Joe had grown so tall that the teacher and school administrators were afraid he would hurt the smaller children when he had seizures. They asked him to leave the school, and it broke his mother's heart to see him singled out.

Gust became a stranger to his family, coming home only eight to 10 days a year. He hated being an absent father, but he had to make a living, and his family incurred many expenses. He lived in boarding houses and hotels and missed being with his family and eating home-cooked meals.

Lissie wasn't good at budgeting, and she opened numerous charge accounts when Gust was away. Elsie couldn't hold a job because of her epilepsy, so she kept going back to school, where she was an excellent student. But tuition was expensive. There were ongoing medical consultations and expenses for both Joe and Elsie.

To make matters worse, one of the pastors at Lissie's church told her that epilepsy was punishment for her sins. That ended her church attendance, causing her to feel even more isolated and alone with her problems.[108]

On Gust's infrequent visits home, sleeping arrangements became awkward in the small house. Joe and Uncle George shared one bedroom, and Lissie slept in the overstuffed chair in the front room. In the other bedroom, Arthur and his father slept in one bed, and Elsie slept in the other. Lissie's insistence on sleeping in the chair even when her husband was home reminded Gust that she had not forgiven him for going away.

Lissie's circulation was poor from sleeping in a chair for so many years, and she struggled with leg ulcers. She made many trips to the doctor in Fort Frances, and there were constant expenses for bandages.

Gust couldn't control his family's expenses. He was proud and never wanted to ask for help. Finally, in desperation, he wrote to Lissie's brother, George, and asked that he pay rent to help the family make ends meet.

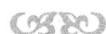

Uncle George became the children's father figure. He took an interest in Art, treating him as a son because he had known him since he was born. Eventually, George taught Art photography, training him in both slides and prints. Later, he gave Art a camera.

Lissie's dreams had crumbled into a heap of lifelong worry about her children. Elsie continued to strive for a normal life but kept running into roadblocks. In 1940, she took college courses in the Falls. Then, in 1942, Elsie moved away from home and enrolled in church-sponsored Northland College in Ashland, Wisconsin, where she occasionally was able to see her father. From there, Elsie went to the University of Texas, graduating with a master's degree in sociology.

Epilepsy continued to interrupt her life. She got a job teaching in the Ozarks, Missouri, but she didn't stay long. In Warren, Minnesota, she lost her job after only one month because the administration found out she had epilepsy.

---

[108] Edith Holmstrom interview

Determined to work, she joined the Women's Army Corps (WACS). She went to Milwaukie to be examined and sworn, and on her way to the swearing ceremony, she had an epileptic seizure. She collapsed and hit her jaw, breaking it in two places.

Elsie spent months in a Chicago military hospital. While there, doctors discovered that she had contracted tuberculosis in one lung. She had a lobectomy—removal of the lung—at a hospital in Anoka, Minnesota, but the staff deemed her an uncooperative patient. She was released as soon as medically possible, and the hospital was glad to see her go.

As Lissie received letters of Elsie's plight, she ached for her daughter. Elsie was intelligent, yet she struggled to fit into a society that refused to accept the things it didn't understand.

Joe's life was even more discouraging. He had never been allowed to lead an ordinary life. He lived at home until he was 46, then he moved into a facility at Moose Lake. Because of his bad temper and epilepsy, the administrators asked him to leave after only one year.

He then moved to cottages for the disabled. When doctors determined that he was not a mental patient, he could not stay there, and he moved to the private home of a former Moose Lake ward attendant and his wife, who cared for four men on the second story of their home. Next, Joe moved to Cromwell, a county facility for the disabled, where he lived for eight years. Then officials decided that non-mental patients should live as close as possible to their homes, so he was moved to Ah-gwah-ching, the former tuberculosis sanatorium at Walker. Even though it was the closest facility, it was more than 150 miles from his family's home in International Falls, making visits nearly impossible. Eventually, Joe moved to a nursing home north of Bemidji, where he lived out the rest of his life.

Chapter 26
Art Holmstrom, Student

Art was 13 years old and in junior high in 1939. He had a busy school schedule, and he strove to do well. The pressure of always trying to excel caused him to have a nervous stomach. He had to hurry to school at 7 a.m. for band practice Monday, Wednesday, and Friday before school started at 8 a.m., and he had orchestra practice Tuesdays and Thursdays after school, plus studying every night. His expectations for himself were high, and nothing but the best grades satisfied him.

He vomited every day on the way to school. Once during his years in junior high, Art fought back vomit when he had to give a speech. He always required himself to perform better than any of the other students, but when it came to giving speeches, he didn't feel he measured up. He kept working at it and did better in high school, but in junior high, the idea of giving a speech was sickening.

His mother, concerned that epilepsy might be the reason her son vomited, took him to Dr. Withrow's office, a place that had become familiar to Art over the years. Every time he had a fever or a sniffle, Lissie needed the doctor's reassurance that it wouldn't activate epilepsy.

"I don't think the nausea is connected to epilepsy at all," Dr. Withrow told Lissie. "Do you drink milk for breakfast, Art?"

"Every day," Art replied.

"Stop drinking milk, and start drinking orange soda pop with every meal," the doctor advised.

Art beamed. He didn't drink soda often, and now he would have it every day. Soda pop was a luxury for some of his school friends. It was hard to believe that for Art, it was doctor's orders. It didn't help his condition, but he was happy to enjoy the treat.

Art was well over six-feet tall, and people tried to get him to join the Falls high school basketball team, but he always offered an excuse. To explain why he wouldn't play basketball, Art told little fibs to his friends, saying he had a hernia in his stomach from his brother, Joe, falling on him. Dr. Withrow's earlier warning that a blow to his head could trigger epilepsy was enough to keep him at his books instead of roughhousing and playing ball with the other boys. He didn't participate in physical education, and his family didn't allow him to play school sports.

Art had seen enough prejudice against his brother and sister because of their epilepsy that he was determined to do whatever it took to avoid having seizures himself. It hurt Elsie and Joe—and the whole family—when classmates and sometimes even thoughtless adults made fun of them for having 'fits.' "Oh, that dreadful word!" Art exclaimed to his mother. "How can people be so cruel?"

Art liked to ice skate on the city ponds, the one physical activity his mother allowed—probably because she enjoyed ice skating herself. Dressed in layers topped by a heavy wool coat, he glided smoothly over the ice, exhilarated but always cautious, never quite feeling the freedom of his youth.

Beginning in 1934, the family sometimes rented a cabin across the international boundary in Canada. It was nestled in the trees at Bull Moose Lodge on the shores of Crow Lake—called Kakagi in Chippewa—just north of Nestor Falls. The road to the lodge was like a cattle trail. Indians lived between Crow Lake and Lake of the Woods, and the Holmstroms sometimes hired an Indian guide named Big George to take them fishing.

When they went in winter, Art skated between the ice-fishing houses and fish-smoking shacks with soft swishes of his sharp steel runners, catching the aroma of fresh coffee and smoked fish as he skated by. He was careful, never skating with abandon or taking chances.

Chapter 27
The Summer Job

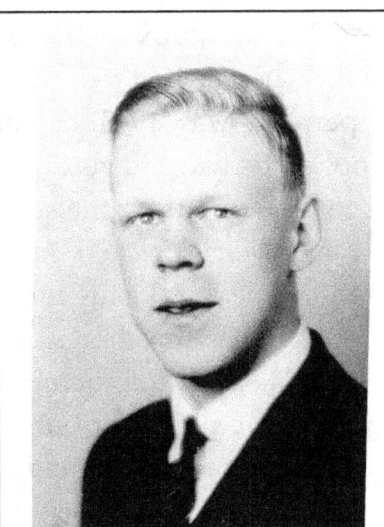

Lissie and Uncle George were proud of Art. Gust was too, of course, but he didn't often see his son. Not only was Art's mother happy that their son had made it to age 17 with only two epileptic seizures, but she was proud that he would graduate in June as valedictorian of his class. With any luck, she thought, he'd have a scholarship to go to college in the fall.

"Art, your future looks as bright and shiny as a new penny," his mother declared. She loved his brother and sister and was proud of their achievements, too, but she was especially proud of Art. She believed he would be the only one of her four children who would have a chance for a prosperous future, and she wanted at least one of her dreams to come true.

*Art's graduation photo taken in late 1943
Art Holmstrom collection*

Art had seen a little sickness among his classmates, but most seemed strong and healthy. A few had come down with tuberculosis, but after a quick hospitalization, they had returned to school. Like other people Art's age, he had no worries about catching a disease. His only concern was about epilepsy, and he generally lived cautiously to avoid it.

⋅⋅⋅

During WWII, there was a shortage of workers at the pulp and paper company. Therefore, the mill was willing to hire some high school juniors 17 or older if they passed the physical, which included the Mantoux test to check for tuberculosis. Art was tall for his age, lithe and wiry, the picture of good health.

He'd had many Mantoux tests in school to test for TB. The tests were administered by Dr. Mary Ghostley, who continued to make time to conduct them even though she ran the TB hospital 108 miles away.

There was nothing to the Mantoux. Students stood in line with their classmates, and one by one got a prick in the arm. Then, after a few days, Dr. Mary would look to see if there had been a reaction to the tuberculin. For Art, there had always been just a small red dot, nothing of significance.

The students considered the Mantoux test an excellent way to miss class for a few minutes, and except for those who were afraid of a prick in the arm, most welcomed the interruption of class time.

The Mantoux at the mill was Art's first to be taken for work instead of school. When he had it done as a condition of employment at the Minnesota Paper Company in May 1943, he completed his physical, and everything seemed fine. He looked forward to getting the formalities out of the way so he could earn some college money during the summer.

Dr. Mary pricked Art's arm, and he stepped forward to allow the next person in line to take his turn. He just had to wait a few days for the test results, then start work. But things didn't go as Art had planned.

"Ma," Art stammered one morning after the Mantoux, "my arm itches like mad. I've got a big, hot bump!" He pulled his arm out of his pajama sleeve and stared at a massive, inflamed swelling—red as a beet and the size of half an orange.

When Art went back to have Dr. Mary take a look, she exclaimed, "Oh my, that's a big one! But I think it looks OK, not like tuberculosis. I'll sign off so you can start work."

"But why did I get this big lump?" Art asked.

"It seems to be just an odd reaction to the tuberculin," replied Dr. Ghostley.

Dr. Mary Ghostley had doctored in the Falls for years. Everyone knew her or at least knew of her. She was a state authority on TB. Every student for miles around, in several counties, knew her because she did all the Mantoux testing to check for tuberculosis in the public schools in the northern quarter of Minnesota. Many folks believed she knew more about TB than the male doctors.

Art displayed the prominent bump to friends and family; it was a novelty. Despite it, he would be allowed to start work the following week in the Kraft mill.

The summer was sweltering, and in mid-August, after nearly three months of work, Art was glad when the job ended. He had worked hard, doing a man's job and had built up muscles and a nice chunk of cash. With graduation coming the following June, Art was happy to have some money for college. After laboring all summer, he welcomed a vacation at the cabin across the border in Canada, where he stayed until school started in September.

Chapter 28
Illness Strikes

Art's vacation had been restful—swimming, fishing, and reading—and just as it was ending, he caught a cold. He started his senior year with a red nose, sore glands, and a cough. It ran its course, as colds do, but he couldn't get rid of the cough. It just hung on, all through the fall and into the winter, and it became more pronounced when Christmas vacation started in mid-December.

As soon as school was out for Christmas break, Art went with a friend to chop Christmas trees for their families. Trudging through deep snow while dragging the trees home, he tired more quickly than usual. Sweat poured from him, and he couldn't stop coughing. That night, he went to bed at 9 p.m., exhausted from the effort of getting the trees and from his constant cough. He propped himself up on his pillows. His mother put a kettle on the stove, but the steam did not quiet his cough.

The next day, he didn't feel like helping her decorate the tree. She brought him a long thread on a needle and bowls of popcorn and cranberries. "Here, Art," she said, "I thought we could sit together and string a garland."

Art just wanted to rest. He lay there and coughed as his mother softly hummed Christmas carols and strung the decorations.

In the afternoon, Art coughed and cleared his throat, and his mouth filled with liquid. He recognized the familiar taste of salt and iron, remembering the nosebleed his brother Joe had accidentally given him the year before.

Warm moisture seeped out the corners of his mouth as he got up and ran for the bathroom, a hand cupped beneath his chin.

Art spat blood into the toilet and watched red swirls form on the water. He coughed more and more—sat on the bathtub coughing and spitting, coughing and spitting—blotting the blood from his lips. After deliberately suppressing his cough as much as possible, he finally had some relief for an hour or so. His stomach muscles ached. He went to the kitchen for a glass of water and told his mother what had happened.

"Back to bed with you, Arthur," she lectured as she handed him a neat stack of pressed hankies, still warm from the iron. He gladly returned to his bed.

His mother wanted to call the doctor immediately, but Art didn't want to spoil Christmas. "No, Ma, it's just a cold. If I'm not better by the day after Christmas, call him then," he begged.

Art was drenched with sweat during the next night but awoke without a cough. He felt better. He knew his mother always counted on his help at Christmas. Still, she wouldn't let him do much, so he mostly stayed in bed and studied. His graduation as valedictorian was only a few months away, and he didn't want his grades to slip.

Art, Joe, Lissie, and Uncle George spent a quiet Christmas together.

"I'm not very hungry," Art protested when Christmas dinner was on the table. His mother fixed him a small plate and sent him to his room, where he picked at the food.

The next morning, Lissie called Dr. Chermak. He was new and had replaced Dr. Withrow, Art's doctor since birth. Withrow had come on the first train to the area in 1907, the very first passenger to ride from Duluth to Ranier, and was the first doctor in the area.

Art heard his mother say to Dr. Chermak, "Thought I should call—probably nothing—better safe than sorry—seems a little better."

Dr. Chermak asked Lissie to bring Art in right away. Art was exhausted by the time he entered the exam room. It had been an effort to get dressed and then to go to the doctor's office. Art noticed that Dr. Chermak was younger and taller than Withrow, who had become stooped with age and had failing eyesight.

Dr. Chermak examined Art and explained, "Son, I think you've got yourself a bad case of pneumonia. I don't have the equipment here to take X-rays, so I'll send you over to Littlefork to see Dr. Hanover."

"I'll have my brother drive us," Lissie explained.

"Art, you rest on the way," Dr. Chermak cautioned. "It's 20 miles from here, and this pneumonia could tire you."

At Littlefork, Dr. Hanover examined Art and listened to his chest. "Did Chermak take any sputum samples?" he asked.

"No," replied both Art and his mother.

"We'll take an X-ray of your chest to satisfy Dr. Chermak, but I'd also like to get some sputum samples while you're here today."

After the X-ray, Dr. Hanover ordered, "Spit into these bottles. Just spit sputum—no food, no saliva—and bring up several samples for each of these three bottles. Sputum is the product of your cough, and it comes from your chest, not from your mouth like saliva. I'll come back shortly with the preliminary X-ray results."

Art hoped he wouldn't embarrass himself by spitting blood. He cleared his throat repeatedly, pulling up thick phlegm with difficulty and spitting the skimpy results from his chest into the bottles. His throat felt raw from the effort, and he sweated profusely.

As Dr. Hanover entered the room with the X-rays, Art noticed the worry on his mother's face as her dream cracked every which way like the crazing on her china plates.

"I've read your X-ray," Dr. Hanover stated, "but I'll have to send it, along with the sputum samples, to the State Board of Health for evaluation. We'll have results in a few days, but it looks like you have pneumonia, as Dr. Chermak diagnosed."

"Just pneumonia," Lissie whispered, letting some of the lines in her face relax. She had expected worse.

"Well, we hope that's all it is," Dr. Hanover said. "Dr. Chermak will call when he has results. Meanwhile, Art, you stay in bed and don't do much, and no school until Dr. Chermak releases you, even if you're feeling better."

On January 6, Dr. Chermak called Lissie. "Come to my office at 2:00," he ordered. "Leave Arthur home in bed. I've got additional findings on his illness."

Art wished he could have gone with his mother to comfort her. Because his father was away, the family burdens all fell on her frail shoulders. He lay at home, imagining her twisting her handkerchief into a tightly wound rope as she often did when she was nervous.

"I have here the results from Dr. Hanover and the State Board of Health," Dr. Chermak told Lissie. "I was correct about Art's pneumonia, but I'm sorry to tell you he also has tuberculosis."

"Tuberculosis?!" Lissie asked, stunned.

"It's probably just a light case—didn't show up on the X-ray, only in the sputum," replied Dr. Chermak, "but I want you to take him to Lake Julia, the TB sanatorium over by Puposky, for a full and thorough examination."

"Is he contagious?" asked Lissie.

"Yes, he is," replied Dr. Chermak. "He needs to be kept isolated, away from the general population. I've already contacted Dr. Ghostley, and she is ready for him. I want you to take him there Saturday and leave him for a few days."

"He won't have to stay long, will he?" asked Lissie. "I've heard of folks with TB who have had to stay in a sanatorium for years."

"We just want to have plenty of time for thorough testing," assured Dr. Chermak. "He probably won't be there long, maybe just a couple of weeks. I've diagnosed a few other Falls students with TB in the past year, and they were all back to good health in a wink."

"Will you tend to him at the sanatorium?" asked Lissie.

"No, I'm afraid the San's too far away for that," replied Dr. Chermak, "but Dr. Ghostley is a wonderful doctor. Dr. Mary Ghostley. You probably know of her from her work here in the Falls—she's known as a top-rate TB doctor, and Arthur couldn't be in better hands."

"I don't understand how it could be TB," puzzled Lissie. "Just last June, he passed the mill physical over at Backus and Brooks."

"Yes, Dr. Ghostley forwarded his Mantoux results to me. His chart here shows that he did react strongly to the tuberculin when he had the Mantoux," explained Dr. Chermak, "though she didn't suspect tuberculosis."

"But you told me his chest X-ray looked fine, except for pneumonia. How could he have TB?"

"Sometimes people out in public have an initial tuberculosis area, and they seem to weather it without being detected," replied Dr. Chermak. "The body makes a kind of encasement, like a jail, for the tuberculosis germs and the area they are affecting. People can go through life with that little encapsulation, or even several of them over the surface of the lung, trapping the tuberculosis."

"Then what causes it to become active?" asked Lissie.

"A severe blow to the chest or running down one's health, or a bad case of pneumonia similar to Art's might cause the TB to escape and become active. I suspect the TB was present when Art applied for work at the mill, and this case of pneumonia probably allowed it to escape. Many of us test positive, and the TB never becomes active; but unfortunately for Art, it has. We'll want to test you and everyone else in the household, too, to be sure no one else has contracted it."

Upon returning home, Lissie's face showed concern, and her eyes were stained red. She walked into the bedroom with the news for Art, her eyebrows drawn together and her knotted hanky clutched tightly in one hand.

"That means I must already have had TB when I got tested for the mill job," Art voiced after learning of his diagnosis. "If so, I was sick all summer. I've exposed everyone I was around."

"Dr. Chermak told me the pneumonia might have allowed the TB to become active," Lissie explained. "Before that, it wouldn't have been contagious."

"Oh, Ma, you'd better take good care of yourself. Don't get run down. You and Uncle George—and Joe and Elsie, too. Father's the only one in the family who I haven't been around."

"They will test all of us," she replied.

Art lay in bed, wondering. If it was TB, how did he get it? Was it from Albert Johnson, the family friend who had emigrated from Sweden? Mr. Johnson worked in the insulate mill and had become sick about three years earlier. Every day, Art's mother had sent him over to Mr. Johnson's with a hot meal. Art hated seeing the poor man lying there, so he would sit with him to ease his loneliness.

Mr. Johnson had had a bad cough, and when it didn't get better, they tested him and found tuberculosis. He'd spent a little over a year in the San, then had gone back to the Falls as a house painter. Before his diagnosis, Art had never thought of the possibility of contracting tuberculosis from Mr. Johnson.

After several days of bed rest at home, Art felt better. It wasn't good news to find out he had TB, but he was sure he could recover quickly, as those few others in his school had done, and like Mr. Johnson.

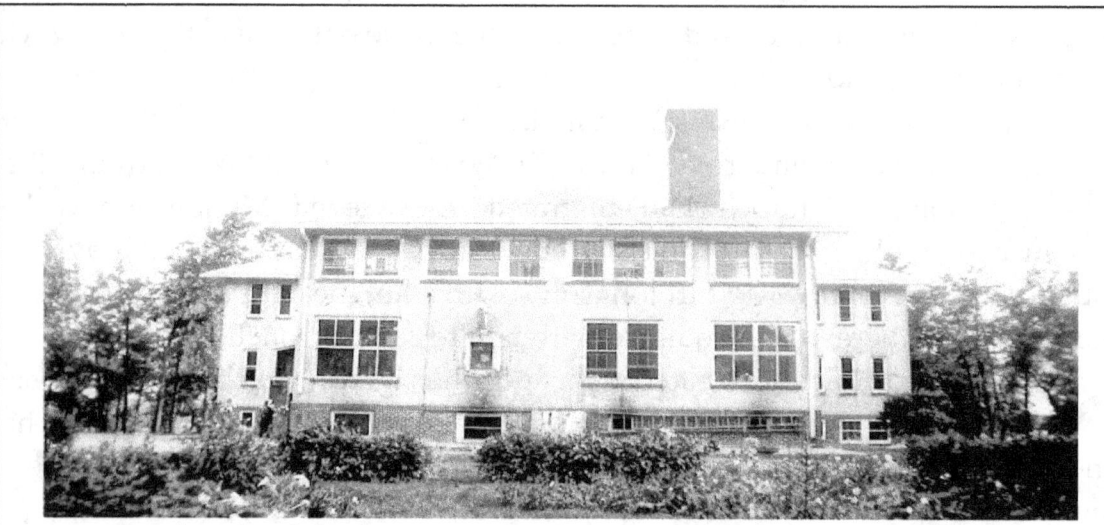
North side of the San as seen when driving in through the gates
Photo by Pat Nelson

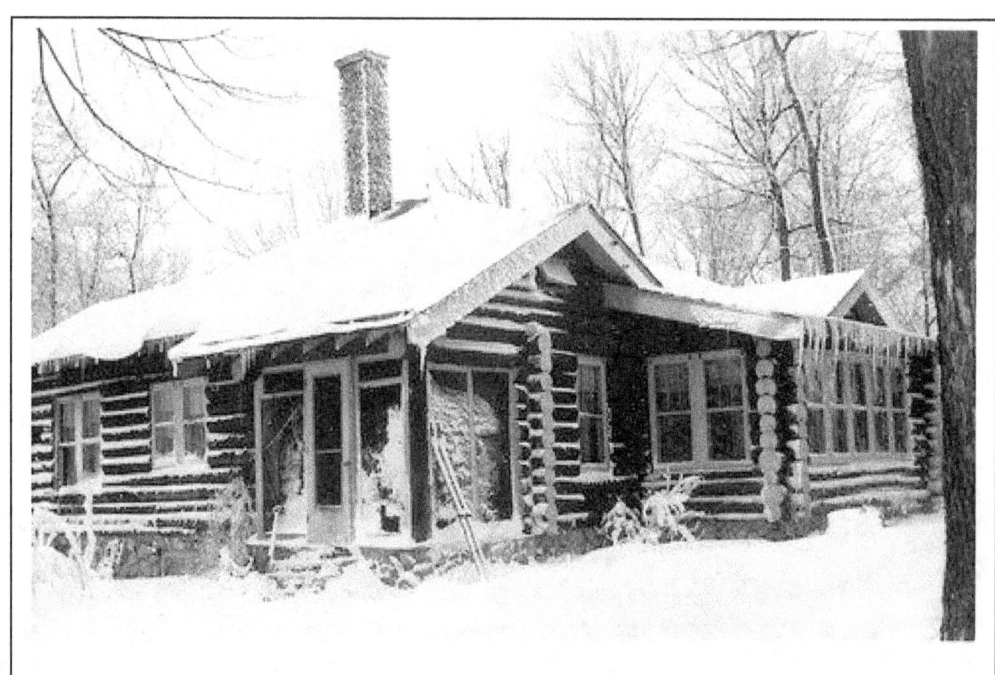
Dr. Mary's log house at the San
Art Holmstrom collection

Chapter 29
Sanatorium Admittance

Art continued to rest at home until Saturday, the day he was to check in at the Lake Julia Tuberculosis Sanatorium for evaluation. He looked forward to recovering quickly and getting back to school to pursue his quest for scholarships and a college education.

On January 8, 1944, Art's family traveled to the San in the family's 1937 Pontiac. Lissie, her brother George Goransson, and Art's brother, Joseph, accompanied him. As usual, his father was working out of state. His sister, Elsie, was in college at Northland in Ashland, Wisconsin.

Lissie bundled Art in blankets and packed a stack of handkerchiefs in his travel bag. She fussed over him, asking if he was all right. That felt awkward to Art because he felt better than he had for days.

Art didn't know what to expect as he headed toward the San. *Will there be anyone my age? How many people to a room? Am I allowed to wear my own clothes?* He had packed pajamas just in case. *What about the food?* There were many foods that Art refused to eat. *How long will I have to stay?* Question after question raced through his mind.

He had never been to the Lake Julia Tuberculosis Sanatorium. As they approached Puposky, a drive of more than 100 miles from the Falls that had taken several hours on the frigid 15-degree day, Art tried to ease his mother's nerves. "I shall try to eat everything on the tray, Mother, even olives and pickles, and I will start drinking milk again," he promised. She hated it when one of her children embarrassed her, so Art told her that he would not do so with his picky eating. At home, Art had refused to eat tomatoes, leafy greens, cheeses, many vegetables, and a whole list of other foods. As he rode toward the San, he was determined to stop being finicky.

"But what if the milk doesn't agree with you?" asked Lissie. "You might have to stay longer if you begin to vomit again."

"At school, I learned that TB patients must drink a lot of milk," Art stated. "It's full of calcium. If it helps me get well, I will drink it."

They passed the Turtle Lake School on their left, a one-room schoolhouse at Buena Vista with a hand-operated pump in front for water and a big stack of wood to keep a fire going when school was in session. Soon they passed the Buena

Vista Ski Slopes on their right. He had never seen downhill skiing. They drove along through quiet country roads, then past one end of a beautiful lake on their left that they decided must be Lake Julia—and on, closer and closer, to the sanatorium.

There were a few houses, most with barns and outbuildings, but not much else. At a sign on a white wooden post, they took a left-hand turn. After a short distance, they came to a set of fancy wrought-iron gates opening onto a long drive. Looking down the driveway, they saw the large, two-story facility perched atop a basement. It didn't fit in this rural setting of farmhouses and barns so far out in the country.

"This has to be the Lake Julia Tuberculosis Sanatorium," Lissie declared.

"It's bigger than I expected," Art replied.

"It's a hotel!" exclaimed Joe.

Lissie, sitting next to Art, quickly smoothed his hair into place, then touched up her own as they approached the massive structure.

"Ha, brother, since you're going to live in an institution," Joe joked, "I'm going to take over your bed at home." Joe felt nervous about the threat of institutional confinement because of his epilepsy. He fidgeted and talked too much, easing his tension. It did not help Art's.

Lissie sat quietly, alternating between twisting her hanky and rubbing her index fingers over the deep grooves in her thumbnails—lines earned by washing, scrubbing, canning, and other never-ending household labor. *Elsie and Father are lucky to be away from home and missing this trip*, she thought.

As they reached a log cottage on their right, with a snow-covered roof and icicles jutting down like long, crooked fingers, out stepped a woman Art recognized as Dr. Mary Ghostley. She wore snow boots and a long, gray wool coat. A knit hat covered her hair.

Uncle George slowly pulled the car to a stop so as not to skid, and Joe and Lissie cranked their windows down with stubborn squeaks. Dr. Ghostley, with a warm smile, approached the car, pulled off a wool glove, and extended her hand—not to Lissie or to Joe, who sat closer to her, but beyond to Art, making him feel special. For a moment, he felt like an honored guest. A deep cough reminded him of how he had earned this honor.

"Welcome, Arthur. I'm Dr. Ghostley."

"Hello, Doctor," he greeted, leaning toward her across the car and reaching his hand past his mother. He tried to shake the doctor's hand with a firm grip to show his manliness—and his healthiness.

"You probably remember me from your Backus physical."

"Sure do," replied Art, "and I remember you doing the Mantoux tests at school, too."

"Well, I certainly remember you, Arthur, with that reaction you had to the Mantoux when I tested you over at the mill."

"Yes, it was a whopper."

"I was happy that I wasn't finding any positives," Dr. Mary told Art, "and then I came to your arm with that big bump. It didn't look like the usual positive reaction, but it did look odd, so I can't say that I'm surprised to see you again."

She turned her attention to the adults and extended her hand. "You must be Mrs. Holmstrom."

"Pleased to meet you," Lissie said, "and I'd like you to meet my brother, George Goransson, and my oldest son, Joseph. Mr. Holmstrom is away working in Wisconsin."

"I'm pleased to make your acquaintance," Dr. Mary said, smiling and shaking hands with each of them, then quickly slipping her hand back into the warmth of her glove. "I'd heard the name Holmstrom in the Falls but had never met any of you except Arthur. Just pull your car up by the front of the San there. I'll run in through the kitchen door on this side to leave my wraps and then I'll meet you up at the front door. Do you feel well enough to walk into the building on your own, Arthur? Can you climb a few steps?"

"Yes," Art replied, "I'm feeling quite well today." He wondered how one would get inside who could not walk up the stairs. *Dr. Mary was slender, and she certainly couldn't carry a patient up the steps*, he thought.

They trudged through a few inches of snow and climbed a half dozen wide steps to the large double doors. Someone had cleared the snow from the steps. Dr. Mary pushed one of the doors open from the inside and held it as the Holmstroms walked into a large room with gleaming, spotless terrazzo floors and a fire blazing in the fireplace. Beyond, in the dining room, white cloths covered tables decorated with red and green paper bells. A tall, decorated Christmas tree stood in one corner. Art remembered his recent Christmas-tree expedition and shuddered when he saw the size of the San's tree. The tree he dragged home had tired him out, and it was only half the size of this one.

The dining room reminded him of one that he'd seen only through windows at a fancy restaurant in Falls. He smelled freshly baked bread and realized he was hungry.

"You'll be on the second floor, Arthur," Dr. Ghostley told him. "Take your time going up those stairs over there. Rest when you need to, for as long as necessary. There's no hurry. I'll be right there to steady you if need be." She turned to Art's family. "I'll be back for the rest of you when I get Arthur settled in his ward. Just have a seat there in the dining room, and the waitress will bring you some sandwiches and milk—we have a dairy farm, and the milk is fresh! Or you can have hot coffee if you prefer."

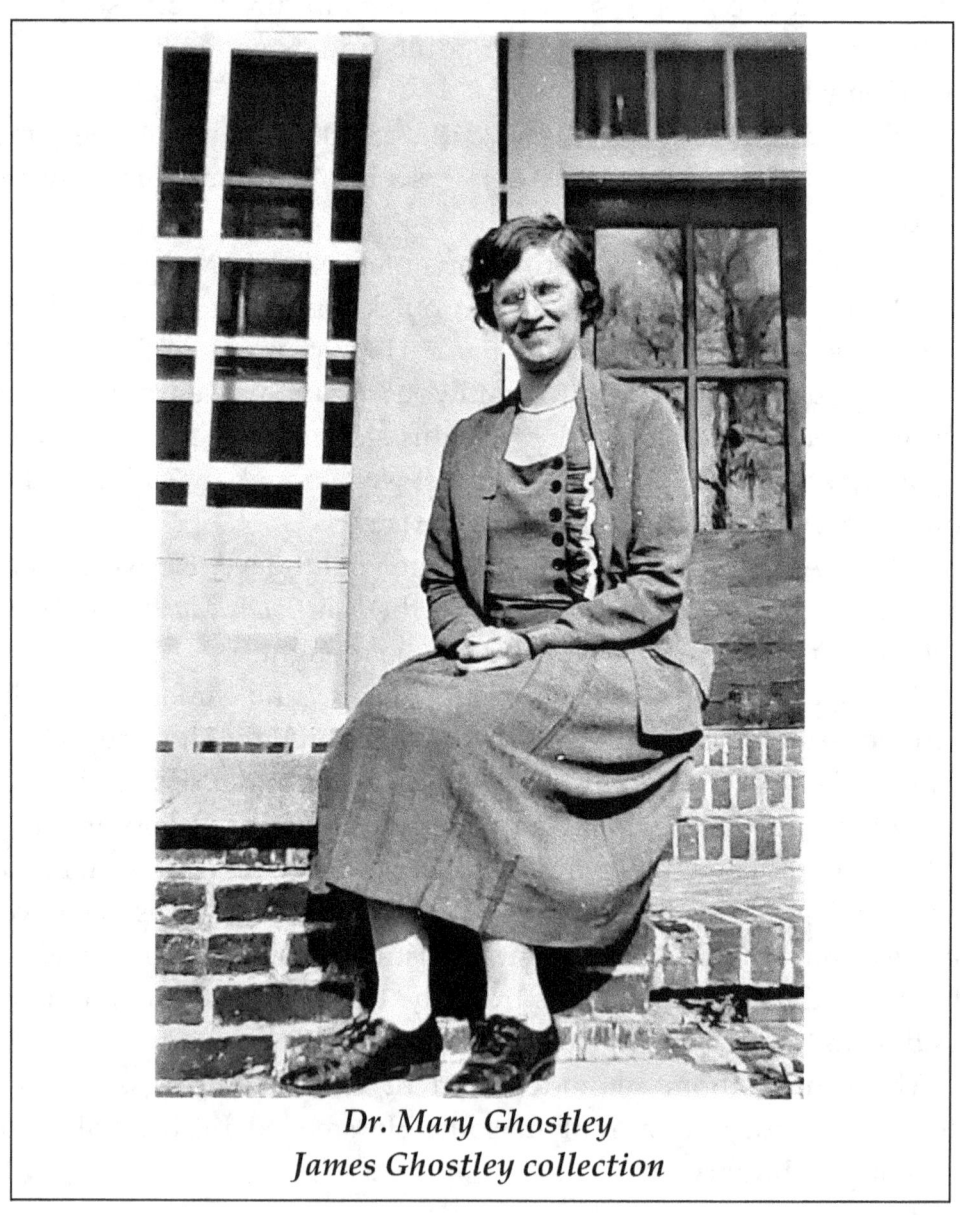

Dr. Mary Ghostley
James Ghostley collection

Art and Dr. Mary moved slowly up the stairs, stopping every few steps so Art could rest. What probably was only a one-minute climb for a healthy person took Art nearly ten minutes. Dr. Mary showed Art the locker room and assigned him a locker before he changed into pajamas and used the bathroom.

When he came out, Dr. Mary took him to the ward. "Be quiet," she whispered outside the doorway. "It's rest time." She showed him his bed, and he crawled up under a fresh, crisp sheet and two blankets. He noticed four men in the ward. Two slept, and the other two nodded and quietly mouthed hello. The men appeared to range in age from 20 to 60.

Dr. Mary told Art, "Remember, this is rest time, and we'll speak quietly so as not to disturb the others. You will be on complete bed rest for now. That will allow the formation of a web of calcium that will help trap those spots of tuberculosis."

"Do you suppose I had TB all summer while I worked at the mill?" Art whispered.

"Possibly," Dr. Ghostley replied quietly. "But I suspect your body trapped the tuberculosis in an encasement of calcium so that it wasn't active and then it probably broke loose recently when you got pneumonia."

Art didn't like the idea of being restricted, but he was tired from the trip, and the bed felt good. He'd sweat the night before, but had woken refreshed. The long ride to the San had drained his energy, leaving him weak. His cough returned, burning his chest. Goosebumps raised on his arms. He lay back, taking in the high ceilings, dull green walls, and huge doorways and windows of his new home.

Uncle George quietly led Lissie and Joseph into Art's room. "Please stay just a few minutes," Dr. Mary cautioned. "This has been a tiring day for Arthur, and he needs to rest. Our patients have just finished quiet time, so it's all right for you to talk with Arthur."

"He'll probably prefer to be called Art," Lissie told the doctor. "That's what everyone calls him at home."

Uncle George interrupted. "We'd better be on our way before we have more snow. We're lucky we had just a sprinkling on our drive here. No telling how deep it'll be before we get back to the Falls."

"Stop back in the dining room on your way out," Dr. Mary said. "I had my staff prepare some sandwiches for your return trip."

After hugs and parting words, Uncle George led the family out of Art's room. Even Joe had stopped cracking jokes and had tears in his eyes. Lissie resisted leaving Art's side, but she finally kissed his moist forehead and took a step backward toward the door. Art didn't cry. He knew he would be home in a few days.

When the family left, Dr. Mary remained in the room. "Art, I need to explain to you about privileges."

"All right," he replied. He was an achiever, and he wondered what type of privileges he might earn.

"Here, we don't base privileges on good or bad behavior; we base them on your progress in recovery. For now, you will not have privileges. That means you will eat your meals in bed, and you will not be allowed out of bed to use the bathroom."

"What?" asked Art, a deep furrow crossing his forehead.

"Beginning next Saturday, though, I might allow you to go to the locker room to use the bathroom, just there and back once if you are doing well enough. I'll trust you to use good judgment in not abusing this privilege once you get it. I had one fellow who thought he could get up three times in an hour to run to the bathroom, and I had to take his privileges away so he could recover."

"You're saying I can't get up to use the bathroom except on Saturdays? Then only once? I probably won't be here by next Saturday!"

"I'm sorry, Art. Everyone here must earn the privileges that they have taken for granted in their homes. When you're recovering from TB, getting up to use the bathroom is a privilege. It taxes your energy. Until I assess your condition, I'm afraid I can't allow you to have privileges."

"I'm not sure I understand what you mean. I can't wait a week to use the bathroom!"

"I mean you'll have to stay in bed. You will have to learn to use this urinal and bedpan when needed," Dr. Mary explained, pointing to the blue-speckled graniteware. "You won't be allowed to leave your bed until you've earned a privilege. Don't worry, though, you're not alone in having to do this, and you'll get used to it in no time."

A bedpan? A urinal? Art was embarrassed enough by the lack of privacy with four other men in his ward, but worse yet was his location by the doorway leading to the women's ward on the sun porch. *I'll use more energy*, he thought, *trying to hide myself and a cold container behind this sheet than I would use walking to the bathroom!*

"And what will I do to keep my mind busy while I'm in bed all day and all night?" he asked. His nervousness set off a round of coughing, and he spat bloody phlegm into the pan that Dr. Mary held toward him. That frightened him, as he wasn't one to spit up much phlegm, even when he had a bad cold.

"You're ill, Art. You can see that by the bloody sputum you just brought up. Your body has given you a sign of your illness that you can't deny. I want you to do as little as possible so your lungs can rest. Rest is one of the most important medicines in curing TB. That means no walking, no sitting up in bed except for meals, and limited mental stimulation like reading, writing, and visiting. I realize by your grades in school that you are not one to sit idle. Let me assess your condition, and as soon as possible, I'll allow you to do a little more."

After Dr. Mary left the room, Art lay in his bed, staring at the high green ceiling. Reflections from his water glass danced mockingly above him. A mixture of weakness, defiance, loneliness, and despair churned into a nasty porridge in his gut. He didn't want to visit with his new roommates. He didn't want to talk to anyone. Salty tears trickled down his cheeks and into the corners of his mouth. His tears embarrassed him, and he turned his face into his pillow, where he sobbed himself to sleep.

When he awoke, he needed to use the bathroom. He looked around to be sure no one was watching. Everyone seemed to be resting. This call of nature embarrassed him. His pee thundered against the container, but no one seemed to notice—no one but Art.

Art went back to sleep until the supper trays arrived. He was allowed to sit up in bed, propped up by pillows, but just for mealtime. He ate beef and boiled potatoes with tasty brown gravy, and he drank the first glass of milk he'd had for months. The milk was cold, and the rich cream coated the roof of his mouth. *No more effervescent bubbles from soda pop*, he thought to himself. *I'll have to tell Ma I drank milk without making a fuss.*

Art's ward faced Lake Julia. There was a ward on the other end too, and a long sun porch that housed 10 ladies separated them. The entrance to the sun porch was next to Art's bed, and his head was in line with the paper-covered windows of its door. All the other men had their beds on the outside walls near the windows. Since Art was the most recent to arrive and the ward was crowded, he had the least-desirable location, just a little part of the east wall that had no window to the outdoors.

There were no radio earphones above his bed like there were above the other beds in his ward, either. He didn't care; he wouldn't be there long.

The men in his ward introduced themselves. A couple of them ate their meals in bed, but the other two, who looked perfectly healthy and had dressed in their best clothes, had eaten their supper downstairs in the dining room. Art thought he probably looked healthy, too, but he knew appearances could be deceptive. He had noticed that people equated height with good health, and he was already 6' 3" with still more time to grow.

Over in the corner by the window facing Lake Julia was Elroy Ramstad, who went by the name Eli. He not only had tuberculosis, but he also had progressive diabetes.

There was Ray Knutson, a young Hispanic fellow named Felix Diaz, and also Oscar Berg, who had come from North Dakota. Oscar had been in the U.S. Navy from 1928 to 32, and Art would soon hear many stories about his Navy experiences. A teacher and principal in Red Lake, he had a lot of education and skills. Eventually, Oscar moved to Nopeming Sanatorium to have a surgery that the Lake Julia Tuberculosis Sanatorium could not perform.

The men told Art about various patients whose health had broken down for different reasons—some, too much liquor; others, from the type of work they did, like mining; or many because of a poor diet or crowded living conditions.

It was Saturday night, so after supper, those of his roommates who had privileges, the ones dressed up in their best suits—those with pressed white shirts and neckties and shiny shoes instead of slippers—were ready to go visiting.

"You look like you're going out on the town," commented Art, wishing he could leave his bed.

"It's visitin' night," replied one of the men. "From 7 to 8:30 p.m., we go around and visit the ladies. Don't tell me you didn't notice the pretty ladies next door."

"Oh, I saw them all right, when the nurse opened that door," Art replied. "A couple of them were whispering and looking over at me, and I turned my head away from them as fast as I could."

The next day, Oscar said to Art, "Sit yourself up, Art. Since the door is open to the sun porch, let me make the introductions to our lovely neighbor ladies."

Art pushed himself up in his bed, even though he wasn't supposed to, and looked straight through the doorway at two attractive young ladies with fancy hairdos and pretty dresses.

Chapter 30
Meeting the Neighbors

"**A**rt Holmstrom, may I present Norma Norberg and Anneliese Petersen, your next-door neighbors," Art's roommate Oscar Berg said as he stood near the doorway to the women's ward. "There are other girls down a ways; you probably can't see 'em from your spot."

The young woman named Anneliese waved. She moved over near the doorway, where it was easier to visit with the new patient. "Hi, Art," she said.

Norma giggled.

"Anneliese, a pretty name," Art commented. "When did you arrive?"

"Oh, just last month, and you can call me Annie."

"Hello, Annie."

"I see you've met Dr. Mary. She's a wonderful person, very compassionate. Sometimes she sits with a patient all night."

"Well, I hope that won't be necessary with me."

"Are you still in school?" Annie asked.

"A senior," Art replied. "I'll graduate this year. Valedictorian," he added proudly.

"Same here," she replied. "Graduating, I mean—not valedictorian. Seventeen or 18?"

"Seventeen."

"Me, too."

"I'm from the Falls," Art explained. "You?"

"Over at Solway. Not far from here."

"Well, I hope we're both out of here for our graduations!" Art exclaimed.

"Oh, I'll graduate, whether or not I'm out," Annie declared. "My parents checked with the superintendent, and he told them there would be no problem. They're supposed to send my schoolwork over, but I haven't seen it yet. I'll do the work without actually being required to attend classes."

"You're lucky. Ma checked on my lessons, and the superintendent told her I'd have to make them up when I return," Art said. "He told her they couldn't risk anyone saying I got valedictorian without earning it."

"Maybe I can teach you some German," Annie suggested. "My whole family speaks German. We moved from Germany to Nebraska when I was just 11 months old."

"Nebraska?"

"Yes. My dad's brother told my family there was lots of land for sale, and they sponsored us. We moved to Minnesota later. I hate to change the subject, but ... do you want to meet my neighbor? She's in the little isolation room across from Norma's bed. A big open window looks right into it. It's almost like we're in the same room. You can meet her if you want to."

Lois Olson popped out of bed and poked her head through her window. She waved a quick hello to Art, then she darted back before the nurses could catch her.

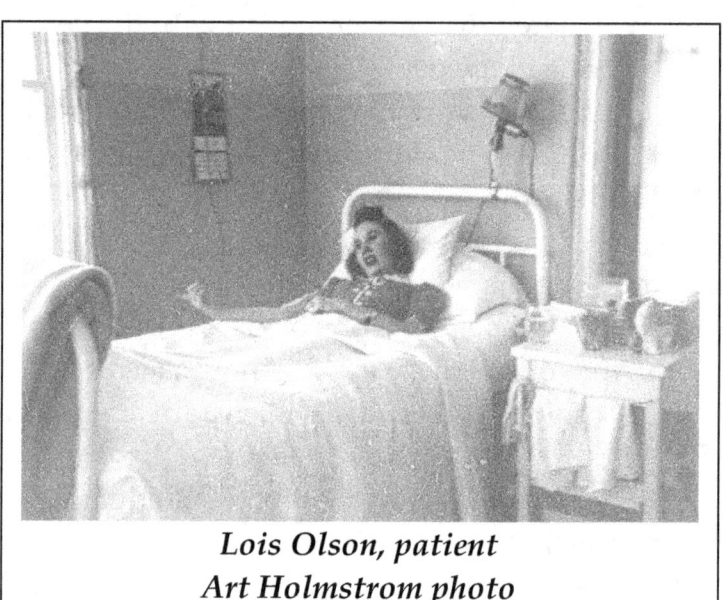

Lois Olson, patient
Art Holmstrom photo

"She sure is sick," Annie whispered, "but she's still spunky enough to sneak out of bed occasionally to see a new face. Lois is a bright light for the other patients, that's for sure, and she writes notes back and forth with the children. Lois is from Nevis and first came here in 1941. She was released, but now, she's returned.

"Irene Taylor's in the room across from the foot of my bed, and Laura Larson's in the third little room. Those three are in private rooms because they're sicker than the others. And this one busy with her knitting is Margaret Phelps. You'll meet the other girls farther down my ward when you get up; there are eight of us right now. They're lying there listening to every word we say. Those girls don't miss a thing!"

Art heard laughter and broke into a big smile. His brief stay at Lake Julia might be fun, after all.

☙❧

During Annie's first days at the San, she didn't have much to do, but one day Dr. Mary told her, "Get busy. You're not going to just sit there." So, she learned to knit. Dr. Mary brought the yarn and needles, and Annie made mittens. She knit so much that her fingers hurt. She and her roommates would knit and talk to pass the time.

Margaret Phelps didn't think the girls should be the only ones knitting. One day, she shouted out to Art, "Hey, Blondie, bet you can't learn to knit." The ladies challenged Art to knit a pair of gloves and told him they would provide the materials. "You're a man; you could never get it done," Margaret teased. She didn't have much faith in him.

"I'd teach you myself," Annie said, but my folks are coming today for visitation. They usually come from Solway once a week. That's why I got dressed up. We like to dress and fix our hair for guests. Or sometimes we wear fancier pajamas. Lois is too sick to get dressed, though. She's been in pajamas since she got here. I suppose your family won't come until next week since they were here just yesterday."

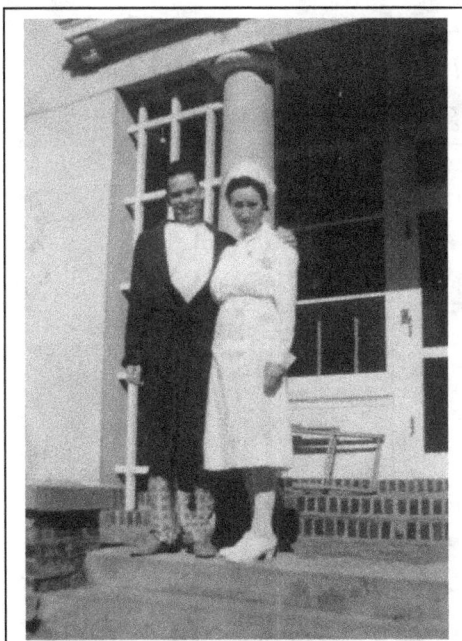

Patient and nurse on the San steps
James Ghostley collection

"Oh, I might be home by next week," Art replied. "If I'm not, they probably won't visit too often; it's a long drive from the Falls and difficult with gas rationing. I don't want to use up all their coupons.

"It must seem strange to your parents to visit you in this place, Annie. And I'm surprised that visitors don't take precautions, like wearing masks."

"Oh, they're used to it here, and they've never worn masks to visit. My brother, Karl, down on the first floor, has been here already eight years. In the summers, I came along when the folks visited, and usually, I went out by the lake while they were in here with him.

When I came here with TB, I already felt familiar with the place. I've seen my brother more since I got here than I have for years, except for waving to him through the window. It's like we're just getting to know each other."

"What does anyone do here for eight years?" Art asked.

"Oh, Karl's one to keep busy. He takes correspondence courses to fix radios—has tubes all over the place by his bed, and can fix most anything. People in Puposky bring their radios over to him, and he earns a little money fixing them."

A nurse walked in, shooed Annie back to bed, and shut the door between the wards. She gently reminded Art that he was not to sit up in bed. That ended the pleasant conversation with Annie, and it left Art anxious for the door to reopen.

⊗

A first-class postage stamp cost three cents, and Art wrote many letters. He wrote the first letter to his family on January 11, 1944, his third day at the San, not knowing that letter writing was a privilege to be earned. He included this postscript: *"Thanks for the letter. I knew you could write if you wanted to. I got it at 11:30 when the 'Star-Journal' carrier came by from Bemidji. They take mail out at 10:30, so we can't answer letters on the same day. It's 3:50 now. I feel quite a bit better. I've struck up a friendship with the girls on the south porch. Those girls have dubbed me 'Blondie.'"*

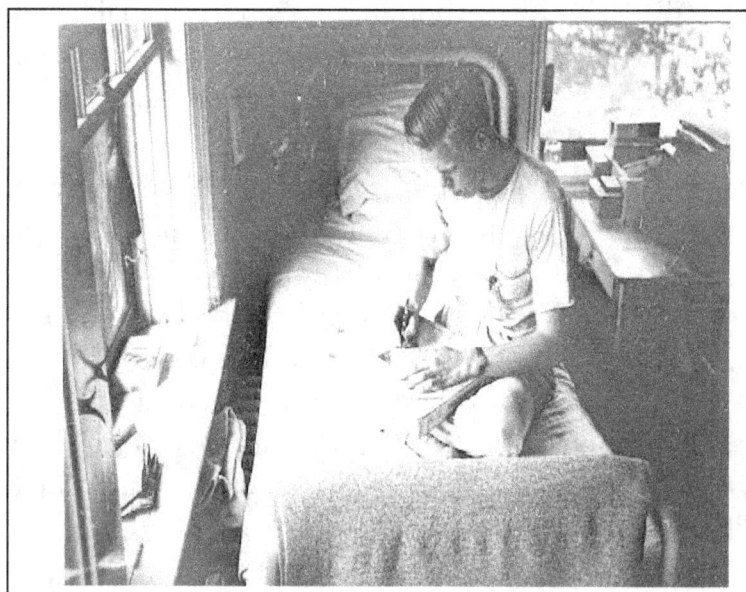

Art Holmstrom writing letters and using his windowsill as a shelf
Art Holmstrom collection

Chapter 31
Treatment Begins

Dr. Mary was anxious to start Art's treatment. "I've considered your case," she said. "Your lung is tearing apart. I'm going to give you pneumothorax, which we call pneumo, a procedure that will allow your lung to rest. We have special treatment and diagnostic areas—the X-ray room, which you've already visited, and the pneumothorax and fluoroscope rooms—all right here on the second floor. I'll take you to the pneumo room after your noon dinner."

After completing 11 letters, Art finally learned that he had not yet earned the privilege of writing. That was a blow to him because he wanted to stay in touch with family and friends, and he wanted to be busy.

სა

When the dinner trays arrived upstairs, Art sat up in bed to eat, then noticed a folded note under his fork. He read, *"Art, my new neighbor, rumor has it that you are headed for pneumo later today. Don't despair. Many of us get pneumo. I still do every few days. It smarts a bit at first, but you get used to it. They take you to a different room for it. Dr. Mary has strong fingers to feel where your ribs are. They use some Novocain to start, so don't worry too much about pain.*

Nurse Thora agreed to pass this note for me. We're not supposed to do it, so don't let on. I don't want to cause her any trouble. She's so dear to do this. Your friend on south sun porch, Annie."

After dinner, Nurse Thora wheeled Art past the small room where she had X-rayed his chest on his first day and into the pneumo room. The nurse had a mischievous sparkle in her eyes, most likely because she'd passed the note from Annie. Art stayed mum about their little secret, not saying a word. Dr. Mary arrived a moment later.

"Here's how I'll do it," explained the doctor. "I will carefully find the space between the two pleurae. I'll use a little needle to inject Novocain to deaden the area where I will insert the pneumothorax needle. I will change the size of the needle, then I'll insert it between the ribs. I'll puncture the first pleura and then put air between the two pleurae, the one that covers the inside of the rib wall and the one that covers the lung. I'll fill the space with air, like filling an inner tube, so that it expands. The air between the two pleurae will act as a cushion. That will force the lung down and restrict its movement, which will allow it to rest."

"What are those bottles?" Art asked as he looked up.

"Those two bottles are filled with fluid. One, as you can see, is higher than the other, and the movement of the liquid from one to the other will force the air through the needle and between the pleurae. We'll do it slowly so it won't get too uncomfortable for you."

Art fired questions one after another. "What will I feel like after the procedure? Will I require some recovery time, or will I feel normal? Will I be able to sit up in bed without pain?"

"You'll be able to function all right once your pleurae have become logged with air, but you'll have some shortness of breath. With one lung compressed, the other will have to do most of the work. Being on bed rest, you won't notice it much once the initial soreness goes away. You're very mature for your age, so you'll be able to handle it just fine."

The compliment made Art determined to tolerate whatever pain the procedure presented.

Art lay on his right side. "Here, Art, place this left arm up in the air and now stretch it upward and over your head a bit. That will help spread the ribs," Dr. Mary explained. "Fine. Now hold that position. I'm going to deaden the area, so you'll feel a little prick."

Art felt something like a bee sting. It wasn't much. Then he watched as Dr. Mary brought out a longer needle—a huge thing—and he pulled back from it.

"Next, Art, as I explained, I will puncture the first pleura and put air between the two pleurae that surround the lungs. I've done this procedure thousands of times, so don't worry."

Dr. Mary's hands automatically felt his ribs and jammed the needle expertly between them. Art winced with pain and drew in his breath as the big needle pushed inside his pleural cavity. Even with the Novocain, he could feel it, but he tolerated it quietly, wide-eyed.

"You're doing fine, Art, you're doing just fine," Dr. Mary comforted. "As I add air, I must calculate that the tissue will absorb some of it. I need to add enough to last until tomorrow."

"I'll need this procedure again tomorrow?" Art asked.

"You'll need it every day for a while; then, as you improve, we can do it less often."

Back in his ward after that first pneumo, Art felt sore. "I can bring you a painkiller," offered a nurse.

"Thanks, but no thanks," replied Art. "I've heard nothing but horror stories of folks becoming dependent on painkillers. I'll tolerate the pain."

Dr. Mary came by later to check on him. "How are you feeling, Art?" she asked.

"Sore, but not too bad."

"I'm sorry the procedure is uncomfortable. I wish it didn't take so long to get patients logged with air."

Dr. Mary came back every day for three days to add air. On the second day, she told Art, "Your body absorbs the air that I put in, so you'll get several refills this week. Then, you'll receive your refill once a week, and later once every two or three weeks, or whatever it takes to maintain the lung so that it doesn't expand again before it has healed. It could take quite a few weeks for the pleurae to become logged so that they will not absorb air from the pleural cavity."

"Several refills this week," Art repeated. "I'm not sure I want to become such good chums with that long needle."

The pneumothorax procedure was something entirely new to Art's body, and as a result, it felt sore. He had chest pain for the first week.

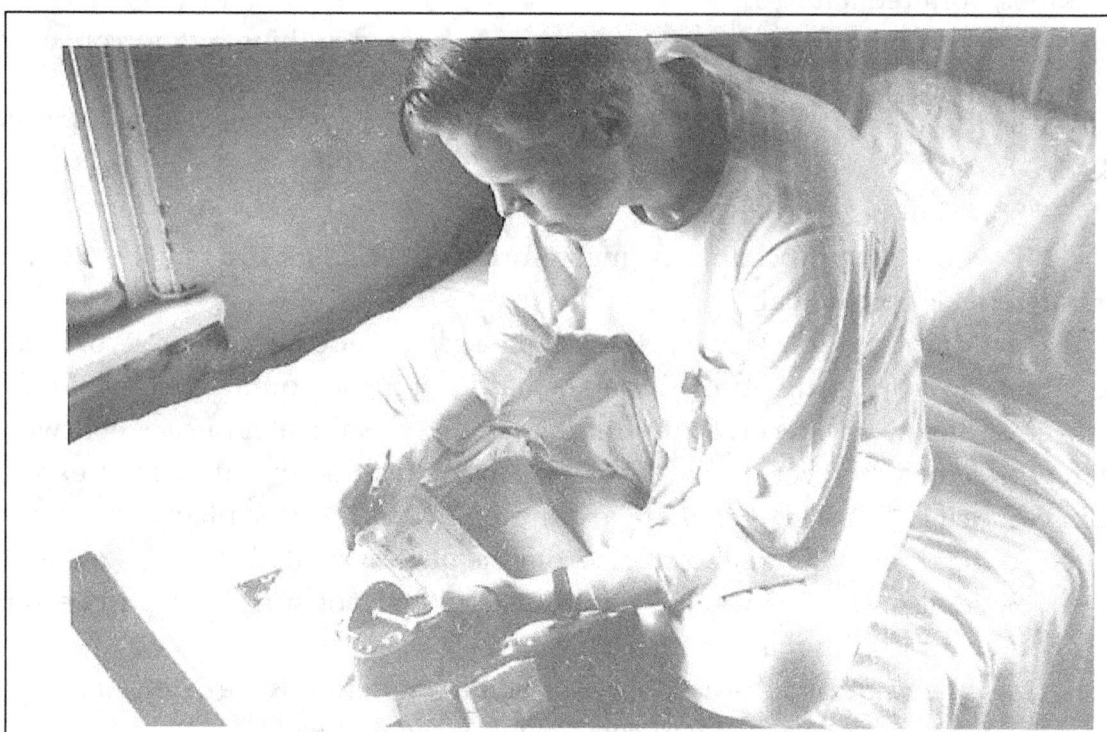

*Art Holmstrom should have rested more,
but he liked to stay busy. He wrote many letters.
Art Holmstrom collection*

Chapter 32
Roommates

On Saturday, January 15, after Art had been at the San for one week, Dr. Mary pulled up a chair by his bed. "If you're careful," she explained, "I'll allow you to try the privilege of walking to the locker room to use the bathroom one time today. If that goes well, I'll add more privileges as your recovery progresses. I think it will be OK if I allow you to read and write some letters now, too. But not too much. You overdid it the first couple of days."

Art treasured that walk to the locker room and made the most of it. He saw that the locker room had three sinks, a bathtub, a shower, and two toilets, plus lockers for the patients.

He strolled the short distance back from the locker room and took in everything he could see along the way. He stuck his head through the open window of a room across the hallway from his ward. Art expected to see a patient in that room. He thought he might be able to strike up a conversation, but the place was empty—without even a bed or a table. The smell of disinfectant alerted his nose, and the terrazzo floors gleamed in spotless readiness.

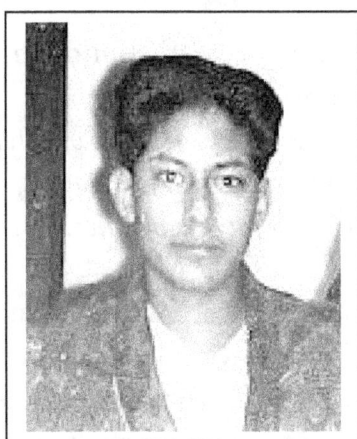

Felix Diaz
Art's roommate
and friend
Art Holmstrom photo

When Art returned to his ward, he commented to one of his roommates, 22-year-old Felix Diaz, "There's an empty room across the hall. It's all shined up, and there isn't a thing inside. I wonder who our new neighbor will be."

Felix, who had been a patient since 1943, looked like he'd seen a ghost. All he uttered was "muerte"—dead—before turning away from Art and sinking into his pillows.

Another roommate pushed himself up on one elbow and said to Art, "That's the dying room. It bothers Felix to talk about it because most of the patients who go there never return. It's empty now, but it sits there with open arms, just waiting for the next one of us to die. And it's not always from tuberculosis. Sometimes it's a heart attack or some other ailment.

You haven't been here long, Art. You'll learn soon enough that when you awake to clanging and squeaking in the night while the janitor and one of the nurses wheel a bed out of the ward, you had better say goodbye to the poor fellow in that bed."

Art sat, wide-eyed, as his roommate continued.

"No one ever tells us what's going on. The fear's more contagious than TB! They take a patient to the dying room. Then, one night, that person vanishes when the staff thinks we're all asleep; but with all the commotion when the janitors move the bed, they might as well just make an announcement. The next day, that's all any of us can talk about anyway."

Felix sat up. "Alto. Stop. You're scaring the boy."

The talkative roommate got quiet. They all remained still for some time as they thought about the dying room. Art vowed never to see the inside of that room again.

The longer the San was Art's home, the more he realized that Dr. Mary didn't think of those spaces as dying rooms, but rather as places of hope where she had one last chance to work a miracle to save her sickest patients. She called those rooms *isolation*. The patients never used the term *dying room* around her. She wouldn't have liked it.

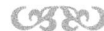

Art was eager to be more active and to stay in contact with friends and family. He wrote to his brother, Joe, on January 18 after a treatment:

"I got another pneumo today—400 cc. I didn't feel a thing before, during, or after. Have only spit once in 92 hours—I got a puzzle and a book from Victoria a few days ago. I haven't had time between eating, resting, and writing to read or put it together. I still could like it better at home."

He kept busy and had so many projects that he had to be creative to make good use of his small space. The 6-feet-tall lockers were for the storage of clothing, shoes, and other things. Patients couldn't store belongings underneath the beds because the floors had to be kept clear for cleaning, and there were no shelves on the walls. Each bed had a small bedside table with one shelf below a drawer. There was a box on one side, too, where Art accumulated things. Patients often stored a radio and earphones on top of their boxes. Art carefully hung supplies from his bedside table and organized his locker so that it would hold as much as possible.

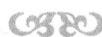

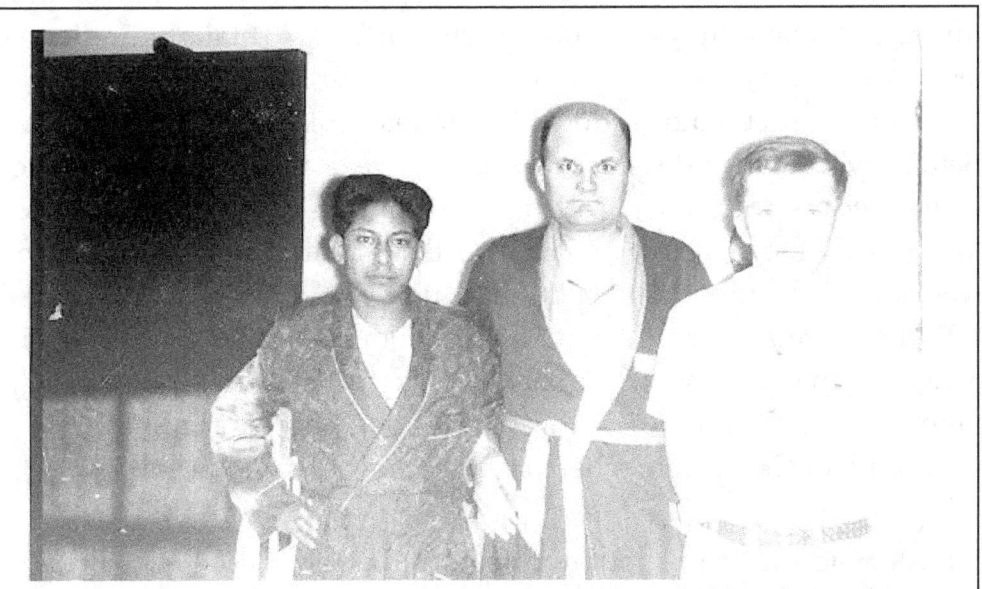
Felix Diaz, Raymond Knutson, and Elroy (Eli) Ramstad
Art Holmstrom photo

Elroy Ramstad (Eli,) the young fellow over by the window facing the lake, had been a carpenter and painter at the Bemidji Box Factory before being drafted into the service. The Army physical found his tuberculosis, and he entered the San on September 2, 1942. He left there and went to the hospital on May 9, 1944, where he died six days later from diabetes and tuberculosis.[109] That meant Art got Eli's bed by the window, a location with earphones. He felt guilty for being happy to get a better spot in the ward. He wrote to his family, *"There isn't really a pecking order as you become a more senior member of the room, but as you saw, my first bed had neither a window nor earphones. In the new spot, if they open the door into the women's ward, I can see around the corner, and if I am quiet, I can hear some conversations. The move has also put me closer to Felix Diaz, and we get along quite well."*

As time went on, Art met many patients and employees. A Catholic divinity student named Eddie Hissler, from St. Paul Seminary, was only six months older than Art. He was a patient from December 1947 to July 1948 but returned every 10

---

[109] Minnesota History Center, Lake Julia Tuberculosis Sanatorium Patient Register

days for pneumothorax refills, so Art had an opportunity to see him on those visits. They discussed many things, including religion, and Art taught Eddie to knit and crochet.

Because of tuberculosis, Eddie had to leave his priesthood studies at the St. Paul Seminary. He was a deacon in his second year of education when he came to Lake Julia. Because of their friendship, Art had an opportunity to meet Bishop Shenk from Crookston, about 88 miles northwest, and priests from both Solway, just over 20 miles from the San, and Blackduck.

Eddie originally came from Shooks, about 40 miles northeast of Bemidji. When he left the San, he went back to his training and became a priest in Blackduck. Then, he served in the Crookston diocese and a couple of other locations south of Crookston, where he was known as Father Ed.

ଔଞ

Lester Gibson spent about two years at the San, 1947-1949. "I was so ill," he said," that I had to be moved around in a wheelchair, and I was in an isolation room. On Sundays, if no one came to visit, I felt like no one cared about me. When I first went to the San, I was a junior in high school, and I was in poor health. Dr. Mary gave me pneumo treatments every eight or nine days."

For the first couple of years, Lester had his meals in his room, but he was finally able to go to the dining room. Like Art, he was about 6'3" tall, but he weighed only just over 100 pounds. "Eventually," Lester said, "I started to gain weight. I began to get better and was then able to move into the room with Art and his roommates. I enjoyed the food and weighed 200 pounds when I left the San. "

A nurse commented to Lester one day that it looked like he and Art had become good friends. "I get along well with Art Holmstrom," Lester replied, "even though Art is a little different, being so smart." After spending three or four months in Art's ward, the doctor transferred Lester to the other end of the hall and then he and Art seldom saw each other.

Lester learned to knit while at the San, and he knitted a sweater for his little sister. "Many young family members wore that sweater over the years," Lester said.

During his hospitalization, his family moved to Wyoming because both parents had TB, and they hoped the dry air would be better for them. His dad refused sanatorium admission because he had a family to support. After Lester's release, he joined his parents in Wyoming, where his mother eventually went into a sanatorium. His father did not, and he died from TB.

In one letter, Art's Uncle George asked if there was much friction between roommates. Art replied:

"We do argue and debate different things. One man, Ray Knutson, an ironworker from Bagley, on the iron range, is very much pro-Tito. He grew up knowing Josip Tito, the leader of the Communist opposition forces in Yugoslavia. If we want to get Ray riled up, we just say something against Yugoslavia.

"Tito developed the Yugoslav Communist Party into a powerful organization. The Germans are in Yugoslavia, so Tito is leading the opposition. There is another guy too, Draza Mihajlovic, who runs the resistance movement.

"Two of the guys in my room take joy in arguing with Ray about politics and other subjects but especially about Yugoslavia and Tito. When they get a report that Tito has done something effective against the Nazis, then they downplay it and boast about what the other guy has done. That causes a lot of arguments. They finally had to remove Ray from our room because the other guys got so worked up, and Ray got excited and had coughing fits.

"There is often a lot of fun in our ward. Sometimes the men feed the chipmunks. Someone trained one, and it came in the window.

"Sometimes when the patient isn't well, but the family wants to have a get together at home, a patient goes home for a visit and refuses to return. When that happens, he is sometimes forced by the authorities to go back to the sanatorium. Wayne Shunkweiler, from Park Rapids, would leave Ah-gwah-ching to return home, so they moved him to the Lake Julia Sanatorium to stop that practice. Here, he chose to walk around independently instead of staying in bed, so the staff tried to persuade him to stay in his bed and out of the women's wards. He left one day, and they tracked him down at his home in Park Rapids. They returned him to the State San and housed him in a locked ward downstairs.

"Eli Paatalo, a Finnish fellow from Nashwauk, is the second Eli to stay in my ward."

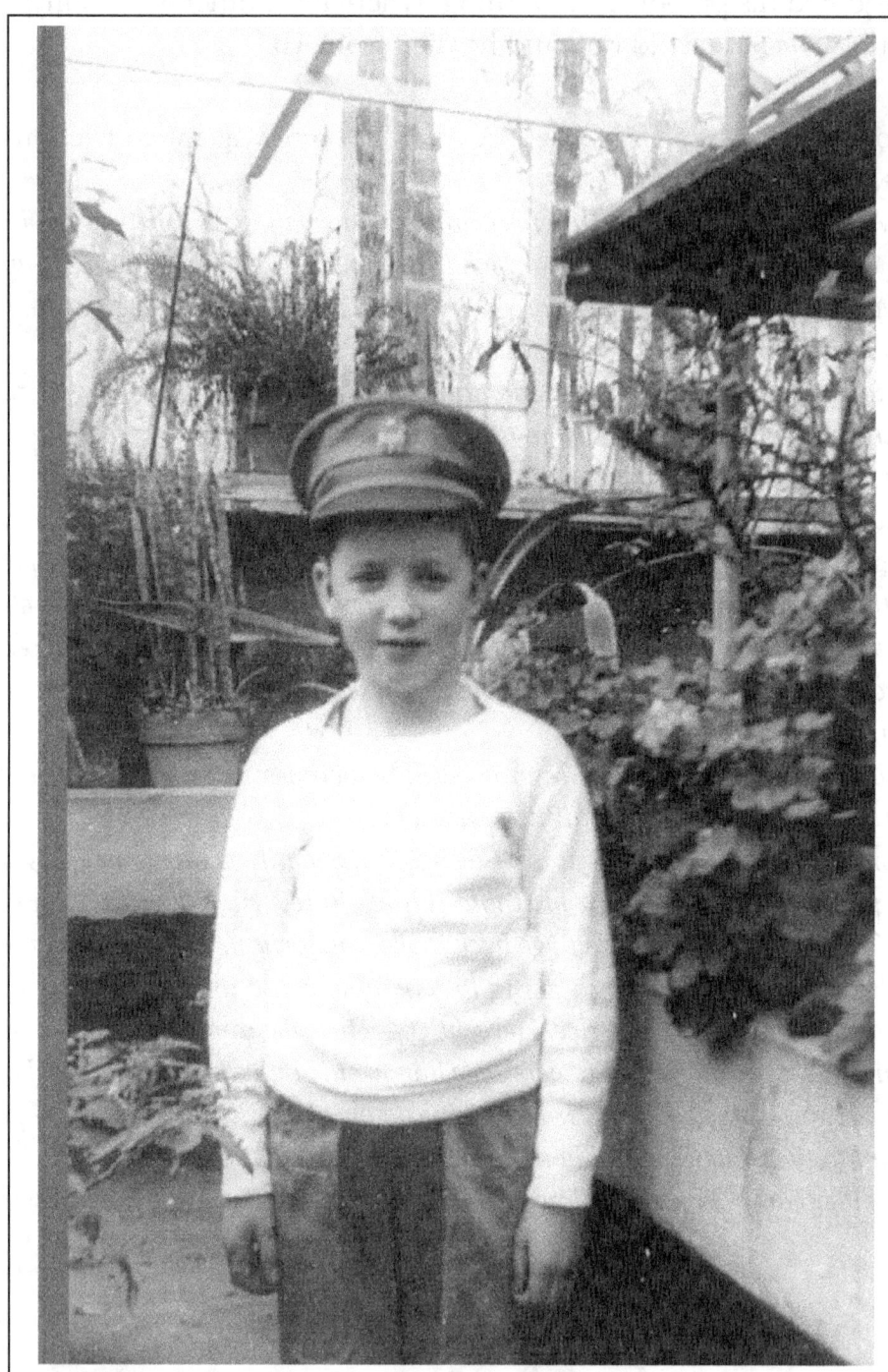

Ken Nordstrand at the San
Art Holmstrom photo

Chapter 33
A Young Patient

There weren't many children around while Art was in the San, but one was 10-year-old Ken Nordstrand, a kid from International Falls.

Ken had always felt like he was sick with a cold. He never tested positive for TB, but he suffered from pleurisy and breathing problems. His school nurse, Gertrude Rennell, and Dr. Mary Ghostley both thought Ken had water on the lungs.

On his first admission, he rode from the Falls to the Sanatorium with Dr. Mary and another lady. Dr. Mary often drove back and forth between Puposky and the Falls because of her TB duties and her cabin at Rainy Lake, so it wasn't uncommon for her to give patients a ride.

"On the way to the San," Ken said, Dr. Mary told me she wanted to get something to eat. No cafes were open, but there was a basketball game going on at a school—in Blackduck, I think— so we stopped there. The ladies took me way up high so I would not be near the spectators in case I was contagious. I felt weak from climbing the stairs, so the ladies had me lie on a bench while they got some food for us. It was my first time at a basketball game, and, even though I was sick, I had fun."

After Ken spent the night at the San, Dr. Mary stuck a needle into his lungs and tried to withdraw fluid, but to no avail. When that failed, she knew he had pus instead of water on his lungs.

Ken went back to the Falls, where he went into the Northern Minnesota Hospital for surgery. Ken said, "I remember a rag with ether that the doctor placed in my mouth before surgery. The doctor stuck a tube through my side to let my lungs drain."

His younger brother, Bob, was in the hospital at the same time for the same problem, but he was not as sick as Ken. The boys' parents watched and worried. When Dr. Craig slapped green salve on Ken's chest and wrapped him in a warm towel, his father asked, "What are you doing to 'Sonny?'"

The doctor replied that he was keeping the boy's chest draining.

Day after day while Ken was in the hospital, his bandages had to be changed when they filled with blood and nasty pus. Ken said, "My folks came to see me one last time because the doctor didn't expect me to live. But I recovered and finally returned home after an extended stay in the hospital." When Ken and Bob left the hospital, they each had an identical long, deep scar where a drainage tube had been stuck into them.

In 1924, Ken's parents had lost a 4-year-old son to scarlet fever. Another son, Eddie, was deaf and could not speak. Their parents, like Art Holmstrom's, had experienced a lot of worry with their children.

"I left the hospital but started getting worse again," Ken said. "I went back to the San, where Dr. Mary took me under her wing. At first, I was kept in a bed in the nurses' home, on the top floor where the nurses slept and where Dr. Mary could keep an eye on me. After a while, she transferred me to the main building, where I stayed for several months in the basement with five older guys—the janitors and engineers—where Dr. Mary could keep me away from the TB patients. The men treated me well. I slept on a top bunk in a corner."

When he got better, but not yet well enough to go home, Ken pretty much had the run of the place, except for the areas where those with active tuberculosis lived. The janitor, Bill Masterson, watched out for the youngster. Ken followed him all over—had lunch with him, helped him stoke the furnace—and even went fishing off the dock with him and caught a sunfish. Ken especially liked a wonderful grandmother-like woman by the name of Mrs. Cross, who was Dr. Mary's sister. Dr. Mary's other sister, Anna Brown, was also a nurse at the San.

Ken ate a lot of oatmeal in the San dining room, and he took his time because he had a crush on Dr. Mary's daughter, Cathie, and her friend Patsy Maher, who worked as summer waitresses. "I ate in the large dining room," Ken said. "I remember that the terrazzo floors were always shiny, and I watched as girls scurried around putting place settings on the tables."

Cathie and Patsy told Ken that they sometimes rode their bikes to Bemidji on their days off and spent the night with nurse Thora Bakken. "It seemed like a long way to ride," Ken said, "but they thought nothing of it."

He played *In the Mood* on the piano in the big room just inside the front entrance, and the help gathered around, laughed, and clapped.

At night, as Ken tried to fall asleep in the basement, he could hear patients moan and groan. Ken lay in the dark and listened as some screamed. "Someone died while I was there," he said.

Years later, when I visited the San, the basement looked foreboding with its dark corridors, rooms full of accumulated parts and pieces, most of them broken, and the upheaval of its concrete floors. It was sobering to remember that the basement had been home to many, including my father and this boy.

Ken enjoyed his days at the San because he was the center of attention. The janitors and engineers kept him company. They liked to play jokes on him. One man told him he had a visitor, but it was just an April Fool's joke. He never did have visitors while he was there, but he got to know some of the patients, like Art Holmstrom.

There was a room full of jigsaw puzzles, and people often brought more because Ken was good at putting them together.

When Dr. Mary discharged Ken, he rode back to the Falls with another patient who was leaving. He didn't know if his family even knew he was coming. He was dropped off on 11th Avenue and 15th Street in the Falls. As he walked through the neighbor's yard and up a long path to his house, he heard his dad say, "Here comes Sonny."

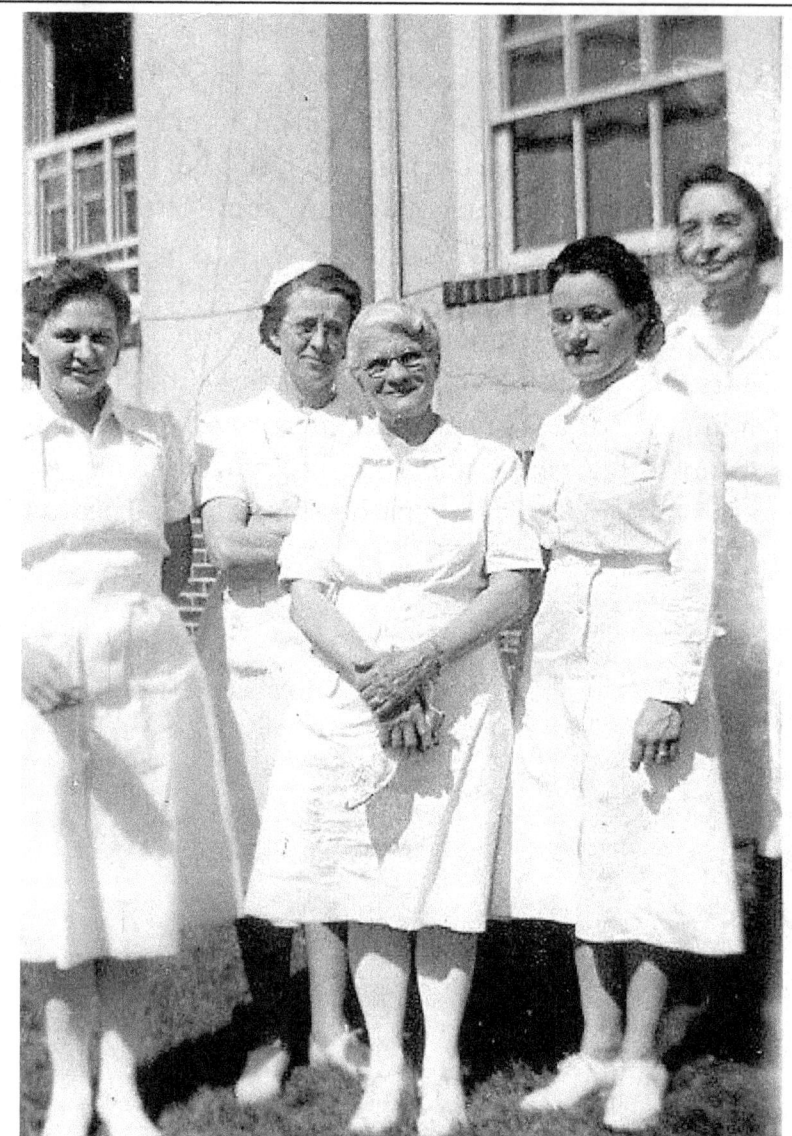

Peggy Cross, center. Wilma Watts, far right.
James Ghostley collection

Together, let's continue to collect history on the San.
If you can identify others in this photograph or in photos
that I will post from time to time on my website,
www.OpenWindowTB.com,
please contact me through the website or email
Contact@OpenWindowTB.com.
Do you have Lake Julia Sanatorium photos to share?

Chapter 34
The History Lesson

With Art's 18th birthday coming up in a week, he wrote to ask his brother to have Uncle George go to the draft board on his birthday— not before—and also to the Clerk of Court's office to renew his driver's license. At 18, young men had to register for the draft for possible military service.

"I've written 50 letters since I came here," Art wrote. "*I hope you've taken care of the gas—and remember and use all points out of the ration books.*"

During World War II, many items were limited or rationed: meat, fats, sugar, processed foods, fuel oil, gasoline, shoes, coffee, cigarettes, tires, and others. Ration stamps were required to purchase a limited quantity of restricted items.[110]

Art felt a little envious when a patient from the Falls told him his family planned to visit in a week or two. On Sunday, while some of the other patients had visitors, Art wrote his brother Joe another letter.

"*A visit from home would be nice, but I don't want the family to feel obligated to make the long trip. Stay home and go fishing, and use the gas wisely.*"

But he really did want company, so he added, "*Don't come on a Sunday, come on a Saturday, so Uncle George won't have to lose time-and-a-half pay; he needs it. Visiting hours are 10 to 1, 3 to 6 and 7 to 8:15, but these may be stretched, seeing you come such a distance.*

"*There's a typewriter here, but I haven't had a chance to use it yet. It needs a ribbon. Could you bring me one when you come? And I'd like my camera. Pack it good. Better yet, have George do it, and see if he'll send my films from the hall cabinet. I need the 116-120s and the 620-616s.*

"*Dr. Mary told me I could start my schoolwork, but I'm to take it easy, so easy that I barely graduate, and she told me not to try for scholarships or valedictorian-ship. That's a big disappointment, but my health is the most important thing now. So, you could bring along some schoolwork or ask to have it sent.*"

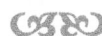

---

[110] http://www.lakesnwoods.com/BlackduckHistory2.htm

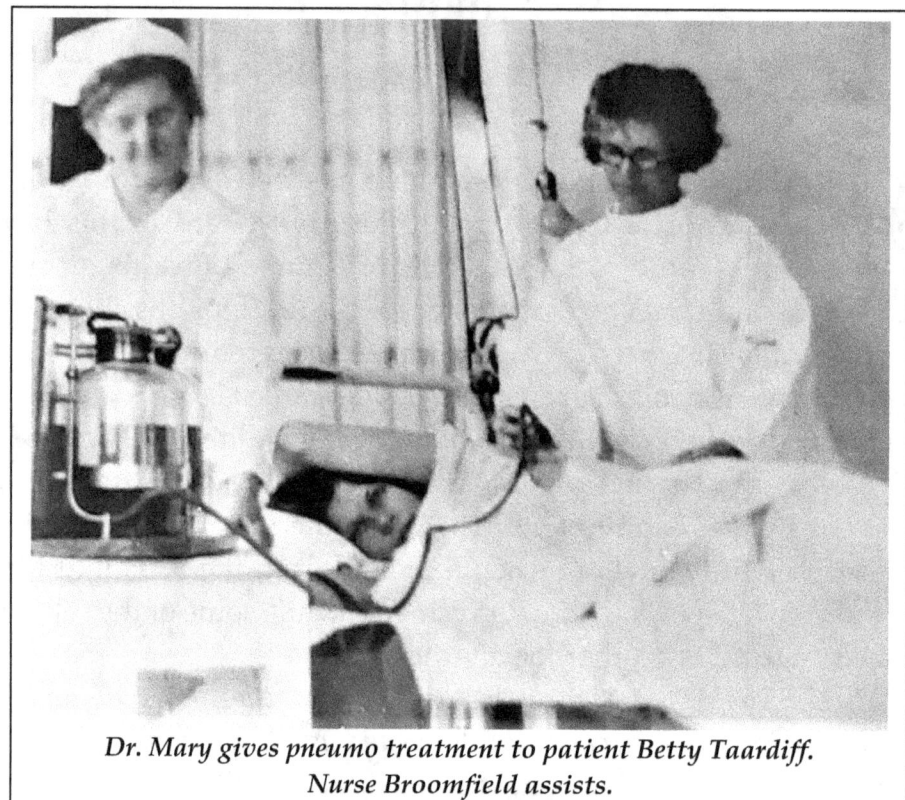
*Dr. Mary gives pneumo treatment to patient Betty Taardiff.
Nurse Broomfield assists.
James Ghostley collection*

After a couple of weeks, outside of feeling the first poke of the long needle, Art didn't think much about the pneumothorax treatments. He had gotten over the novelty quickly.

He no longer felt the initial apprehension, and he settled in. In time, he got so accustomed to the refills that he received them in his bed, not needing to go to the pneumo room. He rested, ate well, adapted to his new surroundings, and began his recovery.

One morning, Dr. Mary stood at Art's bedside and explained, "I'm going to allow you the privilege of getting up to walk to the bathroom and back to your bed one time every 24 hours."

"So, for 23 hours and 50 minutes, I stay in bed."

"That's right."

"Thank you, Dr. Mary. That's a big improvement," Art declared. "I won't abuse the privilege. I'll do anything to get well. And—I'm sorry I questioned you before."

"I understand, Art. Everyone's nervous and a bit frightened when they get admitted," she empathized. "I'm responsible for your health, and that's why I have to be firm. You've done a good job of following the rules, and I can see that you're doing your best."

※

Nurse Thora came in the next day and pulled up a chair by Art's bed. "Well, young man, it looks like you'll be here a while, so you might as well learn the history of the place."

"Have you been here long?" Art asked.

"Oh, yes, I've been here since the late-1920s. I came first as a patient. I was here back when we had a doctor named Laney. It used to be that the windows in the San were open day and night, summer and winter; in fact, there was no glass in the windows, just a heavy canvas shade to pull down. The cold, fresh air was supposed to be the cure. In winter, patients woke to snow on their blankets, ice in their water glasses, and frozen urine in their pots."

"It doesn't seem like that cold air would be very healthy."

"The thought at that time was that the cold air was therapeutic for assisting people in breathing and that it had some remedial effect. People often went to Colorado to cure their consumption—that's what people called TB back then—back in the latter part of the 1800s and early 1900s. That's what attracted people to Northern Minnesota; they could come and live in the cold fresh air and the pines to arrest their consumption. We didn't close windows until Dr. Mary came," Nurse Thora said. "Dr. Mary took special training on treating tuberculosis, so she made some big changes here."

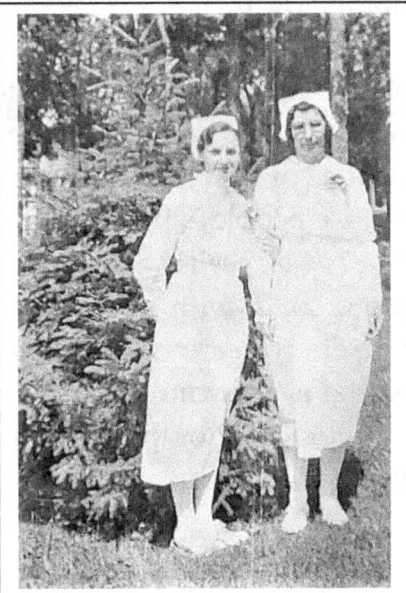

Opal Christianson Falk and Thora Bakken 1935 James Ghostley collection

"Was the San new when you came in?"

"No. It was built in 1916, and I didn't come until 1927. Oh my, I wasn't even 30 years old.

"You're pretty much confined to your bed now, Art, but when I came into the place, we were all outside a lot, year-round, if we were able."

"That sounds nice," Art commented.

"No, no. We were too sick to be out like that. Even if we had a temp and a terrible cough, we were out there tobogganing or going for sleigh rides. Often, we had to work on the grounds splitting wood or doing other chores."

"When you were a patient, where was your ward?" Art asked.

"Right there, through that door next to you, on the sun porch. That porch had been just a place to roll the beds during the day so that the patients who were too sick to go outside could get some sun, but as the population grew, it became another ward.

"Having no glass in the windows was OK in the summer, but it was bitterly cold in the winter. The radiators did add some heat to the room during the day, but the engineers turned them off each evening so we would breathe the cold air. The idea of the cold air was to improve the breathing and open the bronchial tubes because people experience congestion when temperatures are warmer.

"My head was right by the window. The water next to my bed was often frozen solid, with snow on the table and the floor and sometimes right on my blankets. Then, in the morning, the radiators would come on, but the cold kept coming in the windows. Snow and ice melted all over the place. That made quite a mopping job for the janitors, and everyone had to watch their step until the floor dried.

"Earlier, you asked me about the window openings in the walls of the interior rooms."

"The patients in those rooms would stay warmer without them," Art stated.

Nurse Thora explained, "The open windows allow airflow through the entire building. Air goes right through this place, from the front to the back—in one side of the building and out the other."

Goosebumps raised on Art's arms. "So, with this type of disorder, when the air is colder, it is easier to breathe," Art clarified.

"That's right. There are big furnaces in the basement, and they run 24 hours a day. Those steam radiators function even in the summer. There is a valve to stop

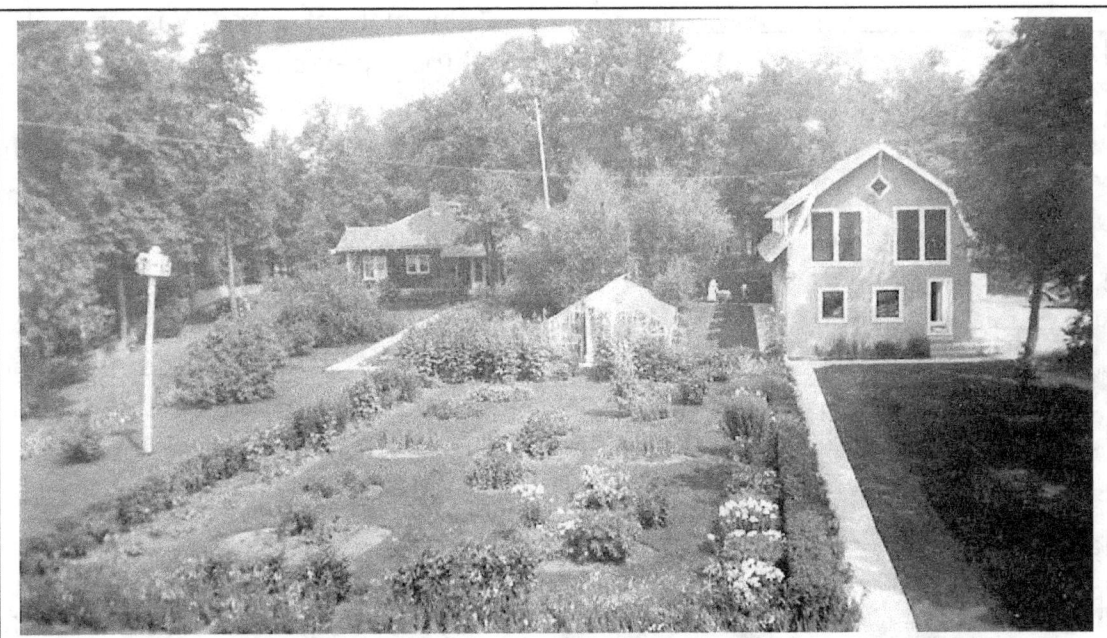

Dr. Mary's log house (left), the greenhouse and flower garden (middle), and the garage (right), where Dr. Mary and Lucy Barrett's offices were located upstairs
James Ghostley collection

After the San closed, Leroy Graham, who had operated the boilers, bought the garage and moved it. Eventually, it was destroyed by fire.

the steam from coming through, and it's that valve that shuts off the heat at night and fires it up again in the morning. The steam goes to each building on the grounds, in addition to heating the San."

"And how many buildings are there?"

"Oh, let's see. Well, there's Dr. Mary's cottage and the garage—that's where Dr. Mary and Miss Barrett—the one with the red wig—have their offices upstairs. There's another house where one of the employees lives, the greenhouse, the nurses' home next door, and the dairy farm. Raw steam goes out to the garbage house. That's where we steam the garbage cans to kill the bacteria. Cans get cleaned with the hot steam right to the bare metal.

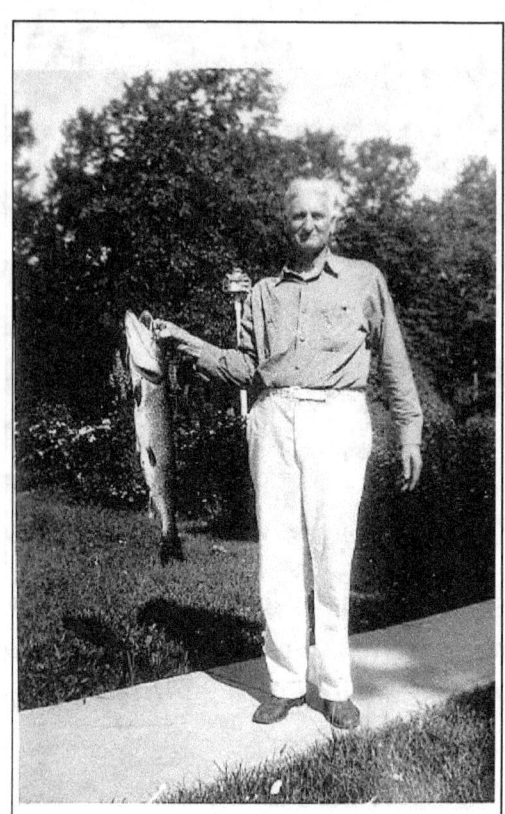

Pops Warner
Art Holmstrom photo

"One patient, Pops Warner, walked over to Puposky every day for the mail; that was his chore then, as a patient, and he still does it today as an orderly. Orderlies deliver meals and water, tidy up rooms, take out the garbage, make beds, and help patients organize their clothes. You've seen them around. They help wherever they can, and Pops is a fixture around the place. People joke that he sat outside on a stump, waiting for the San to open."

"Were you a nurse when you came in?" Art asked.

"No. I was discharged on June 6, 1927, with instructions to continue resting at home. I didn't know what I would do or where I would go when I got well. I felt kind of lost, so when Dr. Mary showed up here on the board, she insisted I needed a skill."

"Then, she hired you as a nurse?"

"Oh, not right away. In November 1927, I took the job of dishwasher. I worked 7 a.m. to 3 p.m., six days a week. Later I was a maid, and when Dr. Mary took over, I started training as a student nurse. I had skills when Dr. Mary got done with me—she saw to that! After training me as a nurse, she taught me to be her X-ray technician, and I never left the place. It's the best job I could have, meeting friendly folks like you. I wonder where I'd be without this place."

"That's a lot of X-rays, taking them of all of us patients."

"I don't just take X-rays of you patients. Every six months, I take X-rays of the employees, too. And sometimes, I take X-rays of people who are not patients or employees, like I did in the winter of 1933. One Sunday, 33 people, mostly pupils and teachers, came from the Baudette and Williams schools, about 95 miles away, for X-rays because each one had registered positive on a Mantoux test. After we took the X-rays, we sent the plates to Dr. Myers in St. Paul, and he returned a report," explained Nurse Thora.

Those folks all rode the Spooner school bus, and they made quite a day of it. After the X-rays, they went to Bemidji for dinner and a motion-picture show."[111]

"How could so many people afford to come all this way?" Art asked.

"Mrs. C. H. Dodds, who had been chairman of the Christmas Seals campaign for several years, organized the project. The Christmas Seals campaign funded it."

"I've seen Christmas Seals on envelopes for years, but I don't know much about them," Art said.

"Christmas Seals came about when a Delaware sanatorium needed to either raise $300 or close its doors," Nurse Thora explained. That's when Emily Bissell, a veteran fundraiser, designed and printed special holiday seals and sold them at the post office for a penny each. She and her volunteers raised 10 times the amount needed, and that was the beginning of the American Lung Association Christmas Seals program to support the fight against lung disease. Since tuberculosis primarily affects the lungs, this screening was the perfect program for Christmas Seals to sponser."[112]

---

[111] *The Baudette*, Lake of the Woods County, Minnesota, December 1, 1933
[112] American Lung Association

200

Chapter 35
Patient Visitation Night

On the evening of Art's third Saturday at the San, when patients were allowed to visit with one another, Art was disappointed that he had to stay in bed. His frequent communication with the girls on the sun porch consisted only of a short visit when the door was open or of passing notes. He was surprised when Annie and Norma stepped into his ward. Both had curled their hair, and they looked like they were going out on the town or to church.

"Hi, Art," Annie said. "We thought we'd pay you a little visit. Usually, the men call on the women, but we know you're restricted to bed, so we're calling on you."

"How's the pneumo going?" asked Norma. "It's kind of hard to get used to at first."

"Oh, I'm doing OK," Art replied. "The chest pain lasted most of the week, and I noticed a little shortness of breath, but it wasn't too bad since I just stayed in bed."

"My father had pneumo," Norma commented. "He had tuberculosis, too. In those days, they pumped oil between the pleurae because it was heavy, and it settled, forcing the lung to rest. Sounds strange, doesn't it?"

ೞ೩

After Annie visited Art in his room on January 31, Art couldn't wait to tell Joe about their conversation. He wrote, *"Anneliese Petersen, the girl from Solway, Minnesota, who is going to teach me German, has a mother 51 years old. Her Papa is 50 years old. She's about 18 and probably will get out for graduation. She came here on December 27."*

Art and Annie visited whenever they could. At night, if the doors between wards were open, they communicated by making shadows on the walls with their hands.

Art learned that Annie had lived in Bemidji during her senior year of high school to take care of children for the folks who ran the Gamble store. That's where she first had night sweats, causing her to wake up wringing wet. When her brother, Karl, heard about that, he insisted that their parents take her to the doctor for an examination. Sure enough, she, too, had TB.

While visiting, Annie and Art both spoke highly of their woman doctor, and Annie mentioned that she liked the distinct white streak through the doctor's gray hair.

"Dr. Mary's a great person," Art remarked. "I don't know how she can work so hard with so little rest and still be so even-tempered most of the time."

"Oh, if something isn't right, she'll tell you," Annie responded, "but it can't be easy to keep this big place running smoothly. She's a kind person, very compassionate. I once saw her sit all night with a little girl who was a patient in one of the isolation rooms behind our sun porch."

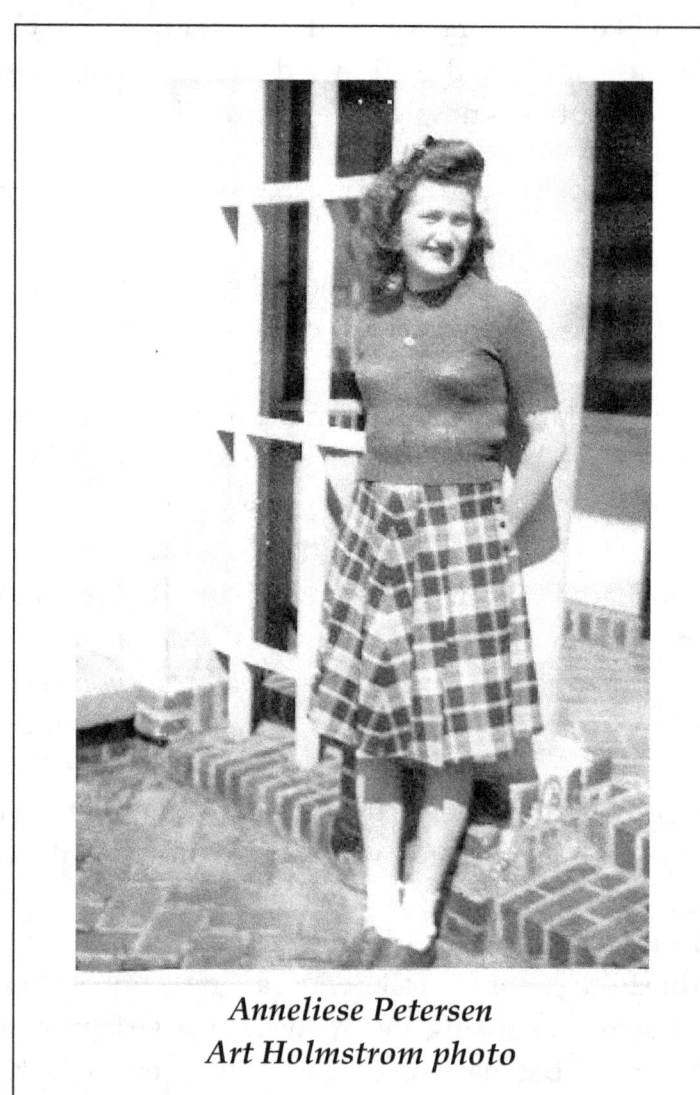

Anneliese Petersen
Art Holmstrom photo

Chapter 36
A Change of Plans

Even though Art had tested positive for TB in January at home, once he arrived at the San, he tested negative. That sometimes happened. There were no tuberculosis germs in his sputum. He tested negative for active tuberculosis again at the end of February.

Dr. Mary announced, "Well, things look so good that you can go home in May. You'll be able to attend your graduation, after all!"

"Hallelujah!" Art exclaimed. He wrote to tell his friends and family that he would soon return home. He'd stayed longer than he had anticipated, but it was good to be well. He started to say his goodbyes in preparation for leaving. He knew he would miss Annie, but he planned to keep in touch with her after his discharge.

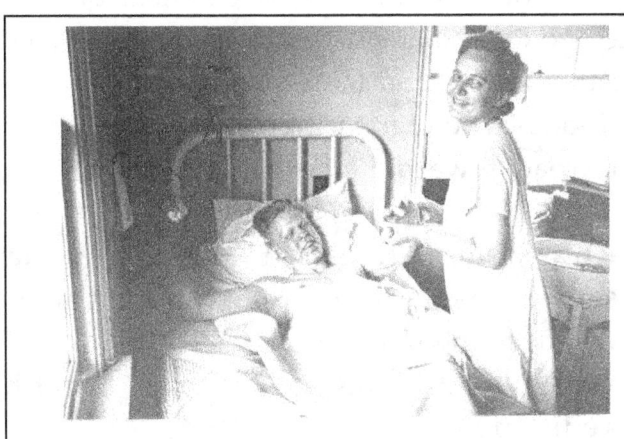

Art Holmstrom and nurse Charlotte Zimmer
Art Holmstrom collection

Most patients were able to spit up their sputum and capture it in a bottle to be tested, but, for Art, it was nearly impossible to bring it up. Dr. Mary thought that during the night, he probably swallowed anything that came up from his lungs. It became necessary to run a tube down his throat to his stomach, pump in some water, and pump it back out for testing. That was the only way Dr. Mary could get a sample of his sputum so that she could be sure he was, indeed, negative.

After a March 10 washing of Art's stomach, tuberculosis germs again showed up in his sputum. He wasn't going anywhere. Art had to endure many of those washings, and as difficult as it was to accept that tube the first time, he soon learned to swallow it without difficulty.

He had hoped to graduate as valedictorian, but his illness forced him to give up that dream. His school and family were disappointed, too. Many school officials and parents debated whether Art should be allowed to graduate while completing his studies at the San. And if he was allowed to graduate, should he still be named valedictorian? There were hard feelings, both from those who thought it unfair to grant the honor to someone who was not attending school and those others who believed Art had earned the honor. Finally, the school decided not to name either a valedictorian or a salutatorian. To avoid being in that position again, they did not do so for several years.

Dr. Mary reassured Art, "You shouldn't have to remain here much longer. You will probably test negative again soon. But I don't think it's wise for you to leave the San without getting some exercise. The hard part is that you can't start to exercise until you test negative again. Let's aim for you to go home at the end of the summer. That should give you time to become negative and start exercising."

He finally had a string of negatives—he showed no signs of active tuberculosis—, and, in January 1945, he got more privileges. The next privilege was that he could take a real bath, then go downstairs to one meal. Soon he could go downstairs to the dining room for two meals, and then three, and eventually, he could go outside and walk a little. Soon he could go farther, and before long, he could walk some distance down the road toward Maher's place or the other direction toward Puposky and back.

Dr. Mary liked the progress she was seeing. Art seemed stronger every day. She walked into his ward with a big smile on her face and looked straight at him. "Art, you are doing so well that you will be going home soon."

Art felt ecstatic. He couldn't wait to sleep in his bed at home, to eat his mother's cooking, and to continue his education.

The first thing he did was write to his family to report the good news. Next, he started to gather his belongings. To make it official, Dr. Mary called Lissie. "I have good news. Art is doing well. You can pick him up on June 13."

On the 10th of June, a Wednesday, Art had his routine X-ray. He chatted nonstop to Nurse Thora, telling her all the things he planned to do when he returned home. But when Dr. Mary looked at his X-ray, she saw that it spelled bad news. Tuberculosis had spread from the left lung to the right lung, and he wasn't going anywhere.

That day, he lost all his privileges but little of his hope. "While it is a disappointment," Art reassured his mother, "I have progressed to the point of being ready to go home once, so I can do it again." Then, he began having pneumo treatments on both lungs.

While Art lay in bed, Annie received her high school diploma in June. That was bittersweet for Art since his school would not allow him to graduate.

☙❧

As Art continued his recovery, he still turned down a few foods, and he gave food he didn't care for to his roommate Felix. Sometimes, supper was peas over boiled potatoes, and Art didn't think that tasted too bad. A few patients left the food they didn't care for and sent it back on the tray, and if Dr. Mary heard that patients refused certain foods, she had the unpopular items deleted from the menu. The doctor often asked patients what foods they liked and didn't like. Dr. Mary did not want to waste foods that patients wouldn't eat, and she wanted them to be well-nourished to improve their health. Art was frank if he thought the food should be better, but he was no longer picky. After spending some time at the San, there weren't many things he didn't like. There were several cooks, but one lady who had taught home economics in Fargo was his favorite.

It was hard for someone as young as Art to stay in bed. Kathy Saddler, who worked in the kitchen, heard there was a young guy named Holmstrom up on Two, so she broke the rules and sent up an autographed photo on his meal tray. Art was infatuated with her for a while, and Kathy helped him keep his mind off his illness. But his friendship with Annie continued to blossom, and he soon forgot about his crush on the kitchen worker, who he had never met.

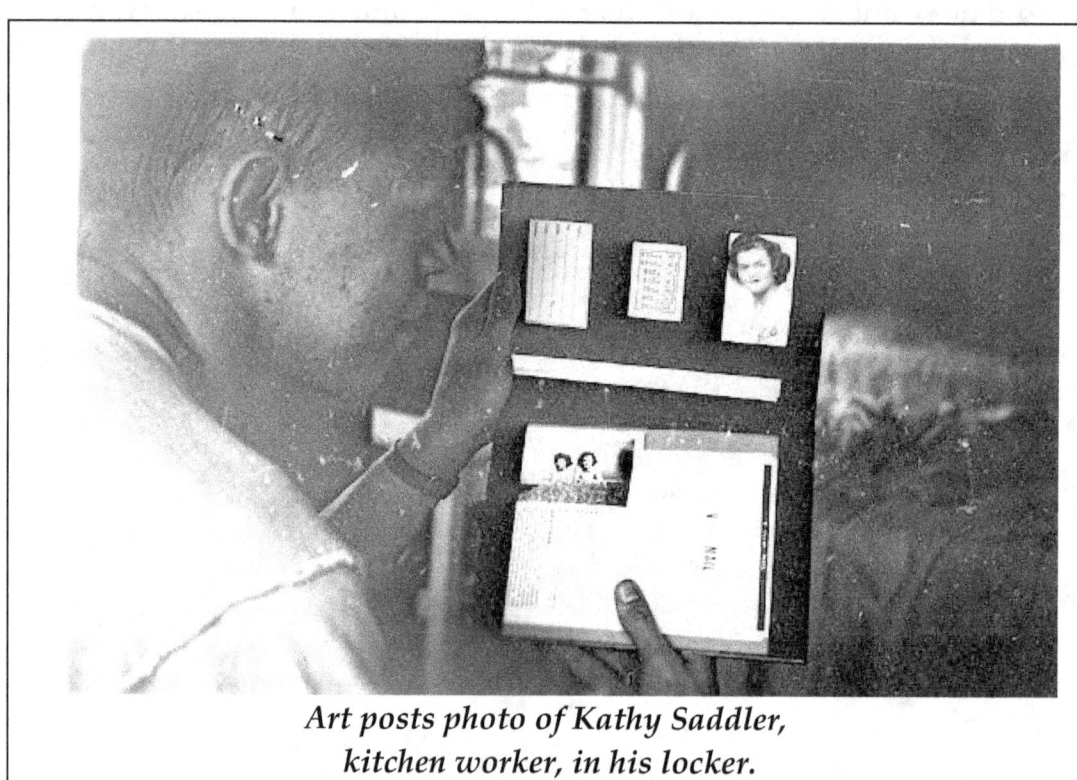

Art posts photo of Kathy Saddler, kitchen worker, in his locker.
Art Holmstrom collection

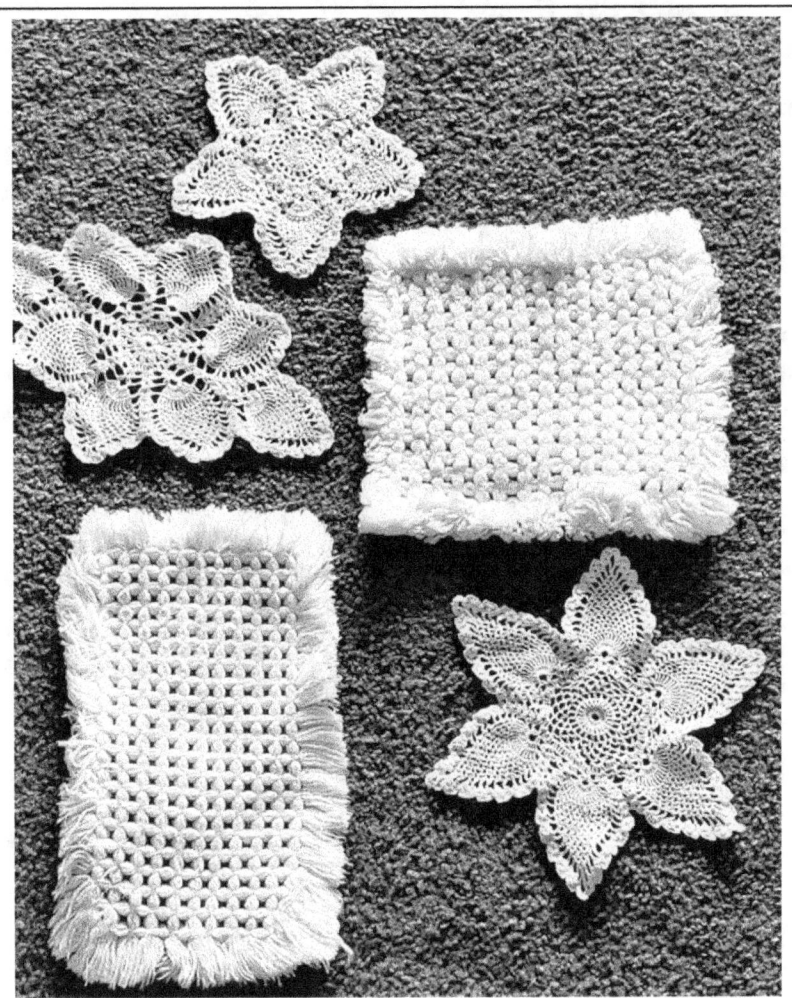
Nurses and patients gave these pieces of handwork to my mother in the 1930s. She treasured these gifts for more than 60 years, and I still have them nearly 90 years after they were created for my mother.
Ella Hedglin collection

Chapter 37
Passing the Long Hours

Some patients felt there was nothing to do at the San, but Art tried to do more than he should. He was always busy.

He found that reading was a great way to pass the time without being physically active, and he was interested in many subjects. Dr. Mary was an avid reader, too, and she wanted everyone to have the opportunity to read books. While she lived in the Falls, and because there was no library, Dr. Mary had opened her home for local people to check out books from her collection. She couldn't bring her extensive assortment of books into the San for fear of contamination, so all the facility had was a small library. Art was happy to read whatever books Dr. Mary provided for the patients. Those who were bedridden had to select from the few that employees brought to the rooms.

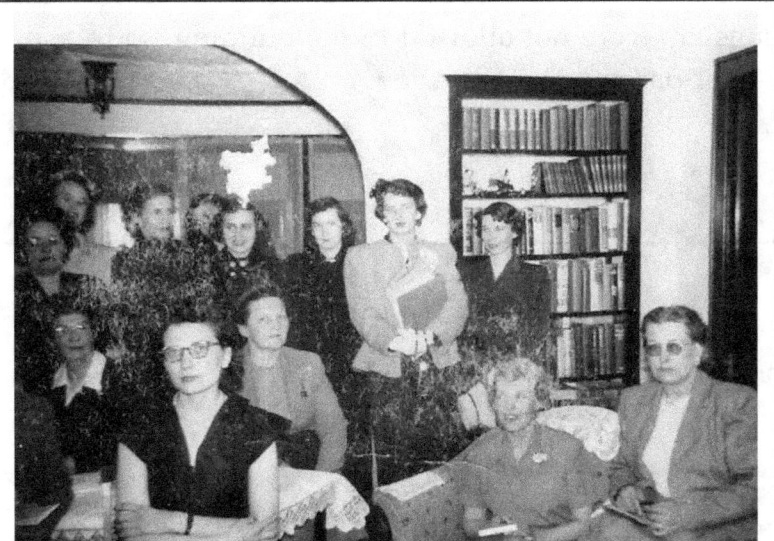

Dr. Mary shared her love of books with many, but she couldn't share her personal collection with patients. One of her bookshelves is in the background.
James Ghostley collection

Art considered using his windowsill for storage of his many hobby supplies, but he needed it for other things. During the time Art was restricted to bed, he took advantage of his location next to the window. He couldn't go outside to feel rain or snow, to touch the plants or to smell the flowers. Art hadn't touched the green grass or dug in the dirt for months, maybe years at that point. With some help, he obtained containers, soil, grass seeds, and flower seeds. There, on his windowsill, a space 48 inches wide and 10 inches deep, he grew grass and flowers.

He loved to touch the grass growing on that small ledge, and he enjoyed its fresh smell. His flowers added a bright touch not just to his space but also for those around him.

"They're cutting the lawn out front now, and the odor wafts in," Art wrote to his family. *"It is so good to run my hands through the grass and to smell it. It represents life and renewal, and it gives me hope."*

He enjoyed watching visitors and their little children playing on the lawn. *"Those chubby little tykes are so much fun as they laboriously go about doing whatever catches their interest."* Youngsters were not allowed in the building, so they often played on the lawn while their parents visited patients.

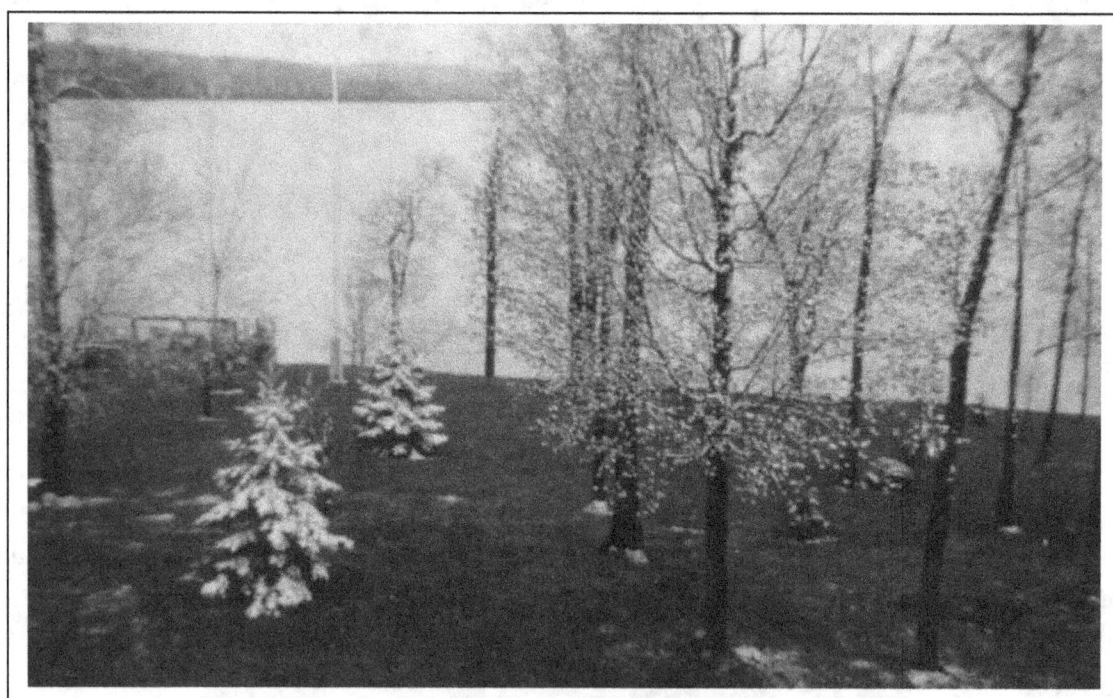

From his window, Art watched the seasons change.
Art Holmstrom photo

଼৪ଓ

Felix Diaz was Art's roommate, and his bed was in the back corner of the room. He was born in Texas to migrant workers. Felix first went to Ah-gwah-ching Sanatorium, but Dr. Mary had an agreement with the head doctor there that if

Lake Julia had patients who required surgery, she could trade them to Ah-gwah-ching for patients who did not need surgery. That's how Felix ended up at Lake Julia. There were many children in Felix's family—six or eight—so hospitalizing him helped to protect the rest of his family.

He had never gone to school or learned to write.

The kitchen help, even the head cook, lived in the nurses' home; all the female help lived in that building. Some of the women walked the sidewalk by Art's room to get to work, and this gave patients in Art's ward an opportunity to see who was there. Soon, Art, Felix, and the rest of the men began teasing with the young employees below.

"Felix is such a flirt, and he is rather good looking," Art wrote to his brother, Joe, *"so when the girls went by from the nurses' home below our second-story windows, it was hard to keep him on task. But I eventually taught him to write. I tutored him every day.*

"Also, there were three teenage girls amongst the women in the porch area, so when the door was open and you could see in, Felix had a very good view right down the line. There was one friendly girl from somewhere down by Laporte, and she was kind and smiled at Felix, so he wanted to communicate. The only way he could do that was by writing a note, so he learned English and learned to spell, then wrote to her. That led him to write letters to other people to show his parents he already knew how to write in English."

There was also a nurse named Miss Annette Miller, who acted as a schoolteacher to Felix or anybody else who wanted to learn.

Felix was a willing student. He trusted Art's advice, and Art became his confidant.

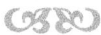

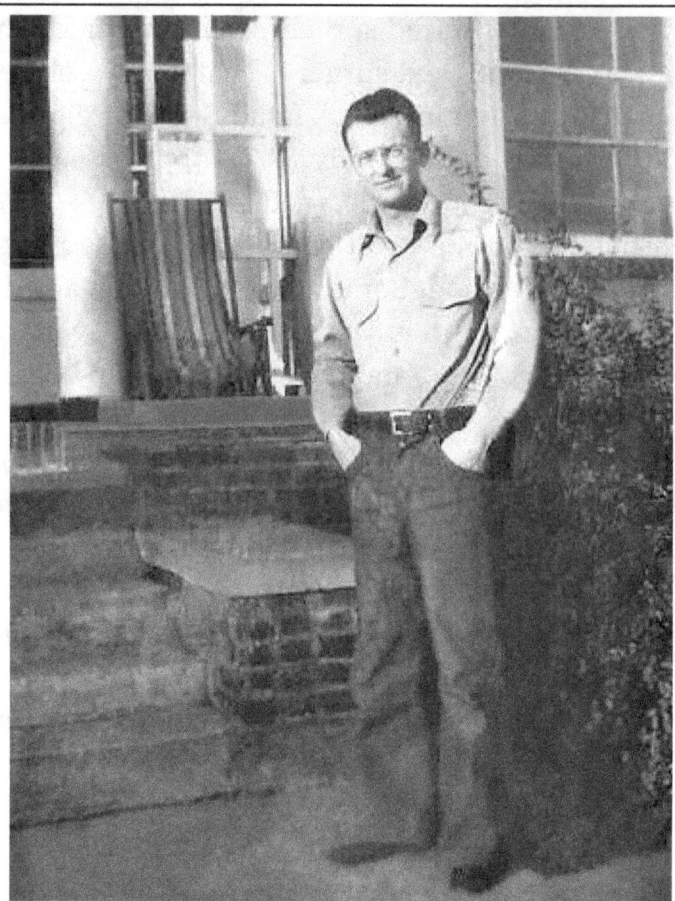

Bill Masterson
Photo courtesy of
Rebecca Tsuji and Jon Langhout Jr., Bemidji, MN

The janitor, Bill Masterson, gave haircuts. Usually, he came on specific days, and he cut hair in the locker room near the bathrooms. One day, Art convinced Felix that he could cut his hair. Art followed Felix's style and was neat, even though he didn't have the best equipment, and he thought he was doing a good job. He had shaped Felix's hair nicely on the sides. Then, Oscar Berg and another fellow berated how Felix looked. They offered lots of disparaging comments, which rattled Felix's confidence. Pretty soon, he told Art to stop. He insisted that Masterson complete the haircut, and Art never tried cutting hair again.

Felix's family traveled to where the farming and agricultural jobs were available, so they could not visit often. When his parents did visit, they brought tamales, which Art was happy to try. Felix's parents rarely were able to visit in the early part of the summer because of their work. They visited Felix about three times per year. He was delighted when the tamales arrived, usually around Thanksgiving or Christmas.

Corn husks wrapped the tamales, and they were spicy, the way Felix liked them. Felix used to carry a little bottle of homemade hot sauce to add some extra heat. For Art, who had eaten bland Swedish food all his life, the tamales seemed extremely hot even without the added condiment.

Felix offered tamales to each of the other three men in the room. All waved their hands in front of their mouths and broke into a sweat and turned red in the face.

Sometimes Art enjoyed just sitting by the lake watching the fishermen or, once, a speedboat that went by. It was exciting for Art to imagine the freedom of skimming along in a boat.

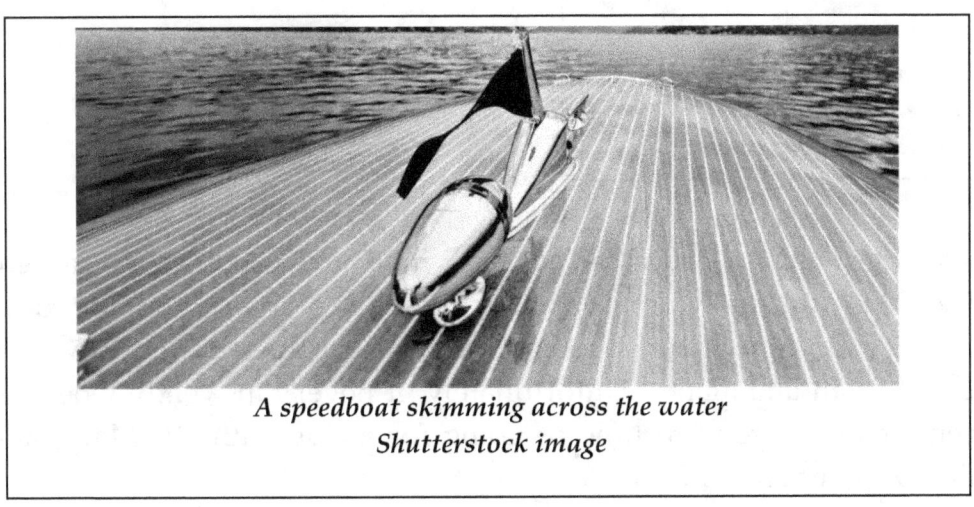

A speedboat skimming across the water
Shutterstock image

Once in winter, he walked out to the lakeshore and watched an airplane land on the ice, something he had never seen. The ice made a good landing strip. The plane he saw carried a visiting doctor from Florida, Dr. Anderson, who had arrived to cover for Dr. Mary while she took a much-needed vacation.

Art had loved seeing that plane and imagining flying off somewhere.

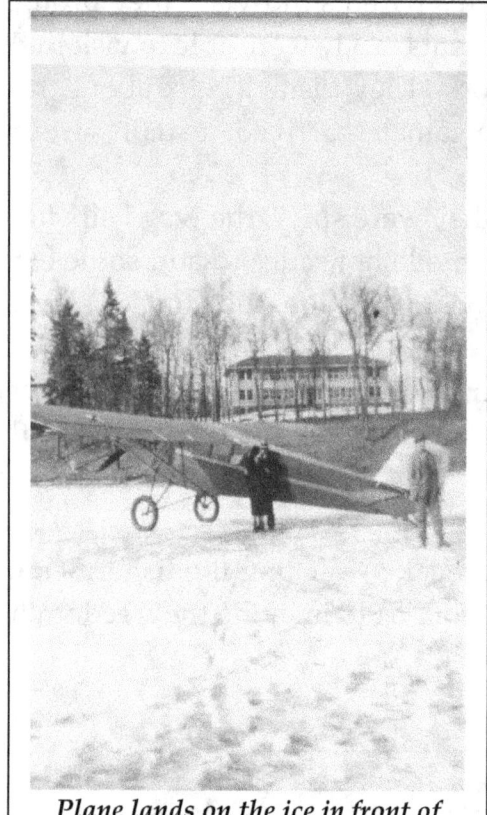

Plane lands on the ice in front of Lake Julia San around 1932 James Ghostley collection

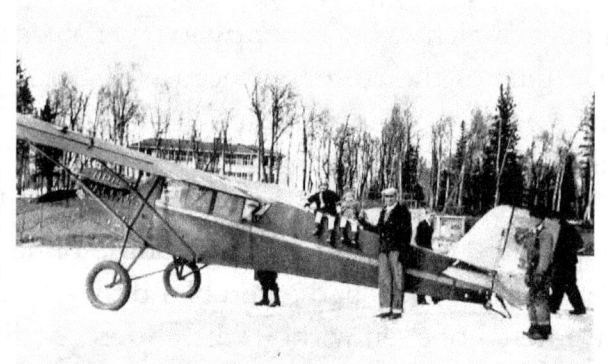

Jim Ghostley is one of the children on the wing of this plane that landed on the ice at Lake Julia in front of the San. James Ghostley collection

Dr. Mary always had a car of her own. The San bought her a vehicle in February 1939.[113] It usually provided an automobile of inferior quality to save the county money. Dr. Mary once bought a Nash because the seats laid down, and she could use it as an ambulance. Unfortunately, it never ran well.[114] One time, five up-patients had the good fortune of going for a ride with Dr. Mary, and they couldn't talk about anything else.

Whether traveling by foot, sled, sleigh, or automobile, Dr. Mary often had to deal with a lack of roads, isolation, swamps, mosquitos, snow, ice, and breakdowns.

---

[113] *International Falls Press,* International Falls, Minnesota, February 8, 1939
[114] Rodney (Bob) Maher interview

At times when Art wasn't well enough to go out, he still enjoyed hearing about the outings of others. Whatever kind of vehicle people were in, he fantasized that he was riding in one of them.

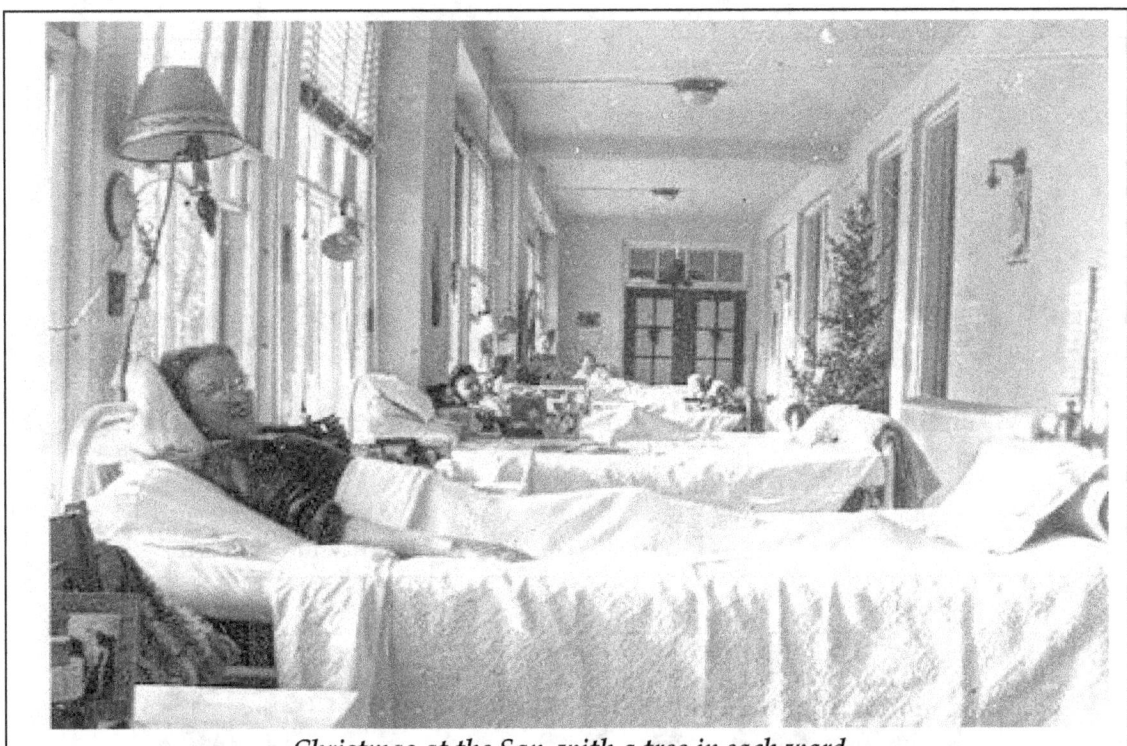

Christmas at the San, with a tree in each ward
Gladys Erickson, Lois Olson, Irene Taylor, and Norma Norberg
Photo by Art Holmstrom

At Christmas, there was always a large, decorated Christmas tree on the first floor for the patients who could go down to meals. For those who couldn't leave their beds, there was a decorated tree in every ward. Patients exchanged gifts. Nurses placed all presents under the trees, and patients opened them in a big celebration on Christmas Eve or Christmas Day.

The patients celebrated whenever they could, whether or not they were allowed to be out of bed. They held birthday parties, and they either made gifts to exchange or bought small gifts—or even a cake—if they had the money. Those who could be up gathered around patients' beds and created a party. Sometimes they also popped corn in the ward, which made the event seem especially festive.

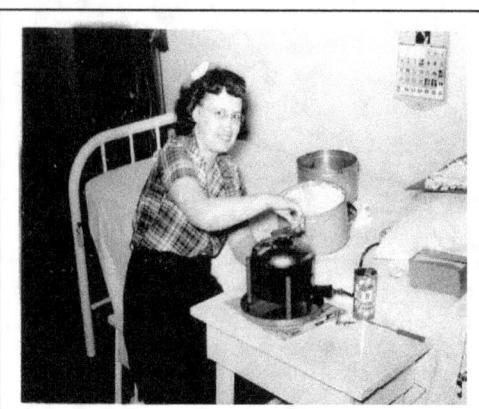

Patient pops corn for a celebration
Art Holmstrom photo

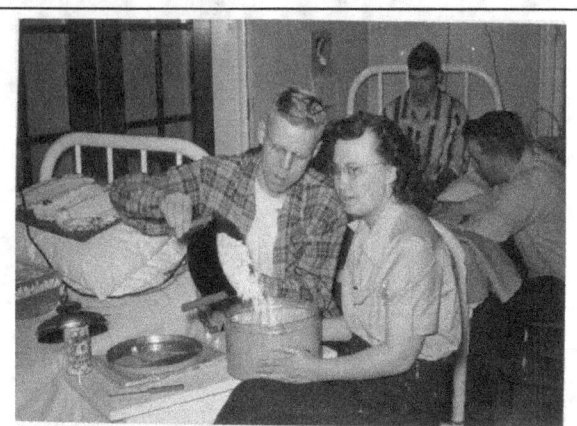

Art and a patient pop corn
Art Holmstrom collection

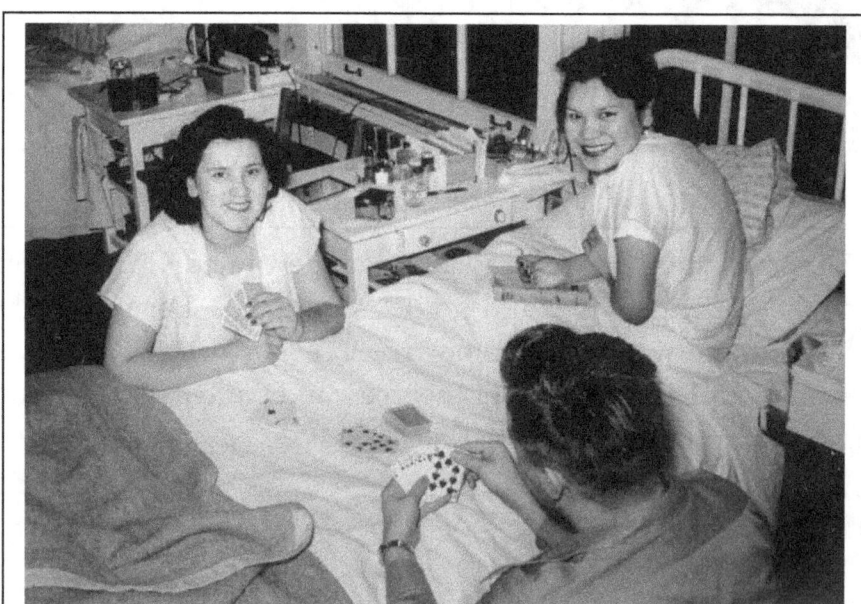

Patients play cards
Art Holmstrom photo

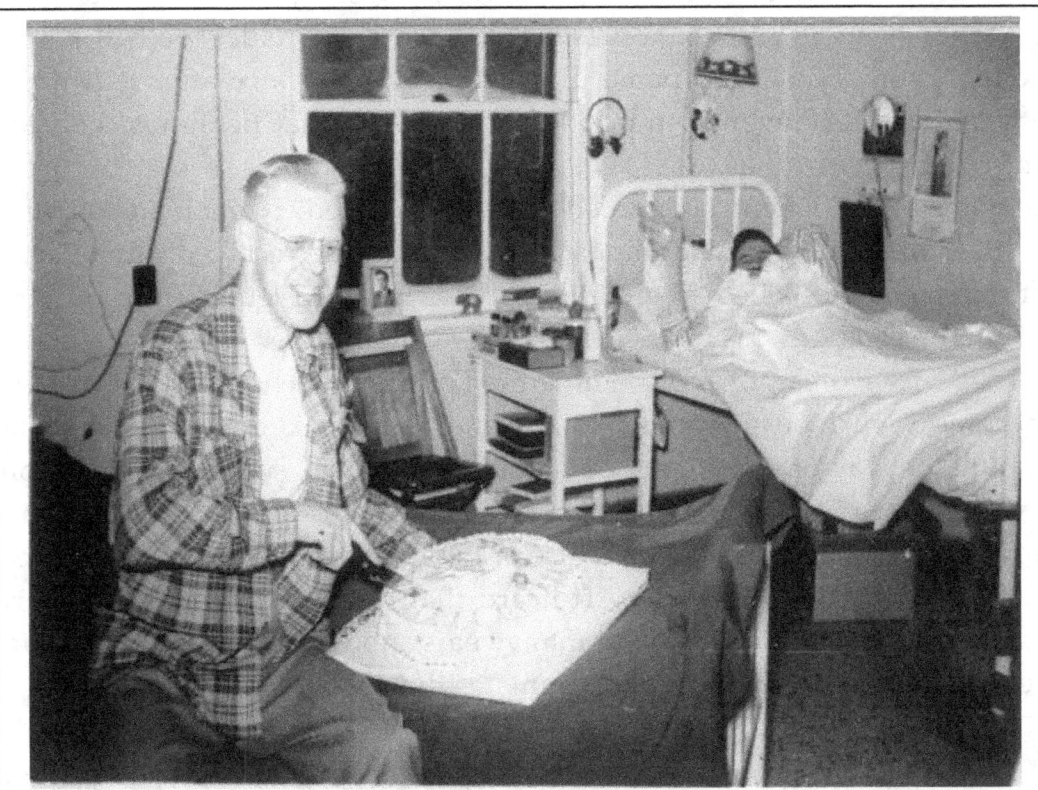

Art Holmstrom celebrates his birthday. Felix Diaz joins the fun from his bed.
Art Holmstrom collection

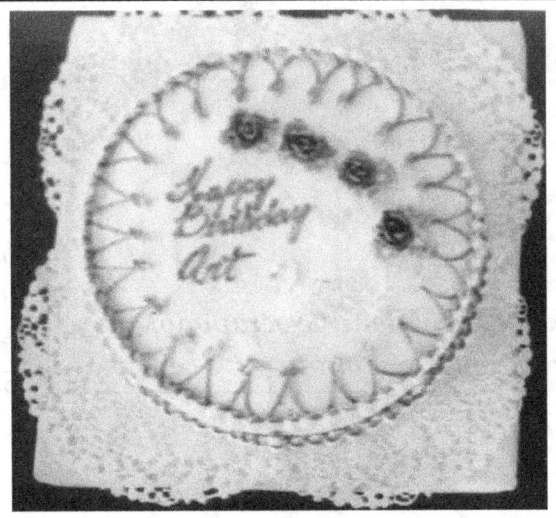

Art's birthday cake

Many gifts given by Art were prizes he had won by entering contests on the radio. Art enjoyed all sorts of contests. Some were to predict football scores for Bemidji, and others were to name different products. Once after listening to a Duluth broadcast, he won so much—close to $500—that he almost had to pay income tax on his earnings.

Some of the patients wondered why Art received so much mail when they received so little. He got mail almost daily because he received advertisements relating to the contests he had entered. He also received letters from classmates, friends in the Falls, and his folks.

Art once won a prize for naming the Forestland School in the Falls, which had become a courthouse. Another prize came from Quaker Oats. They wanted to have a unique way of tempting a person to eat oatmeal, so Art told them one of his favorites was to top it with Lingonberry sauce. He'd eaten it at home. That was a unique enough idea that he won a case of Lingonberry preserves from Sweden.

That was around the time Art heard that his Uncle George had married. George had lived with the family for many years and would always be Art's father figure. Art couldn't wait to tell his roommates that he had a new aunt.

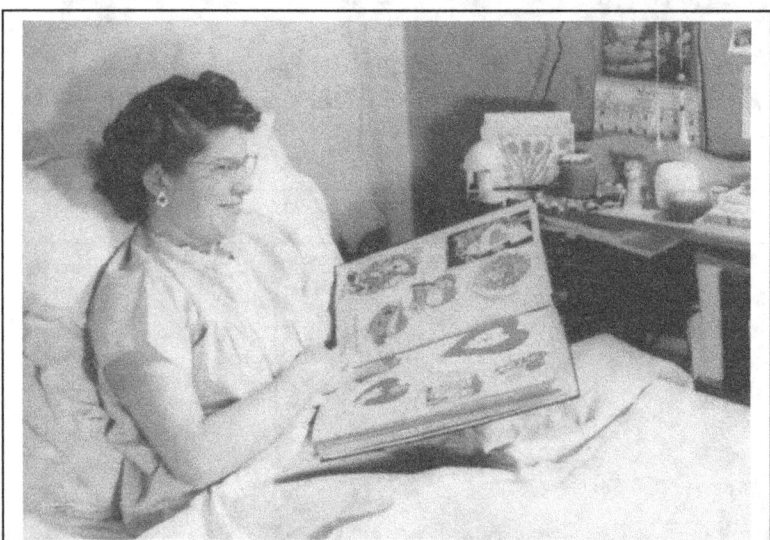

Patient looks at her Valentine scrapbook
Art Holmstrom photo

The patients always had something to talk about or to celebrate when it wasn't quiet time, and they laughed a lot, too. The circumstances that had brought them together were not good, but most of the patients made the best of being confined, and they created new families made up of San friends.

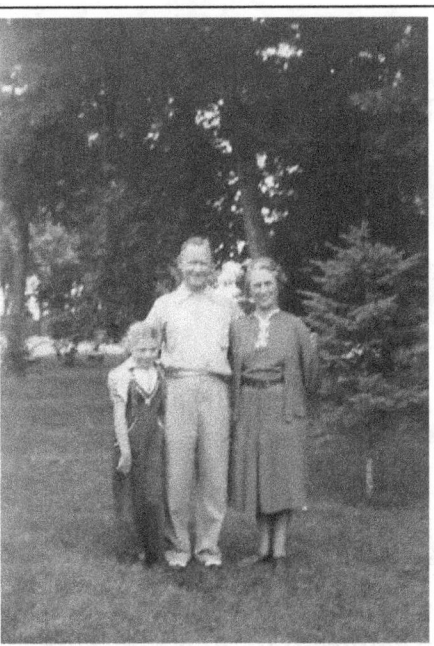

*Cathie Ghostley, Dr. Anderson,
and Dr Mary
James Ghostley collection*

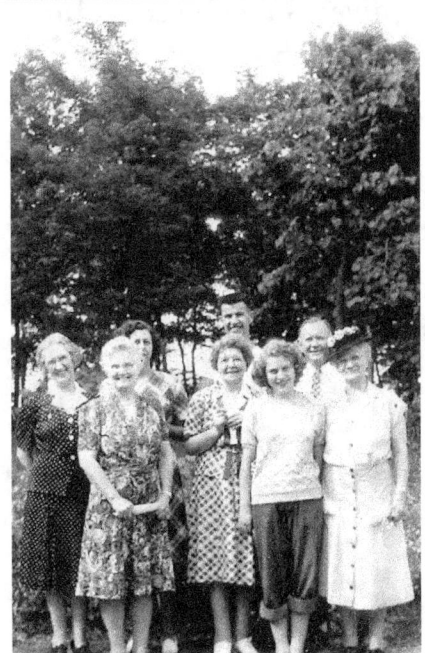

*Dr. Mary, Peggy Cross, Lucy Barrett, Cathie Ghostley, and Anna Brown
Back row: Mrs. Anderson, Jim Ghostley, and Dr. Anderson
James Ghostley collection*

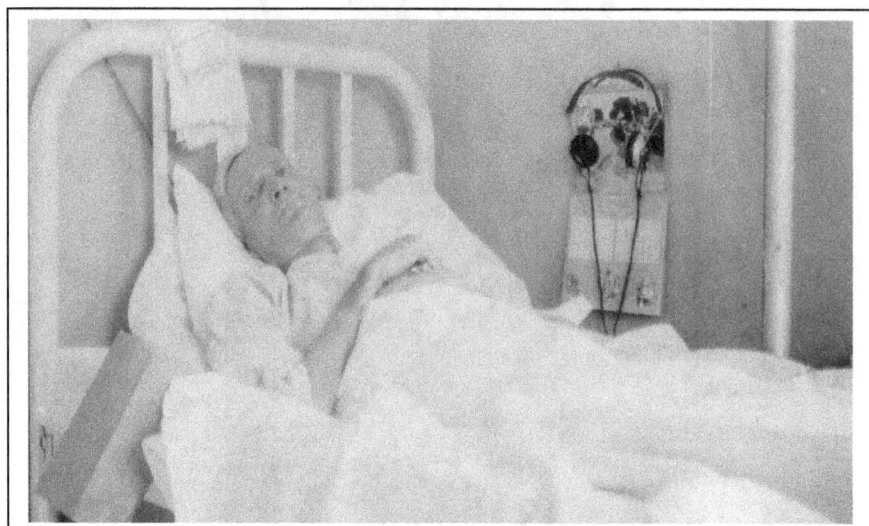

Earphones like those hanging with Anton Strande's calendar were near each patient's bed.
James Ghostley collection

Chapter 38
Big Changes

The war made big news over the earphones in August 1945 when the atom bomb was dropped on Hiroshima and Nagasaki, Japan, ending the war in the Pacific Theater.[115]

By Christmas 1945, things weren't going well for Art, and that was the beginning of a plateau that lasted through 1946 and 1947. Art continued to receive pneumothorax during that time, but in 1945, Dr. Mary gave Art the news that she planned to make a change in his treatment. "It's sort of a waste of time using Novocain to deaden the area before putting the needle in," she explained. "I have a better way. We'll spread the ribs so that I'll know where the space is, and I'll just drive the needle through rapidly. It won't hurt."

That first time, Art squeezed his eyes shut and sucked in his breath, but the fear was worse than the pain from the needle. It was quick, as Dr. Mary had promised, and with just a push, the needle was inside. He preferred the new method, and from that day forward, that's how he received his pneumo treatments.

Art's father wrote to Dr. Mary in February 1947 to inquire about his condition, and she replied that he had not been well recently.

"A week or so ago he had a small hemorrhage, and a few days later he had another. It was only a little in all, and he has had none now for three days. So, I hope that it is over. He had been feeling much better before that happened; but we never know what the effect of a bleed will be. The amount was so small, and his cough was not severe, so I hope there will not be any ill consequences."

Gust struggled with being away from his family and having only limited information on his son's condition. He contacted Dr. Withrow, who had been the family's doctor before his retirement, to inquire about moving Art to another facility, and Dr. Withrow contacted Dr. Mary. She replied to the doctor on March 2, 1947:

"I think Mr. Holmstrom has wanted to move Arthur for some time. And I realize, as you say, that Mr. Holmstrom wishes to do what is best for the boy. He is a fine young

---

[115] http:/www.lakesnwoods.com/BlackduckHistory2.htm

man and, of course, the most promising member of the family. I certainly feel that if there were anything which would hasten his recovery, I would want to do it at once.

"When he came in, he had a cavity in the left lung. I collapsed this lung with excellent results. He became negative, gained weight, and was apparently getting complete control of his disease. I kept him quiet longer than usual as he is a high-strung, nervous boy with a mind far too active for his own good, and I know he would be too active physically as soon as he was let to be about at all. Well, he was promoted gradually until he was walking about outside a little every day. I couldn't, naturally, go with him each time; and he did more than he was supposed to do. Whether that was what caused it or whether his resistance fell off, I do not know; but he got a spread to the good lung. I put him back to bed and have been keeping him as quiet as possible since that time. He remained negative sputum and was symptom-free except for a little temperature at times and an elevated Sed. Rate. It was not high; but high enough to indicate activity somewhere.

"About a month ago, he had a little hemorrhage, and although he was still negative, I was much worried. I wrote his father about it. I had been trying to get the left lung to re-expand a little so that I would dare to partly collapse the right, and when he hemorrhaged, I put in a little air. He has been better, and the cough stopped. But a few days ago, he lost another ounce of blood. The amount is nothing, it is only the fact that the process is active enough to cause it at all that worries me. But he is better again, and I hope this will prove the turning point.

"As for a change of climate, we do not feel there is anything to be gained by it, and in Arthur's case, he would be so excited by new surroundings that it would probably actually do him harm. If Mr. Holmstrom wishes to move him to another sanatorium in Minnesota, that might help. I am expecting some streptomycin any day and think I will try that. It is only in the experimental stage; but has given some good results and might help in this case."

○ঙ৪○

One July morning in 1947, it was again time for pneumothorax, as it had been several times a week since Art's third day at the San.

Dr. Mary and Art had a pleasant conversation. "You always seem to be here day and night. How do you do it?" he asked. Art had noticed how utterly forgetful of self Dr. Mary often was, working until she was ready to drop, then after a brief rest, being up and at it again.

"I can put my mind and heart at ease, whatever the situation," Dr. Mary explained. "If I am tending to someone or taking a trip to go see a patient and can't go home because that person needs me, I get comfortable and doze off for five or

10 minutes until I hear some noise. I displace all my current problems and worries and completely relax. Then, I pick up where I left off."

Art felt Dr. Mary spread his ribs and quickly press the needle through the first pleura. He'd had the procedure done so many times that he seldom paid attention any more. He talked to her about contests he had entered and needlework projects he planned to enter in the fair. This pneumothorax was just one more in a long series of routine refills.

After the pneumo treatment, Art returned to his bed and his correspondence, but he had to put his writing aside. His breathing was labored; it felt to him like there was an anvil on his chest. He lay still, waiting for the heaviness to go away.

If he was to let on that he was having trouble breathing, Art was afraid that he might lose his privileges: his right to go downstairs for one meal a day and permission to get up as often as necessary to use the bathroom. What a treat it was to have privileges rather than staying in bed month after month and using those cold enameled containers. He didn't want to give up the privacy of the bathroom, and he'd even been thinking lately that if he kept progressing, he would soon be home. There was a lot at stake.

As Art thought about the possibility of losing his privileges, his bed felt small, cage-like, and he felt trapped. He dozed for a while. When he awoke, he brushed his hand across his pajama shirt but found nothing to explain the feeling that someone was sitting on his chest, squeezing the air out of him. He slowly sat up and swung his legs over the side of the bed, hoping the heavy weight would drop to the floor and allow him to breathe more easily.

Art forced himself to pull his table over, and he attempted to eat his supper. He tried not to alarm his roommates, who, however well-intentioned, might have jeopardized his privileges by calling for help. Art felt sweat on his brow, and he blotted his face with his napkin.

The food didn't look appetizing, but he knew he had to eat to keep up his strength. He scooped some creamy mashed potatoes onto his fork, first running them through the puddle of butter in their center. As he caught sight of his fingernails, he dropped the fork, alarmed to see that his nails had turned gray-blue. He pushed his meal away and reached into his table for the rectangular mirror he had brought from home three years earlier. He recoiled from his reflection when he saw that his lips matched his darkening fingernails. He looked like a young man who had spent the day in a berry patch.

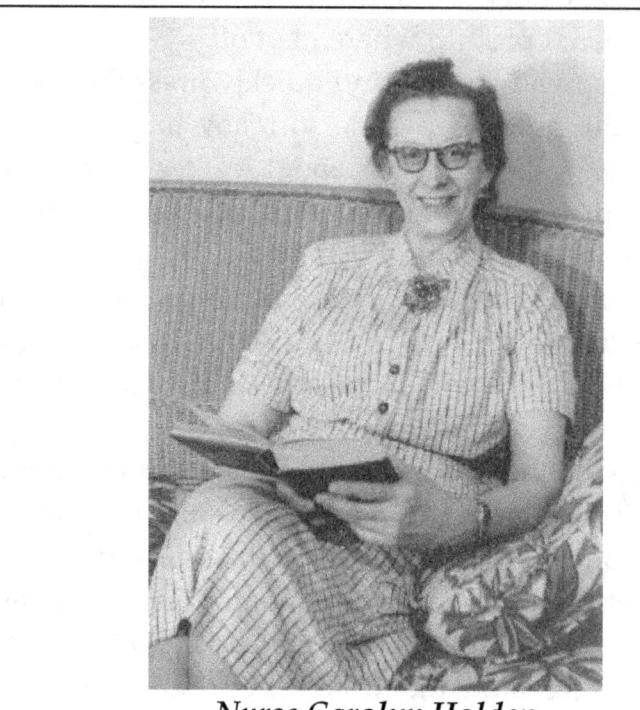
Nurse Carolyn Holden
Art Holmstrom collection

Nurse Holden had gone downstairs to supper, and when she returned, she noticed Art's face and hurried over.

"Something's—wrong," Art told her between labored breaths. "I—think—you—should—get Dr. Mary."

Palms down, Art held out his blue-tinged hands for her to see. Nurse Holden instantly knew that he was in trouble. She turned and dashed out the door and down the stairs to summon Dr. Mary from her log cottage behind the San. Art could hear her quick steps descend the stairs, but he feared he would not survive until she returned.

Even though Art had been in the San since 1944, more than three years already, and had reached the adult age of 21, he suddenly felt afraid and helpless. "I am too young to die. Please, God, let that evil tuberculosis spare me," he prayed repeatedly. "If you don't do it for me, do it for Ma. She's been through too much heartache already."

Dr. Mary took the 170 steps on a run from her cottage to the San. She ran right through her flower garden, toppling hollyhocks in her haste; there was no time to spare. The doctor entered the side door and headed quickly up the stairs. She raced up six steps, past the kitchen at the right, and kept going.

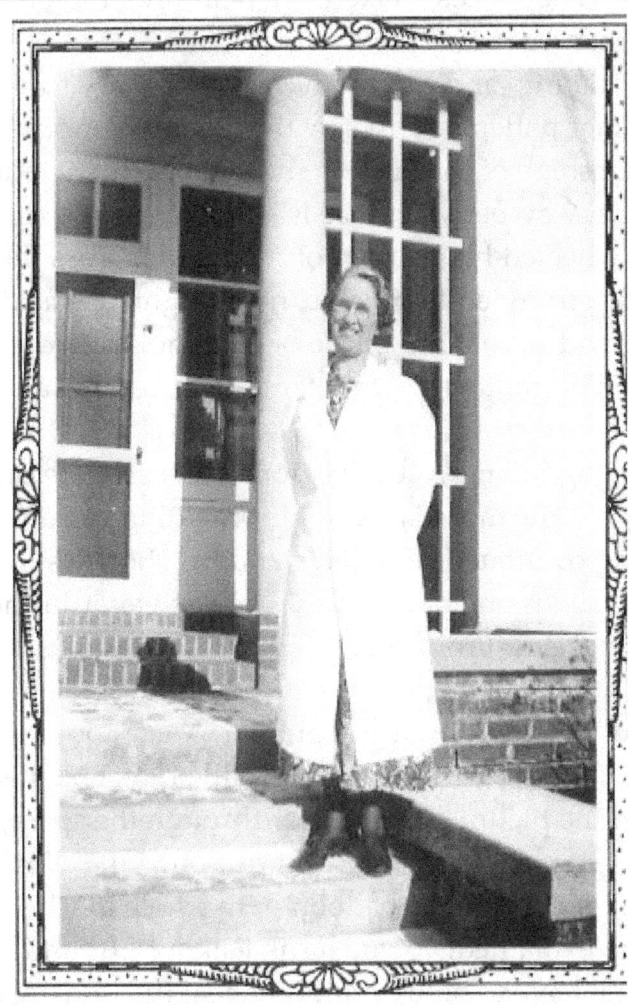

Dr. Mary Ghostley
James Ghostley Collection

Art faintly heard footsteps before Dr. Mary hurried into the room. She hadn't even taken time to put on the long, white doctor's coat that she usually wore. Nurse Holden was a few paces behind, breathing heavily. When the doctor looked at Art, she instantly knew what was wrong. Her typically calm face displayed determination.

She quickly inserted a needle into his chest and sucked out some air, correcting the problem for an hour or so.

Art's lips and fingernails were the first to lighten, then brighten, returning to a healthy pink color. Patients in the nearby beds cast worried glances at him; they sent frantic hand signals to the girls on the sun porch and mouthed messages about Art's condition. Their faces relaxed when his breathing improved but tensed again when his shortness of breath returned.

"Let's move you into another room, Art," Dr. Mary said, "so we won't be a disturbance to the other patients." Art saw the looks of concern on his roommates' faces. He noticed that some of the girls on the sun porch, including his Annie, had crowded into the doorway between wards. As Art gasped for air, Dr. Mary and two nurses quickly wheeled his bed out of the ward, across the hall, and into the isolation room. As he struggled to breathe, he thought, *this is it!*

The clanging and squeaking of the bed sounded louder to Art than it had ever before. It had an ominous tone to it, and his gasps for air added to the eerie symphony.

Once in the dying room, Art tried to force himself to be calm so that it would be easier to breathe, but the more labored his breathing became, the more anxious he felt. His right lung continued to deflate, and his shortness of breath increased. Dr. Mary held out a pill in one hand and a glass of water in the other. "This will make you feel better," she promised, "and after you take it, I'll explain what happened today."

Art struggled to wash down the pill. Dr. Mary took his hands in both of hers and continued. "When I gave you your refill today, I pushed the needle in too far, and it punctured the pleura; it went clear through the space, and then through the next layer of the pleural sac that surrounds your lung. I'm terribly sorry, Art. Your right lung deflated, just like a balloon with a hole in it. That's why you're so short of breath," she explained. "Your air is leaking out and being absorbed by your body. Now we'll have to help your body heal the puncture wound."

She sounded confident and matter-of-fact, but as Art struggled for breath, he still thought, *this is it.*

He wanted to claw away at the invisible beast that strangled the breath out of him, the life out of him. There was urgency everywhere as nurses scurried to keep him going. Everything was a swirl of white as the sedative took effect. He slept, which allowed him to breathe more easily.

Despite the San's design to provide good airflow, not a whisper of breeze came off the lake. A mosquito found its way through the window screens and pushed its way through the still air to buzz a warning into Art's ear.

The medication that had helped him sleep left him feeling drained when he awoke. He wasn't sure if it was the muggy July day or fever that drenched his body. He ran a hand through his hair; it had twisted into damp coils.

He worried and prayed. He thought of his mother. He thought of Uncle George and all he had done for him. He thought of his father, who he barely knew because of his long absences. He remembered other patients who had gone to the dying room—patients who had disappeared in the night.

It was nearly dark, and by looking through the dying room's window opening, then across the hallway and on through the windows of his usual ward, he could see black clouds churning violently. The stillness was gone, and angry clouds pushed a gust of wind through the three sets of open windows, then past Art, through more windows, and out the back of the San. It was a relief to feel the movement of air.

As he watched the clouds, he thought about his young life and wondered why he had to die so soon. Why, he questioned, had his parents had to bear the burden of serious medical problems with each of their four children? Baby Ruthie had lived only a year and a half. Both his brother, Joe, and his sister Elsie were sometimes thought of as freaks because of their grand-mal epilepsy. Elsie had contracted tuberculosis, too, and had needed to have a lung removed. It was impossible to go back to sleep once he started thinking such troubling thoughts.

Art stared out into the darkness. A long, rumbling series of booms and cracks followed a brilliant flash. Then, a bright, jagged streak split his small view of the sky into two uneven sections as it stabbed at the clouds. More lightning followed, illuminating the wards and causing the women to scream in fright.

Art wasn't afraid of thunder and lightning—never had been. Storms fascinated him. He directed all of his attention to the changing kaleidoscope—brief and eerie scenes that lit up the walls and ceilings followed by shrieks of terror that cut through the night and were carried away by the swift-moving dark clouds—just as the storm would soon carry him away.

Unafraid, he was mesmerized as he watched. Like the day he'd heard about when his brother, Joseph, was born, this was one terrific storm.

Chapter 39
Continuing the Cure

When Art began to recover, he wrote to his mother. *"In spite of my vow not to see the dying room again, I was the one being wheeled out of the ward. I wasn't taken far, just to the isolation room, the same one I had shuffled by and peeked into back when I got my first privilege.*

"When I first arrived at the San, you will recall that Eli was in the bed over by the window. He was the young man with progressive diabetes and tuberculosis who lasted only a few months after I got there. We all felt so nervous when Eli was wheeled out to the isolation room. I knew my roommates and the girls on the south sun porch felt the same way when I was the one being wheeled out.

"Whenever anyone is taken to the dying room, it reminds all of us that death is right on our heels.

"I'd felt tremendous guilt when I'd been excited about moving to Eli's spot by the window, where I would have earphones; it was his death that allowed me to take over his spot. I wondered who would be excited to take my corner if I didn't return from the dying room.

"But I am still here, even though I am in isolation, and I will do everything I can to recover again, so don't worry."

On Sept. 16, 1947, Dr. Mary wrote to Art's father:

"I believe there is a great improvement in Arthur's condition. He has had negative sputum now for some time, well over a year. His stomach and digestion are the best they have ever been since he came here, and he seems to have settled down to taking the cure very well.

"If we can only keep him from getting too many interests and engaging in too many activities, I am sure he will get well. But you know how ambitious he is to be doing something. And he always wanted to do too many things until the last year. He seems contented and happy all the time. His mother, uncle, and brother were here for the afternoon Saturday, and he enjoyed that. They showed him some of the movies he had taken and some new ones of the north.

"The right lung, the second to become diseased, is much better on X-ray, and the left is slowly re-expanding. Of course it is slow, tuberculosis always is, but I believe it will be sure this time."

In January 1948, Art was surprised to see Dr. Mary's arm in a sling. She had slipped on a piece of soap and had fallen, breaking two bones.[116] He asked if she was going to take some time off. "No," she said. "Until there is a cure for tuberculosis, I refuse to let a broken arm slow me down."

⊗

When Art was finally well enough to return to his ward, he was still extremely ill. He had no privileges, and he remained on bed rest. Art was no closer to being well than the day he had arrived. And he didn't get to stay in his ward for long.

In March 1948, Dr. Mary stated, "Art, I'm going to transfer you back to an isolation room so you can get more rest."

He didn't realize his condition was grave, even though he was headed back to the dying room. Sometimes, patients went to the isolation rooms for extra care, not just to die. Art hoped that was the case with him even though the room he was being wheeled into was the one most often used just before a patient expired.

He felt weak and afraid as he coughed up frothy blood and saliva. Dr. Mary encased his chest with rubber bags of ice to encourage coagulation. He didn't expect the worst until the hemorrhages had occurred 10 times. Art again began thinking about how the janitor and orderlies would take a patient out of his ward before he would expire, closing all the ward doors and pulling shades so that the person seemed just to vanish. He had asked Dr. Mary about this practice, and she had replied that she wanted to cause the other patients as little anxiety as possible. Dr. Mary always spoke on the positive side, but it didn't stop the patients from being curious. He watched to be sure no one drew the shades on the isolation-room windows.

One day, the daytime nurse told Art that the doctor had been in the isolation room every half-hour during the night to check on him. Art had tested positive for active TB before the hemorrhaging began, and it was not known what stimulus had caused it.

Back in the ward, the other men wondered how Art was doing. Finally, they got word that things had turned around for the better. The last hemorrhage occurred on March 28, and after that date, all his tests were negative. After two more days in isolation, Art returned to his ward. At last, it appeared that he had finally reached a turning point in his recovery.

---

[116] *International Falls Press,* International Falls, Minnesota, January 6, 1948

Some patients were promoted faster than others as they improved or as their TB was arrested, but because Art didn't seem to have as much resistance as some, Dr. Mary took his case more slowly to prevent another breakdown. She was conservative in adding exercise. He got his first privilege on May 26, 1948, allowing him to make one trip a day to the locker room under his own power. He took his privilege in the morning while the nurses made the beds. On June 19, he got his second privilege, which he took in the evening.

He looked forward to working up to full bathroom privileges so that he would be allowed to take a bath, get up as much as he wanted, and eat his meals downstairs again, followed by outdoor exercise.

In August 1948, Dr. Mary shared her excitement with Art and the other patients when her daughter, Mary Catherine (Cathie), married Robert Donn Fuller of Baudette.[117] As a longtime patient at the San, Art enjoyed hearing about outside events and felt that he'd heard so much about Dr. Mary's family that this was like hearing news of one of his own family members.

When Art's health had improved significantly, he and Annie went outside together and had photos taken. They took short strolls on the San grounds, and

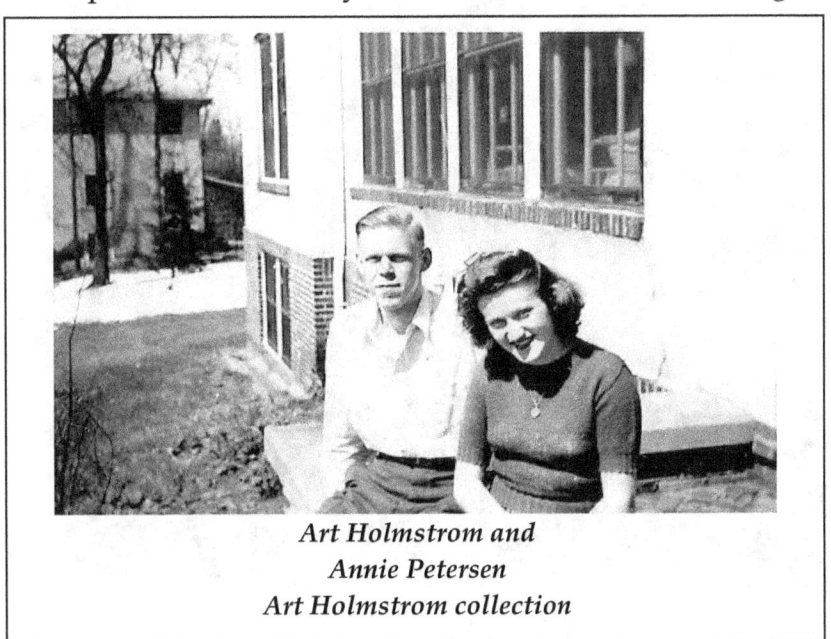

Art Holmstrom and
Annie Petersen
Art Holmstrom collection

---

[117] *International Falls Press*, International Falls, Minnesota, August 16, 1948

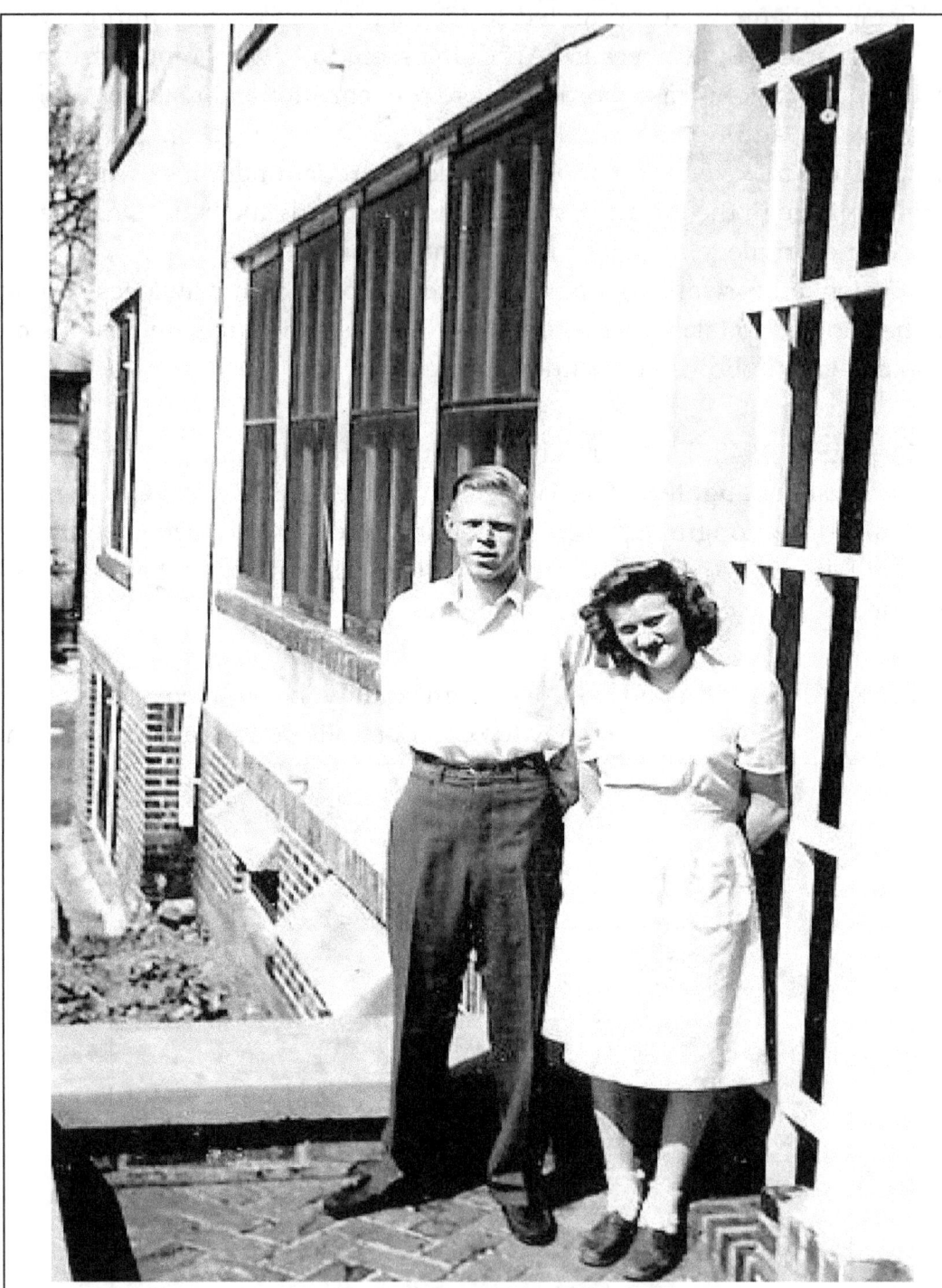

*Art Holmstrom and Annie Petersen
visit outdoors.
Art Holmstrom collection*

they discussed all sorts of things, including food. "How do you like the meals here?" Art asked. "I'm a bit of a picky eater myself."

"Oh, I like the food fine," Annie declared. "But the milk is kind of strong tasting when the cows eat the green grass. Other than that, I think the food is good. I know some patients are fussy. Dr. Mary told one of them, 'If you'd eat like Anneliese does, you'd gain some weight and get well.' But despite eating well, I'm not cured!"

Neither of them had gone home for a visit, and both dreamed of that day. Then, in 1948, Annie announced that Dr. Mary was releasing her. It was a bittersweet moment for Art because he had to stay. *How can I not be happy for her,* he wondered. *Will I ever see Annie again?*

Annie's brother, Karl, had left the San two years earlier to go to Duluth for surgery because he was not improving. He eventually got well and then worked at the Gamble store before opening a repair shop.

With Annie gone, Art put even more effort into staying busy. He still enjoyed going for walks and exploring the grounds and the building when he was well enough, but life at the San was not the same.

Not long after Annie's release, she wrote to say that she got a job with the government agriculture department, starting at 40 cents an hour. Her sister worked there and was leaving to get married, so Annie took a temporary position. Then, the department hired her full time when her sister left. She worked there with farmers for 35 years. Even after she started work, she continued to have pneumo treatments for a while.

Annie did not marry until 1970 when she was 43. She and her husband lived on a Century Farm in Bemidji, where her husband's father had homesteaded.

෬෩

Late in 1948, nearly five years after Art's arrival at the San, Dr. Mary stopped putting air into his left lung, hoping it would expand to full size by itself. She continued pneumothorax on the right side until about 1950.

"*After being put back to bed, we are back on my one-privilege deal,* Art wrote to Annie. *I am aiming to be discharged within the next year.*"

Art had to stay in bed, but that didn't mean his mind couldn't be busy. He got the *Daily Journal* from the Falls, and he read other newspapers that he bummed from patients and staff. He also crocheted.

In August 1949, Art donated a hand-crocheted doily to a Falls fundraising event, the White Elephant Sale. The doily was 24 inches in diameter and contained an intricate pattern, which represented hundreds of hours of work.[118] Eventually, he ordered return-address labels that read, "Handmade Doilies for Sale," above his name and address.

On Mother's Day 1949, Lissie and Gust visited their son. They had been fishing, and Lissie had caught a 34-pound lake trout.

Gust said the fish pulled so hard that he stood behind his wife, holding her shirttails so that the huge fish would not drag her into the lake. Gust took the fish to the San and presented it to nurse Carolyn Holden. When Art woke from his nap, he snapped a photo of Miss Holden holding his mother's fish. That had been an exciting day for him, both having family visitors and seeing his mother's big catch.

For some time, Art suffered from a toothache. Even though there were 14 dentists in Bemidji, most wouldn't go to the San and risk catching a contagious disease. Only one did, but not often. He generally was busy extracting teeth, not filling them, so he did not help Art with his toothache.

As a distraction from the pain, Art devoted a lot of his time

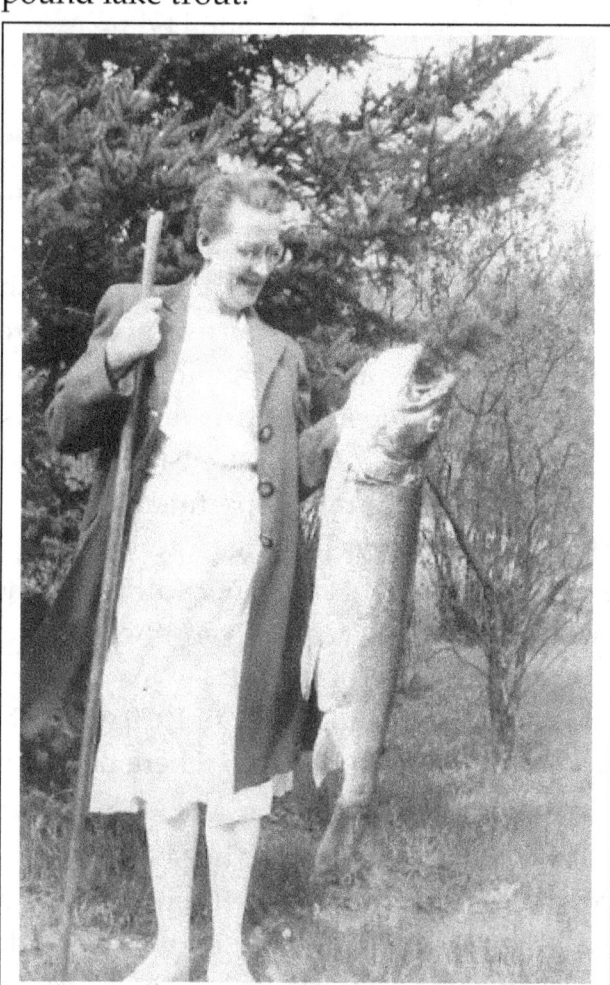

Nurse Carolyn Holden holds 34-lb. lake trout caught by Art's mother. Art Holmstrom photo

---

[118] *International Falls Press,* International Falls, Minnesota, August 19, 1949

to knitting and crocheting and proving to the ladies that he could do it. He used double-ended needles with loops on both ends. He put so much concentration into his work that he didn't pay much attention to the discomfort caused by his tooth.

Art continued to have a difficult time resting. He wanted to be busy all the time, to be useful and to do something of value. Dr. Mary considered that to be his biggest fault.

Art became friends with a janitor, Charles Thoraldson. Charles knew what it was like to be stuck in bed and to have to rest. He had entered the San as a patient on August 14, 1936, at age 17, and had spent 140 days there. Later, the San admitted him twice more.

In 1949, Art figured out how to save his energy when writing letters by duplicating them. He used a hectograph with the help of Charles, who typed the stencils, printed them on a gelatin sheet, then duplicated the news. Art liked the idea of being able to write one letter to many friends to save the time and energy required to write to each one individually. The following is one of those letters:

"August 20, 1949
Here in Bed

"It's been a long time since you've heard from me, hasn't it? My only excuse or reason is the same as ever: Dr. orders me not to overdo, and the effort it would take to write 30 to 40 letters regularly — I love to get letters and hear how those who do not have to 'sit on the bench' are doing, so I hope you will understand my use of this hectograph. Our janitor, a young man around 30 who has been through the mill already (that I'm still trying to get through) has a knack for helping others out, so I got the idea, and he's doing the work for me: typing stencils, or carbon copies I should say, and printing them on the gelatin sheet.

"I plan to duplicate the general news I'd normally have to re-write for each letter and end each letter with my own personal remarks. I know Emily Post is again' it, but maybe I've found an exception to the rule.

"Most of you I've just neglected because of the writing load. I've saved your letters and once in a while read them over. My folks and two others from home have heard from me regularly.

"I spend most of my time on my handwork — the knitting of doilies or woolen goods are almost always as gifts to home or to friends who have had blessed events. I wish I could make lots of things so I could send you all some. I earn most of my pin money from my doilies, and there's a certain amount of satisfaction in that when you're restricted. I've sent doilies to church events and sales and entered them in fairs, as well as sending a doily to

the White Elephant auction sale in the Falls to help finance the Forest Festival. I joy in being useful and doing some good as much as I am able. Dr. says that is one of my faults as I don't take it as easy as I should. This type of letter will make it easier, I think.

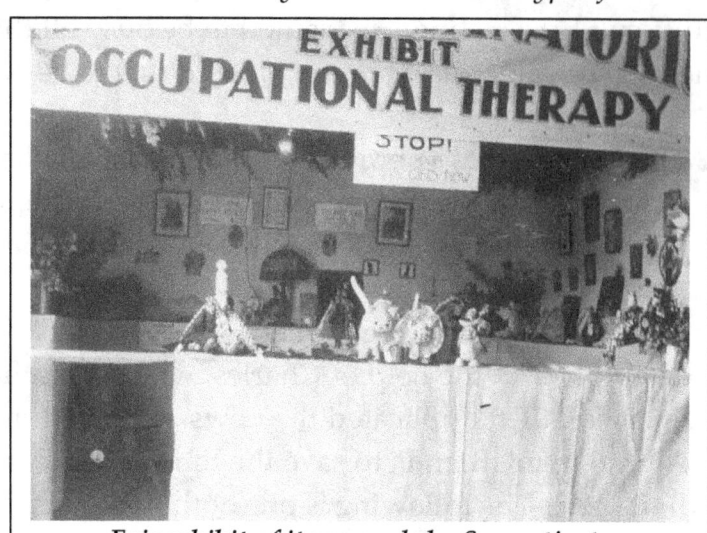

Fair exhibit of items made by San patients
James Ghostley collection

"Fair time is on now. My work is being exhibited and sold now—the 18th to the 21st—in the Itasca County Fair at Grand Rapids. I won two firsts and a second on my work at the Beltrami County Fair in Bemidji earlier this month. Last year it was six firsts and one second for four fairs I entered. This year two of the fairs told me I couldn't enter because, even though the handcrafted items had been sterilized, some of the fair managers were afraid of the spread of TB.[119]

"Several of us here have won prizes at the Bemidji fair. Eight of us got seven firsts and six seconds. We entered Norwegian sweaters, knit sweaters, sox, gloves, mittens, hook rugs, doilies, crocheted centerpieces, and crocheted dresser scarves.

"I had my first taste of embroidery early this week when I was the only one to do the embroidery of the name on a T-shirt to be our floor's birthday gift for a girl patient. Those who usually do it were in her ward, and others were too busy, so I agreed to learn. I drew the letters in script. Even though I feel that it could have been more evenly and roundly embroidered, everyone says it was fine. It was red on white. Now that I find embroidery easy, I'll have to try it more. I like to see work form in my hands or on my needles (knitting needles, that is).

"We had two birthday parties here this week in our clique of 15. We celebrate them together, buy a gift, card, and some sort of refreshment: cookies, cake, ice cream, pop, or something.

---

[119] *Invited and Conquered*, Minnesota Public Health Association, 1949

"There are four in my room now. One, a Catholic divinity student who has been here since Dec. '47, was discharged for good July 27. He returns every 10 days for a pneumothorax refill. He looks good but won't return to the seminary until 1950. We had lots of good times in this room together. He's six months older than I am. We discussed everything, religion included. That helped me a lot. I taught him knitting, and he picked up crocheting and did almost everything I did. He'll be a credit to his religion when he's ordained a priest.

"We have 44 patients here now, 29 on this floor. Eighteen are women. Those in private rooms suffer most from the heat or muggy days due to the poor circulation in their small rooms. I guess I haven't been bothered much by the heat wave as I'm usually busy on something, reading, writing or handwork.

"I understand things are going well with me, that my sputum tests have been negative for a long time and that my X-rays show improvement. I've had a good appetite for nine months now, and it's paid off physically for I've gained to 186 pounds since November. That's 22 pounds—one or 2 pounds every two or four weeks. It shows, too, with the start of a little bay window. I feel good and find my spirits on the happy side most of the time. I was given my first privilege on May 26, 1948 (a privilege is one trip a day to the locker room under your own power). I took mine in the morning when they made our beds. Last June 19, I was promoted to my second one—which I take in the evening. Others are promoted much more rapidly when they are improving or arrested—but Dr. Mary's taking my case slower over the route this time to prevent any breakdown. I guess I haven't as much resistance as others. You work up to full bathroom privileges (take your own bath and get up as much as you want) and then meals downstairs and outdoor exercise.

"You can always hope to be discharged by a certain date, but it doesn't pay to set your heart on it or even think too much about it. The stuff is too changeable—unpredictable. If I don't get out one year, I'll hope for the next. I'll be like a stranger in the world when I get out. I'm one of the old-timers here now. I'm often amused when someone here boasts or complains they've been here 18 months or two years. They haven't even started to get their bed warm. They're the lucky ones, as most here get out in 1 ½ to two years. Several less than that.

"That 186 is my best weight. My most at home was 185 pounds a year and a half before I came here.

"Since I've had trouble in both lungs and the lungs haven't returned to full operation due to pneumothorax treatments, I am often short of breath if I exert myself too much or move too fast. I hope and pray I will recover my effectiveness in the future—that I will be able to use my talents and abilities to fullness in being useful, necessary and productive. In doing good.

"The Bemidji Business and Professional Woman's Club sponsors transportation of entertainment groups to come out here and play or sing for us. They began their project in January and have since brought out four or five afternoons of entertainment. Usually, it's over the earphone system as there's no place or means of gathering the patients here. The latest was the best—they trucked out one of those spinet type Hammond Electric organs—and a young Bemidji man of 30 played it for an hour on the first floor along with requests or anything he thought of. I liked the way he changed keys to play each succeeding piece. They fit together so evenly and nicely. Both he and the instrument were so versatile. They left the instrument here overnight. The next day a good friend of the janitor came out to play the organ for the afternoon of music. He plays the organ as a business in St. Louis. He was up here on vacation visiting friends.

"Several nurses and employees went to The Biggest Show on Earth in Bemidji. The Ringling Brothers Barnum Bailey Circus was there on a one-night stand. I would have loved seeing it as I had never seen a circus before. Another outing I wish I could have gone on was when five patients up on privileges had the good luck of going for a ride with Dr. Mary.

"I enter a few contests as usual—and win once in a while—nothing big—just a dollar or two or some merchandise like a flashlight, nylons, phono records or shaving supplies. They're the small and local contests, radio and other kinds. It's fun to try and apply my efforts.

"Dr. Mary's son is in the Navy as a hospital corpsman. He's stationed at the hospital in San Diego. He's 19 now. He may be home for good before the year is over.

"A few have gone home for good this summer and several others have gone home for a week or two.

"Five of those regaining strength here now are patients who had rib surgery in the past eight months. They're doing good.

"More of the lake, the front lawn, and the road about the south and east edge of the lake in the front. We can watch the cars now, and the headlights of the cars at night shine in when they are on the long straight section parallel to the south portion of the lake.

"Lester and I saw our first speedboat of the season this afternoon when a sleek white and red 16-footer with an inboard motor sped by in a wide arc. It looked so pretty in the bright sunny water with the waves playing follow the leader after the frothy part had disappeared. There was a young man and a big black dog in the boat—probably Dickinsons from the south end of Lake Julia. They're the only ones I know of around here who would have the means for such a boat. Needless to say, Lester and I weren't the only ones in the sanatorium who wished they could be out there with him in the boat. The sight brought back several memories for me.

"Five of the patients up on several privileges had good luck yesterday. Dr. Mary had an hour free after the silent rest hour and took them for a ride to Bemidji, around Lake Bemidji, and the pretty developed areas around there. She regretted it hadn't been a week earlier when all the multicolored leaves were on display. The patients, a boy, a girl, a man and two women really enjoyed themselves. I don't blame them.

"Today was weigh-day. I gained a ½ pound. My appetite is good and most dinners and suppers see seconds come to me.

"Time goes fast. I have a star doily half done on the needles now and I should finish it tomorrow after bath time.

"STOP STOP STOP. (Charlie you can add some if there is space—A paragraph or two—but remember some are older people—some very religious so you can jest or be serious all you like. I guess he knows me."

Charlie, the janitor helping with the hectograph, added the following:

"Note the even paragraphing of the right-hand margin of pages two and three. My typists, Hunt and Peck, are really proud of that.

"Hello you all. I am really fond of older people. Some say I might even become one of them some time. Time will tell. As for the religious ones, let me say that I'm pretty much that way, too. In five minutes I will be off to choir practice, so will say as Art did at the end of the letter:

"God Bless You

"I mean it.

"Charlie"

Art's frequent correspondence allowed him to become a stamp collector. He saved different stamps not only from his mail but also from the other patients and staff. When he entered contests, he received a lot of correspondence and more postage stamps for his collection. With no means for the patients to get out and buy things, the post office did a big business in money orders for goods purchased from catalogs, so Art also received stamps from the packages that arrived.

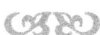

Art made three spectacular 36" Governor's Lady doilies. He blocked them out, starched them, put them on a paper background for contrast, then entered them in the county fairs.

At the Itasca County Fair, a lady who volunteered with display registration wanted to tell Art the reactions of people who had seen his work and wanted to find out if he would make some pieces to sell. As their friendship developed, she came one fall to visit with her family and to meet him in person. The next summer, she started to send Art food packages of cookies once a week. He mentioned the things he missed, like sausage and certain types of fruit, so she sent those things too. He couldn't eat the whole piece of sausage at one time, so he rigged up a way to hang it out the window in nature's icebox.

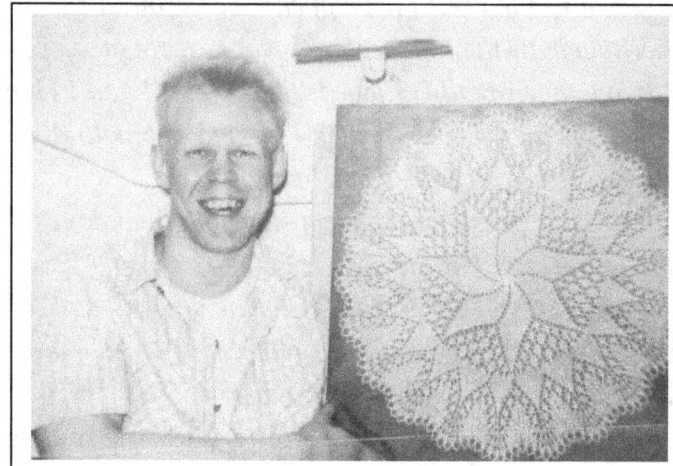
Art with one of his doilies.
Art Holmstrom collection

During the summer that year, she and her family deliberately rented a cottage close to Lake Julia and worked it out so she could take Art in her vehicle to visit with her family in the rented cottage. He napped there and had lunch. She took him back to the San in the evening. The two of them corresponded frequently.

Because of all her gifts and visits, she became like a second mother to Art. His own mother couldn't drive, so she depended on others to take her to visit her son at the San, and therefore, she could not visit often.

Because the San had an intercom system, patients not only used the earphones to listen to the radio and to hear entertainment broadcasts from the first floor but also to hear church services. That way, the ministers could talk to patients who could not go downstairs to attend services.

Rev. Carl Carlson ministered to the patients when he took over as pastor at the Our Redeemer's Lutheran Church in Puposky in 1946. His wife, Mathilda Ronsvold Carlson, had a tubercular lesion that activated when she was given cortisone for another ailment, so Dr. Mary sent her to Glen Lake Sanatorium, where the surgeons surgically removed her tuberculosis.

The Carlson's daughter Connie said that when her family moved to Puposky, they found that the parsonage did not have indoor bathroom facilities. She, a sophomore in high school, had grown up with indoor plumbing. Dr. Mary said Connie could use their bathtub whenever she wanted to. When she spent the night with friends, they teased her that she was just there to take a bath.

Jim Ghostley, Dr. Mary's son, sometimes had a car to drive, so he gave Connie rides to after-school activities until she went to school in North Dakota. The family came back to Bemidji in the summers because they owned property in the area. Jim and Connie corresponded and remained friends. He went into the service, and he looked her up when he got out. She had gone to nursing school at Northwest. They were good buddies, doing many things together, and they eventually married.[120]

Art remembered Rev. Teber Hill, who himself had suffered from tuberculosis before he moved to Puposky.

There was also a pastor from Oak Hills Bible School, south of Bemidji, a very handsome young man, who had some friends he would contact in the San. When he visited, everyone could hear his message. A few other pastors visited the patients while Art was there. A Catholic priest visited Felix, and Pastor J. T. Stolee conducted church services at the San while he lived in the area.

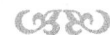

Art used to talk to Jim Ghostley from his second-story window. The doctor's children weren't supposed to be in direct contact with the patients, and she never allowed her son or daughter to go near any of the patients in the sanatorium. Jim and Art were both young, and Art enjoyed being able to visit with someone close to his age.

Jim did artwork in school, and Art wanted to see it. When Jim came home from school, he would stand under Art's window at the west end of the San to visit. Art found a piece of string and a clip and lowered it down. "Here, Jim, clip your pictures to this string and let me have a look," Art suggested. Art got to view many different things that way. The Ghostley children only had friendships with patients at a safe distance through the open windows. Dr. Mary also gave them periodic Mantoux tests to be sure they had not contracted the disease.[121]

---

[120] Connie Carlson Ghostley interview
[121] James Ghostley interview

Jim Ghostley told of visiting with patient Nels Lidholm, a woodcarver. As a child, Jim was amazed at how anybody could create the things Nels did. A Pinocchio figure made by Nels had been in Jim's family since he was young. He treasured that figure. Nels carved gnomes, too. In later years, when Jim was teaching school, he read that Nels Lidholm had carved a whole circus. People traveled from near and far to see it. He was an inspiration to Jim, who also became a woodcarver.

☙❧

Art remembered that Jim Ghostley told him he got his driver's license by mail by sending a quarter in an envelope to St. Paul.

Jim worked on a ranch during the summers to earn money for college. After high school, he joined the Navy and was in the hospital corps.

After being in the Navy, Jim went to college and worked. Then, the Korean War broke out, and the government called the medical corps back into service. After his discharge, he returned to college and became a teacher and later a dentist. Art continued to keep track of Jim throughout his life.

☙❧

Art's Uncle George had both a still camera and a movie camera. When Art was only 10, George introduced him to photography and later gave him a 35mm camera. Shortly after Art went to the San, he asked that his family bring his camera to him. He took many photos during his stay. When Art felt well enough to walk to the neighboring farms, he took photos to make a little spending money. He took wedding pictures for Darlene Quesnel when she married Dick Pearson, and he also took wedding pictures for Andrew Nixler and his bride.

Art photographed events at the San, including the Luther League play in 1951. Rev. Teber Hill often brought young people from his congregation over to the San to entertain the patients with plays directed by his wife, Esther, but unless patients were negative for TB, they could not see the production. It was broadcast throughout the building, so patients who tested positive could at least listen through their bedside earphones.[122]

---

[122] Ella Hedglin

Chapter 40
New Drugs

An inexpensive yet effective cure for tuberculosis was needed. Doctors tested new treatments around 1949. One drug involved taking 27 pills. It was a struggle to down so many. Art remembered well because he could only swallow one pill at a time. He heard lots of complaints from people who had to take so many pills. Experiments with new drugs were done more in Glen Lake or Ah-gwah-ching sanatoriums, or in other states, than they were at Lake Julia. But once there were good results elsewhere from the new treatments, the county sanatoriums began to try them, too.

In 1943, Selman Waksman had led a team to develop streptomycin, the first effective antibiotic against tuberculosis.[123] Streptomycin and Para-amino salicylic acid, commonly known as PAS, brought about dramatic results.[124] That discovery opened the door to using additional antibiotics in conjunction with streptomycin and PAS. Dihydrostreptomycin, combined with the other two, brought better results than using one of the three drugs alone.[125]

Dr. Mary took continuing education courses and attended professional conferences to stay up to date on the latest news in medicine. She kept a close watch as she tested the drugs. Many patients responded well to them and went home. The medicine made the tubercle bacillus extremely hungry. Then, once it was ravenous, another medication was given to kill the TB.[126]

Dr. Mary decided to try the new medicines on Art in 1949. He had a course of the drugs intramuscularly every six hours for 90 days. The nurse did not use any preparatory Novocain when she administered the injections in his buttocks. She had to keep track of where the previous punctures had been, so for Art, that meant 360 pokes over 90 days.

Art's health improved so much that in September 1950, he had his first opportunity in six years and nine months to go home for a visit. At that time, he was eating all three meals downstairs at the San, and he could go for short walks.

---

[123] *Scientific American*, March 2009
[124] *Invited and Conquered*, Minnesota Public Health Association, 1949
[125] *Invited and Conquered*, Minnesota Public Health Association, 1949
[126] James Ghostley interview

"It was quite an experience," Art told his parents, "to see the improvements on the highway—to enter the Falls from the west and to see all the street lights, the areas that had previously been just undeveloped farmland when I left town. The town had expanded."

When Art entered his house, it seemed to him that it had gotten smaller and that he was a giant, but he wasn't a different size from when he'd left, just a few pounds heavier. He was still 6'3", and he weighed about 130-135 pounds. The heaviest he'd been was 194 when he was on complete bed rest.

His mother was tickled to have him home, and she prepared every food he wanted. He had to stop when he was full.

"Don't you like my food?" Lissie asked.

He praised her. The food tasted to him as good as it always had, but he was too stuffed to eat more.

By midwinter 1951, Art could walk to Puposky, 2 miles each direction, and he took many photos. Sometimes he walked the railroad line toward Nebish, with places along the way as his points of reference. He entered some of his photographs in local contests, and he won more prizes.

On June 3, 1951, more than seven years after Art was admitted, he got to write in his diary, "I am going home today."

A June 1951 Falls newspaper article announced his release:

"Joy in Holmstrom Home
Son Returns, Daughter Wins Honors

"There was double reason for joy this week in the home of Mr. and Mrs. Gust Holmstrom, 615 Fifth Street.

"The reasons: A son, Arthur, 25, returned home after a prolonged illness while a daughter, Elsie, graduated from college with special honors.

"Arthur returned to his hometown Saturday from Lake Julia Sanatorium where doctors pronounced him cured after a long siege of illness. Although he has regained his health, he was advised to avoid strenuous activities. He will resume his education after a gradual buildup.

"Miss Elsie Holmstrom recently received a Master of Arts degree for major studies in sociology, social work at the 78th annual commencement exercises at Texas Christian University, Fort Worth, Tex.

"Miss Holmstrom was also awarded membership in the American Association of Social Workers. She is at present a member of the American Association of University

Women and Pi Gamma Mu, national social science honor society. She plans to engage in the field of medical-psychiatric social-case work.

"Both Arthur and his sister attended Falls high school."[127]

◈

Before long, because of the effectiveness of the new medications, patients either started to go home or to other institutions. Virtually overnight, many sanatoriums closed. There was suddenly no longer a need for the tuberculosis hospitals. Auditors and county commissioners that made up the sanatorium district met with sanatorium commissioners to discuss the feasibility of closing the Lake Julia Tuberculosis Sanatorium as the state had recommended. They studied the proposal from all angles.

Commissioners were afraid to lose Dr. Mary, saying, "Dr. Ghostley is the institution," but there was no longer a reason to keep the facility open. Dr. Mary agreed to continue as superintendent for as long as the San remained open. Nurse Thora Bakken also stayed until the end. Some patients were transferred by car to sanatoriums in other parts of the state. Others returned home. The remaining patients transferred to Nopeming Hospital, operated by St. Louis County. The last patient left in December 1952, and the San closed New Year's Eve.

◈

Dr. Mary remained until March 1 to wind up the business affairs. The personal property of the San was sold, with proceeds pro-rated among the counties that owned it—Koochiching, Beltrami, Itasca, and Hubbard. The farm and buildings had not yet been sold when the San closed.

---

[127] *International Falls Press*, International Falls, Minnesota

Chapter 41
After the San

Elsie was not living at home when Art returned. Gust had retired in the spring of 1947, then went to work for a private logging company to run the camps. He did that for one or two years. Then, he retired and bought the Gateway Cabins in the Falls, so Art finally had his father at home. Gust rented the cabins nightly to tourists and rented some monthly during the winter months. Many years later, Art learned that Dr. Mary's son, Jim, and his new bride, Connie, had stayed one night at the Gateway Cabins on their honeymoon.

When Art returned to the Falls, the school district offered him his diploma, but he declined. He wanted to earn his diploma and to attend high school to be sure he could stand up under the rigors of life. Art also wanted to take the classes he had missed—like trigonometry, bookkeeping, shorthand, and calculus. He completed school in four-hour days, then took a one-hour nap, and was home for dinner. He lived a sheltered life. He graduated in the ceremony with the class of 1952 but got his certificate for 1944. The students he graduated with were only in fourth grade when he got sick.

In 1952, Art saw the doctor at Nopeming Sanatorium and asked if he should have surgery on his lung. The physician discussed a left decortication to remove the thick covering of the lung that restricted its expansion. The doctor decided it would be best to do nothing. Since Art's TB was arrested but not cured, the doctor did not want to risk stirring it up. One lung compensated for the other and was much larger than the other.

Art knew he would get his education paid for if he went into the service. He tried to enlist but had no luck. Then, he wrote a letter to request an exemption for medical service as he knew Governor Stassen had done so that he could get into the service. That didn't work, either.

Art enrolled at St. Olaf College in Northfield, Minnesota and graduated in 1956 with a major in physics and a minor in mathematics. He helped his father with the Gateway Cabins during the summers of 1952 through 1956, which gave father and son a chance to get to know each other. He did graduate work in physics at Amherst College in Amherst, Massachusetts. In 1957, Art was awarded a training appointment under the American-Scandinavian Foundation, which took him to Sweden for a year to train in the research laboratory of a Swedish paper mill.

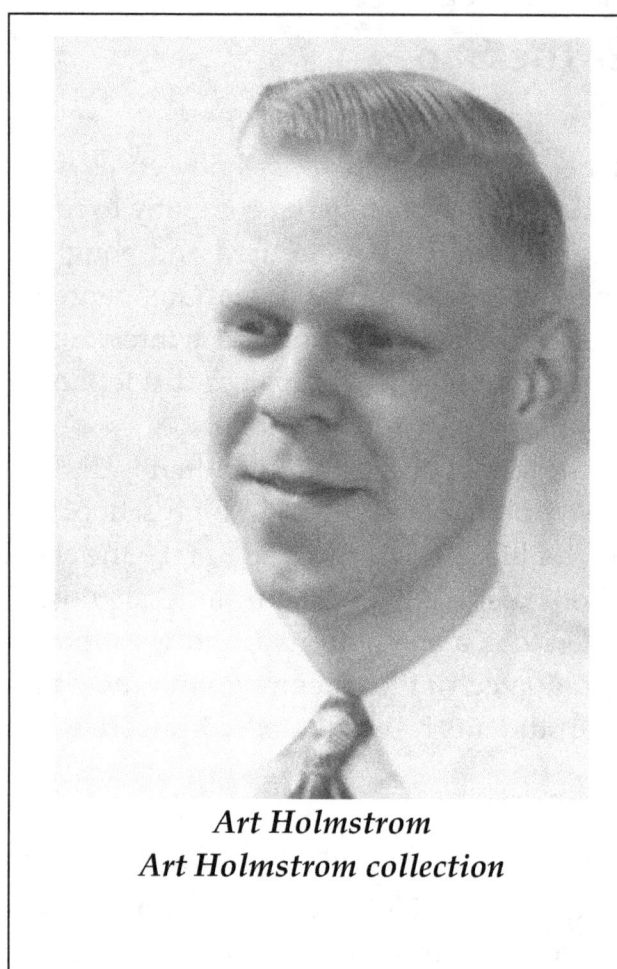

Art Holmstrom
Art Holmstrom collection

After he returned from Sweden, he worked as a night clerk in a hotel for nine months. In September 1959, he got a job in the research laboratory for the Minnesota and Ontario Paper Company, the forerunner to Boise Cascade. He had worked there for two summers while he attended St. Olaf College so they were aware of his potential. Because his training was in physics and mathematics, and they didn't have any specific job title for those types of things, he was called a chemist. He spent his career working in a research laboratory in the pulp and paper industry. His first five years there, he did technical work. He measured the resistance that pulp has for draining water. His tests involved using different additives in the pulp.

※

Eventually, Art met the love of his life, Edith Merry Stillar. Edith had graduated from Falls High School in 1942, then became a registered nurse in the

1946 Cadet Corps at Fairview School of Nursing. By 1950, she had earned her B.A. in English and biology at St. Olaf College in Northfield.

Art met Edith while he was a physics graduate assistant at Amherst College in 1956-57. He did not have a car, and he found out that Edith did. She had a beautiful Oldsmobile, and he liked that it had lots of chrome.

Edith planned to drive home to the Falls for Christmas vacation and had posted a request to find someone to share the driving. Art responded to her notice. She ended up with three passengers, and one of them was Art. Edith thought that meant there would be four drivers, but she was wrong. One passenger was a girl from the iron range—an area in Minnesota with large deposits of iron ore—and another was her boyfriend, an international student from Greece. Neither of them had a driver's license. The girl was taking him home to meet her family. They rode in the back seat, and Art and Edith drove.

The next year, Edith was back in Minneapolis, and Art had gone to Sweden for a year.

☙❧

After she obtained an M.S. in Orthopedic and Rehabilitation Nursing from Boston University, Edith taught those skills to nursing students in Minnesota's St. Olaf, Macalester, and Fairview Hospital nursing programs. She also spent six years in the Army Reserves as a nurse, with a tour of duty in Korea, and she obtained the rank of captain.

☙❧

About three years after Art returned from Sweden, he realized he was alone. He looked through his contact list and decided to call Edith. It was Memorial Day 1962 and 90 degrees outside.

Edith was busy because she worked in rehabilitation, and she had a patient who had been in a tornado in Fargo. The woman was severely injured, and her husband had died. She had run out of funds and had to leave the rehabilitation facility. Edith found an apartment for her. The patient left the facility on a Friday. Edith had promised to see her Saturday morning, and that was the day that Art wanted to visit. Edith was so busy that she barely had time to say hello. Still, Art wanted to get acquainted. He persisted, and eventually, the lady Edith had worked with that Saturday attended their wedding.

Art and Edith married on June 16, 1963. Edith was 38, and Art was 37.

Gust and Lissie were happy for them, and they offered to fix up their best unit at the Gateway Cabins as their apartment. Edith loved them both and appreciated the offer, but she and Art decided to rent a house instead.

◊

In 1964, Art visited the Pulmonary Work Evaluation Unit at his job for pulmonary-function testing. He stated to the doctor that his shortness of breath embarrassed him. Art was concerned because other people could walk faster and perform more physical activity than he could.

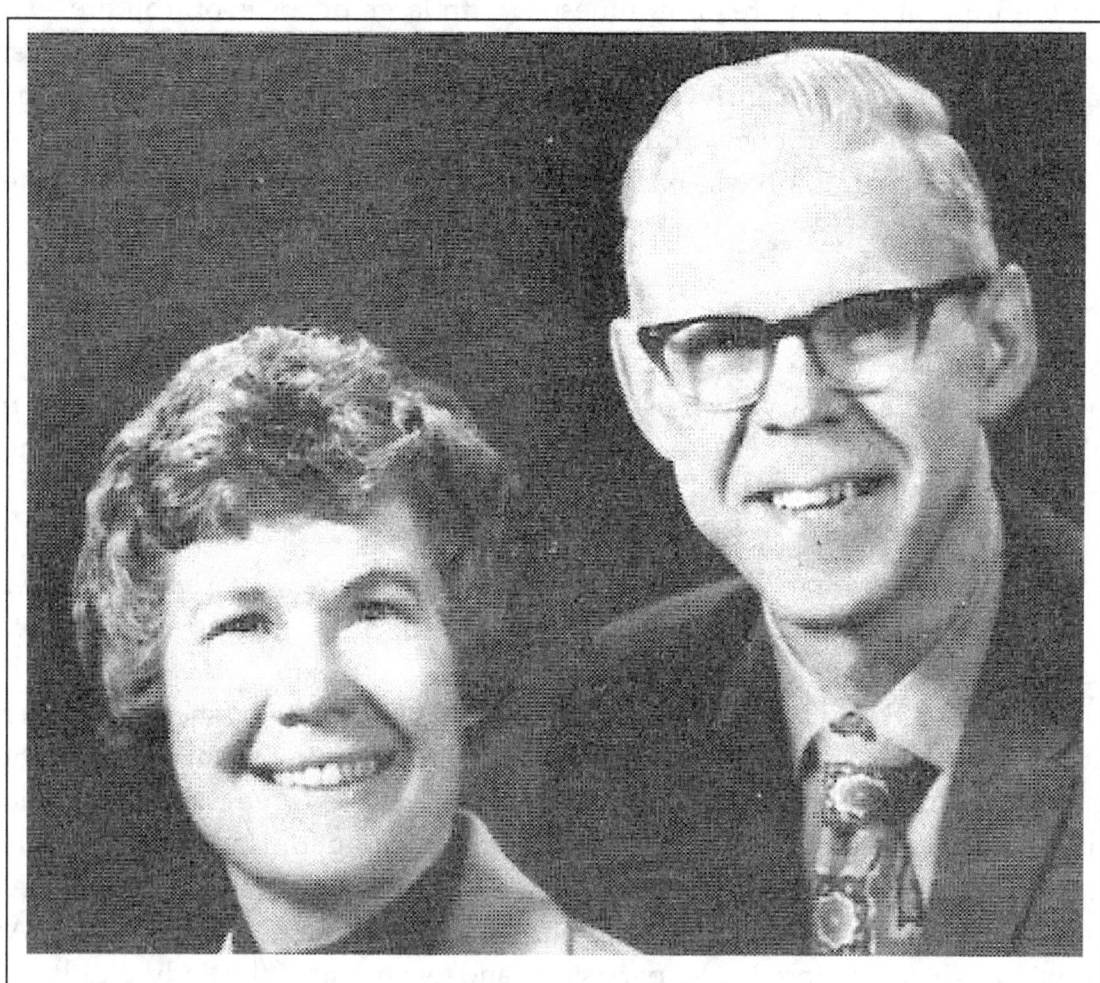

Art and Edith Holmstrom
Art Holmstrom collection

A single chest X-ray taken on March 20, 1964, showed marked pleural thickening of Art's left side, which indicated an unexpanded lung. There was also a fibrous lesion in his left upper lung. His trachea was pulled to the left side. The X-ray showed healed and inactive tuberculosis.

The doctor's report stated:

"This individual has a clinical diagnosis of pulmonary tuberculosis, inactive. His left lung has a great deal of pleural thickening as a result of left pneumothorax. He has shown pulmonary insufficiency of moderately severe degree. It is understandable that he is short of breath on exertion. His vital capacity is cut down to about half, and his maximum breathing capacity is cut down to one-third of his predicted normal. I don't believe that any type of surgery would improve his pulmonary function at this time."[128]

୧୬୨୦

Edith stood by Art through his tests, both as his loving wife and as a nurse. While they waited in the doctor's office, talking about Art's days at the San, Edith mentioned that she was a Dr. Mary baby. Art was truly surprised to learn that Dr. Mary, the woman who had played such a significant role in his life, had delivered Edith.

Edith explained that when she was seven or eight, Dr. Mary had gone to her school to do Mantoux testing. When Edith got to the front of the line, Dr. Mary had commented, "And this is one of my girls." Edith wondered how Dr. Mary had recognized her, especially since she had delivered thousands of babies.

She told her father what Dr. Mary had said, and he confirmed that Dr. Mary had delivered her. "On that snowy day," he reminisced, "I shoveled two tracks in the snow, nearly a quarter of a mile, and a turnaround for Dr. Mary's old Model A. It took me most of the day, then she parked on the old highway by the mailbox and walked instead, not even using my cleared tracks! While she waited for you to be born, she sat and took naps. As things progressed, she would sit and put everything out of her mind and sleep."

୧୬୨୦

Despite Art's medical condition and frequent doctor visits, Art and Edith had a good life together. They became foster parents to 10 local children, and they hosted Rainy River international students from Honduras and Bangladesh. They became especially close to a boy from Bangladesh named Ahmed, their fifth

---

[128] Arthur Holmstrom collection

international student. When Ahmed was only four, he lost his father to heart disease. He felt eternally grateful to find a father figure in Art. When Art passed, Ahmed told Edith, "I still needed him."

Eventually, Art and Edith supported 35 international students, who they considered their children. Their global family later included spouses and children, grandchildren, and great-grandchildren.

The couple traveled the world and volunteered in medical sites from India to Honduras. They visited six of the seven continents. Art and Edith owned a cabin near Nestor Falls, Canada, in the area Art had enjoyed as a child, where they made friends and enjoyed fishing, hosting visitors, and picking blueberries.

Art never allowed the lung damage from his tuberculosis treatments to keep him from living a full and gratifying life.

Section Six: Story Without End

Chapter 42
Moving On

Dr. Mary was proud of the part she had played in taking X-rays and training technicians, but it had taken its toll. After many years of taking X-rays, she lost part of her hand due to radiation.[129] After she had surgery, the doctor, thinking he was doing her a favor by taking off a little extra so that her hand would look more streamlined, received a piece of her mind when she realized her hand would no longer be as effective in her work.[130]

Some wondered if radiation was also what caused her to have a broad white streak in her hair. In a study of X-ray effects in 1926, it was noted that the hair of rabbits became white within areas exposed to X-ray produced at high voltage.[131]

※

Dr. Mary's written procedure for the diagnosis of chest X-rays became the format used by the Mayo Clinic in Rochester and at the University of Minnesota long before radiology had developed into a medical specialty.

Once when Jim Ghostley was on a plane, he sat next to a radiologist who was curious about his last name. "Are you related to Dr. Mary Ghostley?" he asked. "When we took our training," he told Jim, "her letters replying to the different physicians about X-rays were used as a form for us to learn how to respond by mail about X-rays."

Radiology students and male doctors throughout the state sent chest X-rays to Dr. Mary for diagnosis, even though the male doctors were unwilling to discuss other medical issues with her. They were not ready to accept Dr. Mary as their equal, although they used her work and passed it off as their own. Mailbags full

---

[129] Gretchen Wright interview
[130] Jim Ghostley interview
[131] Laboratories of The Rockefeller Institute for Medical Research, 1926

of X-rays showed up at the San for her to read. She gladly did the work but didn't get the credit.

Some said she became more headstrong as the years went on, possibly because of attitudes such as this. She was highly qualified, yet worked in a world in which many still only accepted traditional roles for women. [132]

◈

The Lake Julia Tuberculosis Sanatorium sent home its last patient in December 1952 and locked the doors. Jim Ghostley volunteered to drive the remaining patients to both Nopeming and Ah-gwah-ching Sanatoriums,[133] and Jim was hired on March 14, 1953, to move the records to the Ah-gwah-ching State Sanatorium at Walker, at $4 plus $4.20 for gasoline. From that total, the San deducted $3.05 for a long-distance telephone call to his future wife, Connie Carlson. Lucy Barrett carefully accounted for all San expenses, right up to the end.[134]

In 1954, the facility reopened as the Lake Julia Nursing Home, which operated there until it moved to Bemidji in 1968.[135]

After that, the facility changed hands several times, with various ideas to refurbish it.

◈

Along with the closure of the facility came ghost hunters. Bizarre tales appeared on the internet. Some writers insisted the Sanatorium had been a mental clinic. Others boasted that they had snuck in late at night, and they described their fear. One person reported that the higher he went inside the building, the windier it got. Remember, windows were designed for the air to flow throughout the building, from one side to the other and front to back. Still, some believed the airflow was a paranormal event.

---

[132] Jim Ghostley interview

[133] James Ghostley interview

[134] Minnesota History Center, Lake Julia Tuberculosis Sanatorium, expense records

[135] *The Bemidji Pioneer*, Bemidji, Minnesota, John Eggers, October 1, 2017

Someone insisted there had been a crematory inside. There was no crematory; there was a heating system in the basement that heated not only the San but also all the buildings on the property. One person wrote that the TB patients were housed at the lowest level of the basement. This statement was not valid. The male employees—janitors and engineers—lived in the basement.

Another person claimed to have seen old papers that said more than 11,000 people died there, a considerable stretch of the imagination for a facility that housed slightly more than 50 patients at a time.[136]

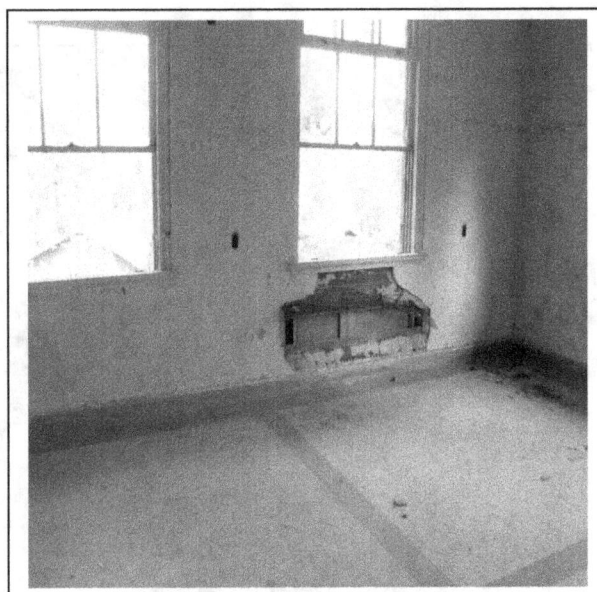

Art Holmstrom's former ward
Pat Nelson photo

And what happened to the San after the nursing home moved? It, and the 360 acres that went with it, sold at auction to a St. Paul Realtor. He sold off some lots and turned part of it into a bird sanctuary. It sold a few more times. As it sat, people took out windows and fixtures. But with 12-foot footings and three- to four-foot-thick walls, the building still stands. It would cost too much to bring it back to life and would be costly to demolish it. Today, it is a decaying shell, still filled with warm memories of its patients and those who dedicated their lives to restoring the health of those who lived within its walls.

It is private property, and the owners take measures to keep ghost hunters and the curious away to allow for their quiet enjoyment as well as for safety and liability reasons. The nurses' home was purchased, and the new owners built their home on top of the basement where my mother, Aunt Bernice, and other female employees once lived.

---

[136] www.ghostvillage.com

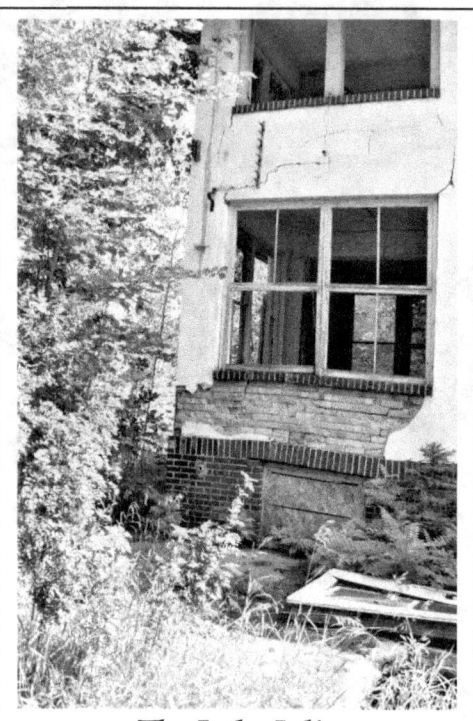

The Lake Julia TuberculosisSanatorium helped many return to good health.
Today it sits in disrepair, the cost too great to either demolish or refurbish.
Pat Nelson photo

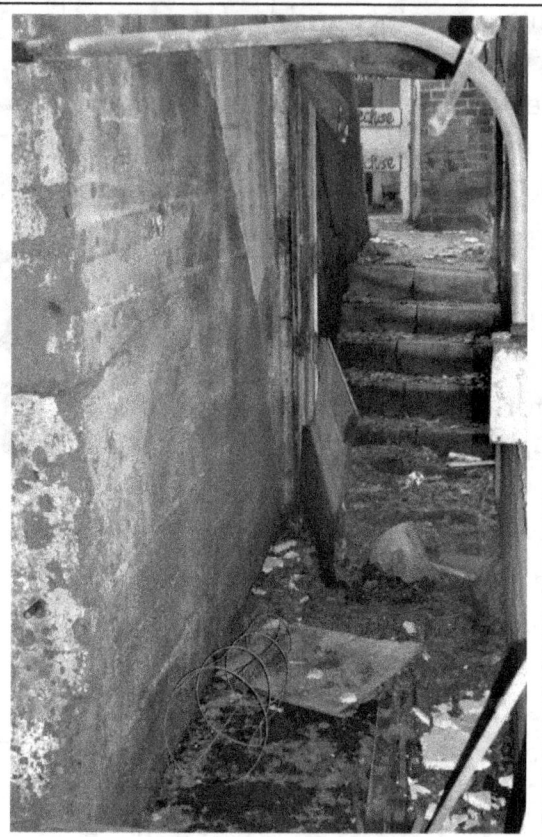

Once considered home by many of the San's male employees, the basement is now in bad repair. Photo shows stairs leading up to the laundry and down to the engine room.
Pat Nelson photo

Dr. Mary, at age 72, left the sanatorium when it closed, but she did not retire. That ended one chapter of her life, but it started another. Her job had not come with retirement benefits, plus she had been generous with her earnings, so she still needed to work. More importantly, she believed there was still a lot of work to be done. "Other people keep retiring me," Dr. Mary often said, "but I haven't retired myself."[137] "Not only have they been 48 years of service, but they have also been years filled with laughter, tragedies, labor, despair, and triumphs."[138]

When she left the San, Dr. Mary moved 12 miles away to Bemidji, where she became the Director of Public Health for Northern Minnesota. She continued to perform Mantoux tests in the schools. Dr. Mary was a wealth of information to the community. When she was in City Hall as director of the health district, the clinic doctors could not figure out what one man was suffering from, and they sent for Dr. Mary. When she entered the back of the clinic, she immediately recognized the odor. Dr. Mary walked directly into the treatment room and grabbed a hemostat, then began to remove a thick membrane from the patient's throat. He was immediately greatly relieved and could breathe again. Dr. Mary had recognized the characteristic odor of diphtheria, a long-past affliction.[139]

In Bemidji, she often visited with the health professionals she had known for years, and the doctor was happy that she was still close enough to Puposky to visit her friends there.

Dr. Mary still owned her old two-story log house on Birch Point at Rainy Lake in the town of Ranier. She had purchased it in 1921 from Rev. Heermance, an early-day Congregational minister. The Birch Point property was her second place on Rainy Lake. In 1914, she had bought property off the north end of Jackfish Bay. That piece of granite extended from Forest Point toward Stop Island, at the end of county road 94, and is still known to navigators as "Dr. Mary's Point." She spent as much time as possible at the Birch Point cabin with family and friends, and she swam to the rock in front of her place every chance she got.[140]

---

[137] James Ghostley interview
[138] *International Falls Press,* International Falls, Minnesota, September 18, 1958
[139] James Ghostley interview
[140] James Ghostley interview

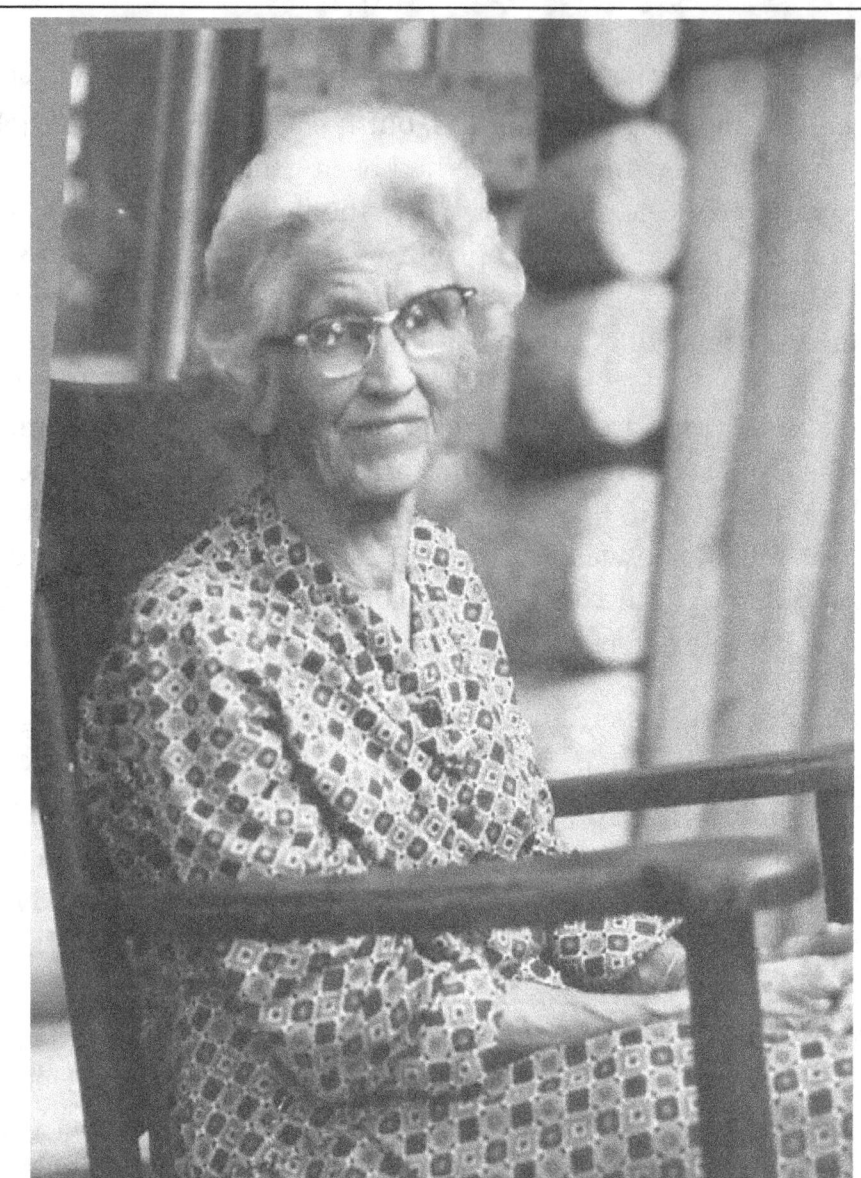
Dr. Mary at her cabin at Birch Point, Ranier
James Ghostley collection

On July 10, 1961, Dr. Mary got up in the night and fell down the steep stairs of her summer home, striking and breaking a mirror on the landing. She suffered a cut on the side of her face and ear, a hip injury, and bruises, lacerations, and abrasions.[141] Her sister Peggy lived with her at the time and got help.

---

[141] *International Falls Press*, International Falls, Minnesota, July 10, 1961

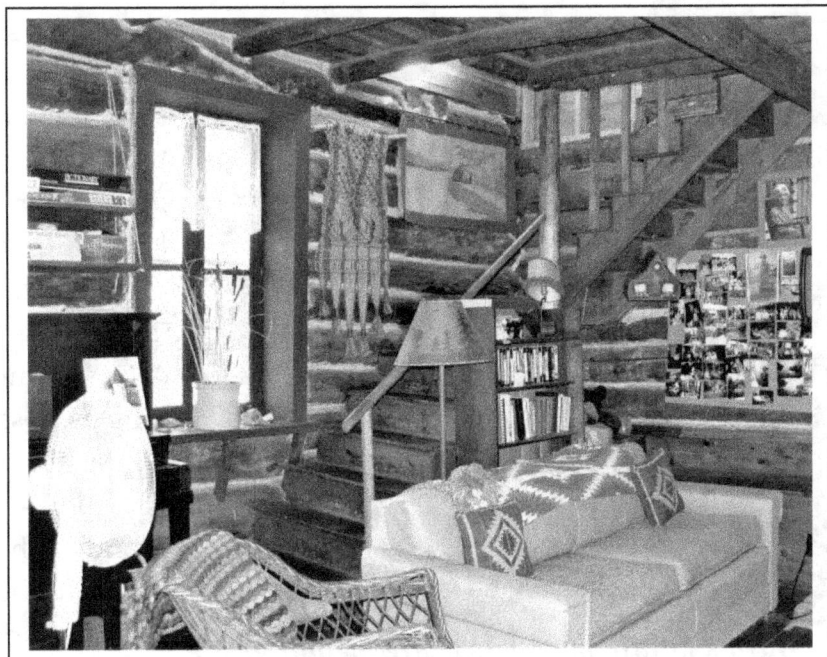

Dr. Mary's cabin at Birch Point in Ranier
Pat Nelson photo

Peck Brown, Peggy's son, and his friend went to get his mother, and his friend donated blood for Mary. She was taken to Falls Memorial for treatment of her injuries. Even then, she wasn't ready to stop working.[142]

At age 85, she finally retired. Dr. Mary had been happy with her work, and she said she would do it all again.[143]

After retirement, she and her longtime friend and former employee Lucy Barrett spent winters in Staples and summers on Rainy Lake until she moved into the Bemidji Nursing Home.

Barrett had been a schoolteacher at both Loman and International Falls for several years. Many in the area knew her. She had also worked at the Koochiching County superintendent's office. Before she worked at the San as Dr. Mary's secretary, Barrett and Dr. Mary had shared an apartment at the Falls in the Montgomery Building and later at the Bacon Apartments, which became the St. Thomas Rectory.[144]

---

[142] Percy (Peck) Brown interview

[143] *International Falls Press*, International Falls, Minnesota, September 18, 1958

[144] Edith Holmstrom interview

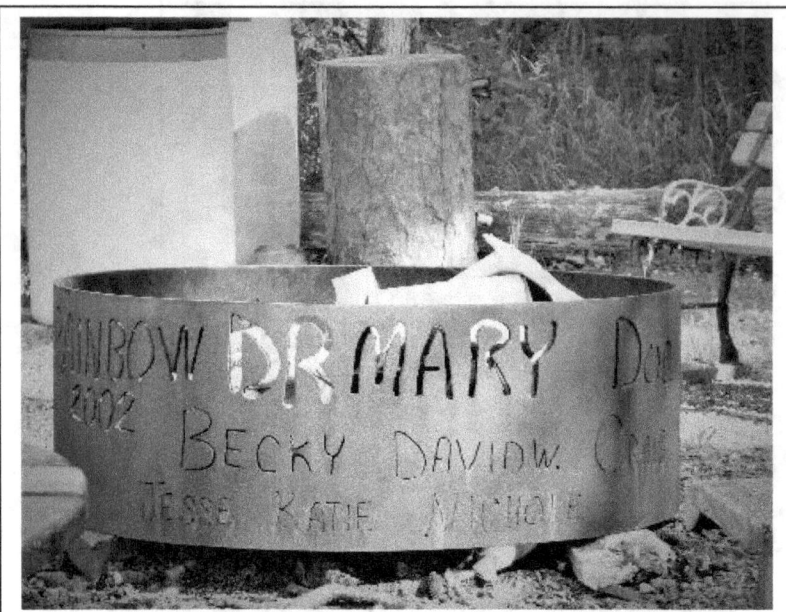

Dr. Mary's family members share memories while they sit around the fire at her summer home. Pat Nelson photo

Dr. Mary's family still gathers around the ring that surrounds the fire pit at the Birch Point cabin. It says in large cutout letters, "Dr. Mary." The family gets together each summer for as long as possible to honor Dr. Mary Ghostley—mother, grandmother, great grandmother, great-great-grandmother, healer, and friend—and to share memories.

Gretchen Wright, a great-niece of Dr. Mary, recalled that when Dr. Mary got electricity in her Rainy Lake cabin, she bought a small freezer, providing the luxury of having ice cubes in drinks. She frugally collected the used ice cubes that remained and put them back in the freezer.

Gretchen loved spending time with her Aunt Mary, Aunt Peggy, Lucy Barrett, and Kitty Peterson. The ladies talked quietly, peacefully telling stories. They giggled a lot. They served tea or coffee on the big front porch at a round wooden table made from enormous purloined logs. It was massive for the cabin.

Gretchen said, "Kitty Peterson had a thick Scottish brogue. Lucy Barrett wore a red pageboy haircut that didn't seem to fit with the powdery wrinkles on her face. My mother told me that Cindy had such beautiful red hair because she always ate her Saturday pills—the iodine pills that I didn't like. I found out later that Lucy's red hair was a wig.

"The ladies loved to read," Gretchen said, "and Aunt Mary had a four-sided oak bookcase that spun. It was crammed with antique books. That is where I first read *Anne of Green Gables*, and Aunt Mary gave the book to me to keep the summer I turned 12."

Dr. Mary's Grandson David Ghostley said, "My grandmother was one of the most intelligent people ever to grace the surface of the planet. She cared equally for animals and human beings and believed that every animal had a soul. Grandmother protested the use of mousetraps in the cabin on Rainy Lake. Grandma was concerned for those little lives and would rather have guests gently sweep the little rascals out the door with brooms."

Back in 1906, when Mary and Fred were courting, Fred wrote this to her: *"In nature, we have to pick out the good and useful from the bad and useless."* She must have seen the mice as good and useful, and therefore protected them.

David Ghostley told about the time a bird successfully nested in the top of the chimney over the fireplace at the cabin. "Grandma promptly decided that the bird had more of a right to nest there than we had to burn fires. She flipped the sofa around with its back pressed against the large fireplace opening. With the sofa situated over the hearth, the family did not use the fireplace for many years."

Granddaughter Barbara Fisher added, "If we let the grass get longer than usual in the summer, forget-me-nots pop up because Grandma sprinkled the seeds all over."

Dr. Mary spent the last five years of her life at the Bemidji Nursing Home with Alzheimer's. She never stopped being Dr. Mary. Even at the nursing home, she went from room to room, checking pulses and visiting patients.

After an incredible career, she died penniless on April 9, 1975, at age 94.[145] She had done everything she could to make a positive difference in the lives of others.

Her memorial service was held on a Saturday at 11 a.m. at the First Lutheran Church in Bemidji, with many in attendance who were Dr. Mary babies or who had received the Mantoux tests performed by her, and others who had been her patients or employees. The Rev. Stephen Knudsen presided. Interment was at the Forest Hill Cemetery in Anoka.

These words found in Fred's letter to Mary of August 28, 1906, had even more impact once he and his beloved Mary were finally together again:

---

[145] James Ghostley interview

"I am here by these falls and yet I am standing by those 'falls of Minnehaha' and you, fair brown haired maiden of the Dacotahs, are standing beside me, and the mist from the water strikes us in the face. It is spring, and the whisperings of love are in our hearts. And they become full. And the world is fair. We have found out that we were for each other and we know that it is best. And we have sworn to love each other for ever, and we know that is best, too. And the land, and the years, and the world are good. O Mary I love you! O the joy and sweetness of it, we, two together for each other forever. Two happy spirits and the stars."

༄༅

Dr. Mary was survived by two children, nine grandchildren, 18 great-grandchildren, and three great-great-grandchildren.

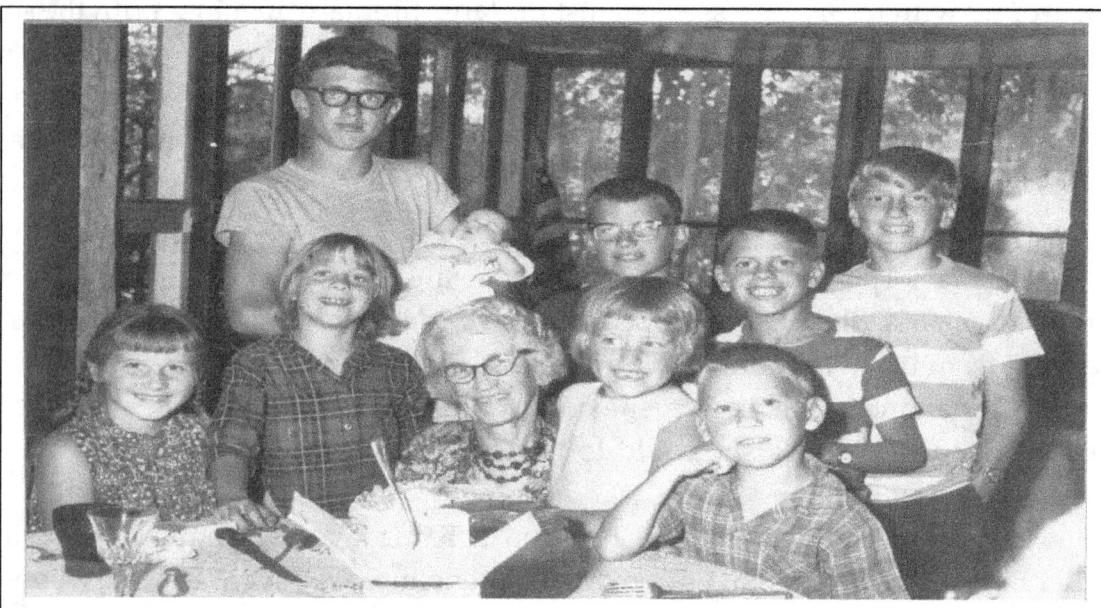

Dr. Mary with her grandchildren
James Ghostley collection

Her portrait hangs at the Bemidji State University (BSU), where she was inducted into the Northwest Minnesota Women's Hall of Fame on March 2, 2002. BSU honored Dr. Mary Ghostley for her many achievements.

Dr. Mary, a groundbreaking female physician, was known as one of the best TB professionals in Minnesota, and she oversaw every aspect of life at the Lake Julia Tuberculosis Sanatorium. She promoted meticulous sanitation, and she administered Mantoux tests to thousands of students. Dr. Mary was known for being second to none at reading chest X-rays. She helped people get a college education, provided clothing to the needy, trained nurses and X-ray technicians, and opened her home as a library filled with books for people to borrow. In short, she helped wherever she was needed. The induction provides permanent recognition for Northern Minnesota women who have made significant contributions to their community. The ceremony was part of the opening for Women's History Month at BSU. Her children, Jim Ghostley and Cathie Fuller, proudly accepted the award. [146]

According to Dr. Jay Arthur Myers in his book *Invited and Conquered*, about the 100-year war against TB, Dr. Mary C. Ghostley is "one of the several women in medicine who has contributed in a large way to the control of tuberculosis in Minnesota. History must record Dr. Ghostley as one of Minnesota's best tuberculosis workers." Myers credited her with keeping up with all new developments in chest diseases and for attending almost every meeting of the State Sanatorium Association, the Minnesota Trudeau Society, the Mississippi Valley Conference on Tuberculosis, and the National Tuberculosis Association.[147]

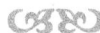

People remember Dr. Mary for her good deeds, and hundreds of the individuals she delivered were proud to call themselves "Dr. Mary Babies." After performing thousands of Mantoux tests for four counties, not stopping until she was in her mid-80s, plus her efforts toward providing meticulous sanitation to help eradicate TB and the care she gave her patients, she would be appalled today to see that tuberculosis is still a considerable threat in the world.

---

[146] Northwest Minnesota Women's Hall of Fame
[147] *Invited and Conquered*, Dr. J. Arthur Myers, Minnesota Public Health Association, 1949

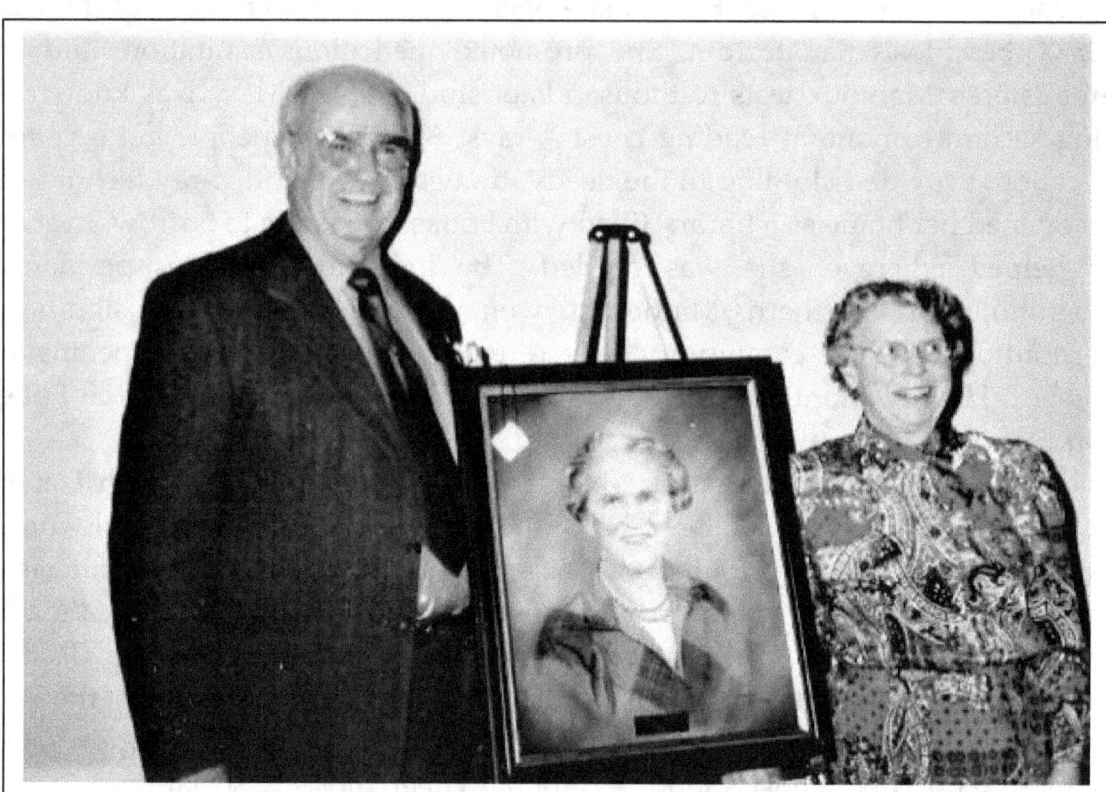

*James Ghostley and Cathie Ghostley Fuller
pose with portrait of their mother, Dr. Mary Ghostley.
Northwest Minnesota Women's Hall of Fame
Bemidji State University
James Ghostley collection*

Chapter 43
Deja Vu

In their later years, Art and Edith Holmstrom lived in the Rivers Edge Apartments in International Falls.

There were many similarities to Art's life at the San. Milk—six glasses a day—was still a daily ingredient in his life. He took a daily rest period, as he had at the San. Art lived on the second floor in an apartment that overlooked the water, and he enjoyed visits with his neighbors. Supplies for his many hobbies filled his apartment, and it was hard for him to make space for everything. He had problems breathing and was on oxygen. He had a nurse (his wife) by his side.

Art's lungs never returned to full operation due to the pneumothorax treatments he'd had at the San. He often became short of breath when he exerted himself too much or moved too fast. His chest X-rays were mottled with specks of calcification and were hard to read. His heart was way over to one side. His windpipe and esophagus were over to the left.

Art had sung in the church choir for 40 years. He loved to sing, but by 1992, he felt he could no longer help the bass section because his lung capacity had declined. That's when he voluntarily left the choir. He found that one way to satisfy his need to sing was to silently sing the hymns—to sing without making a sound.

The tuberculous areas in his lungs could not absorb oxygen, and he had reduced lung capacity because of a smaller left lung. Even though the right lung had expanded to larger than standard size to compensate, the damaged areas still were not productive. After leaving the San, he functioned at about 50 percent, which was enough to allow him to go to high school and college and to work. Eventually, he started to take some oxygen, then a little more, and then he had to have it at night.

He had walked at the college for exercise, 1.7 miles in 34-36 minutes without stress, but eventually, walking became more of an effort.

Art had lunch monthly with the classmates with whom he was supposed to have graduated. He was happy to say, "They still claim me."

In a large frame on his living room wall, he displayed one of his pinwheel designs, and two more lay under glass in end tables.

He was proud of his excellent appetite, and he had never returned to being a picky eater.

At Art's apartment complex, he met Eriga Menzner Hallisch, who was admitted to the San in 1925. (See earlier mention in Chapter 7.) Eriga was quite deaf, but her mind was sharp. She, like many others who lived to tell about their sanatorium experiences, lived a long life. Eriga died peacefully on March 27, 2009, 11 days short of her 99th birthday.

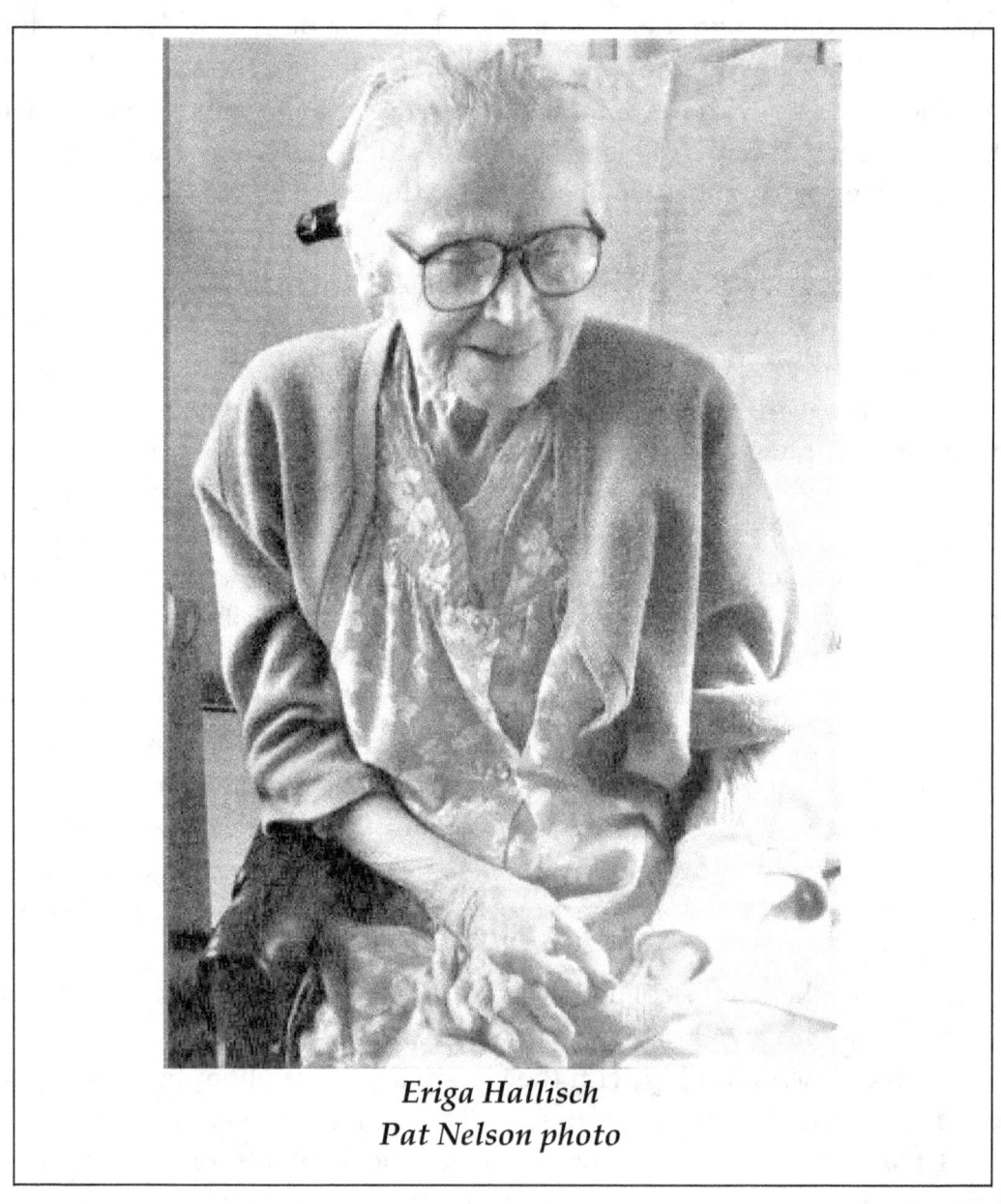

Eriga Hallisch
Pat Nelson photo

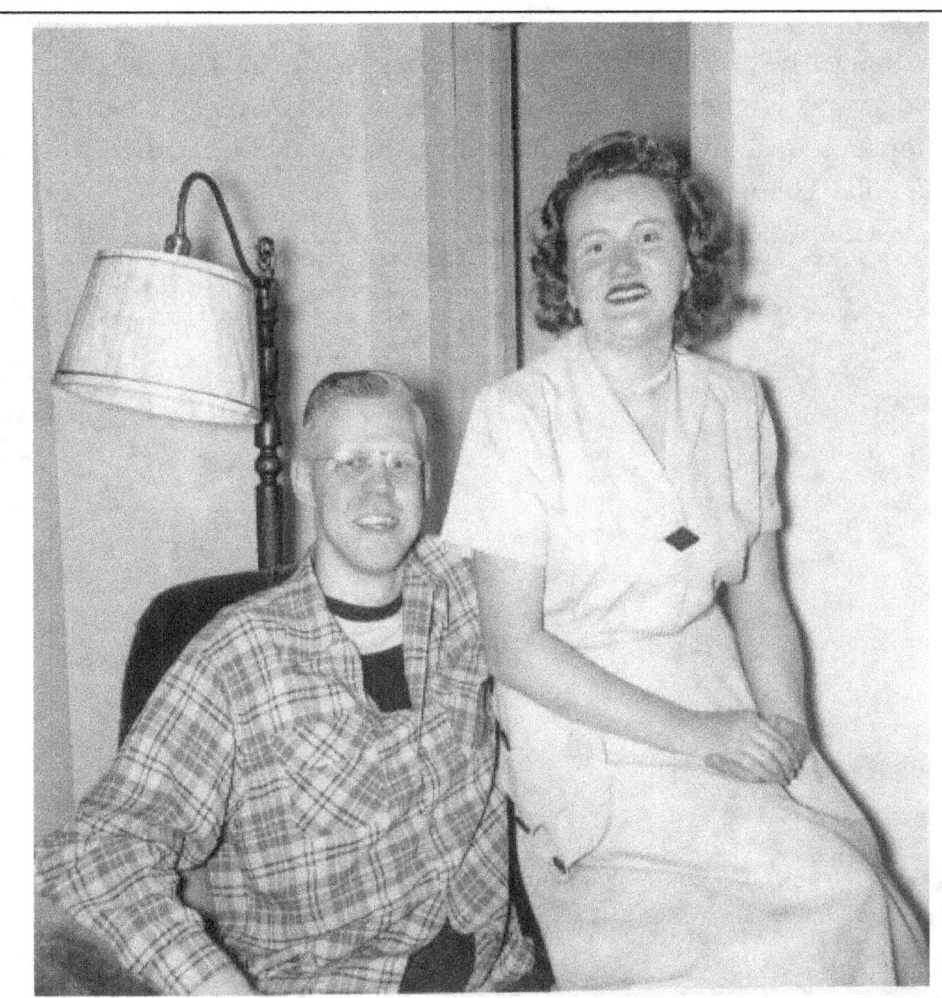

Art Holmstrom and Annie Petersen
visit in 1951
Art Holmstrom collection

In 2008, I drove Art's San girlfriend, Annie, from Bemidji to International Falls to visit Art. She had seen him only once after they were together at the San, soon after his release in 1951, when they were both 25. This time, in 2008, they were 82.

Art's wife, Edith, greeted us downstairs at the Rivers Edge Apartments and walked us up to their unit. Art opened the door and stared at Annie. He didn't say a word, just looked at her while squinting his eyes. Finally, Edith interrupted the embarrassing silence. "Art, it's Anneliese!"

"I know it is," he responded. "I'm just trying to see her." More than 60 years had passed since he'd fallen in love at the San with the 17-year-old girl called Annie, and he no longer recognized her. Once the shock of seeing each other passed, they had an enjoyable visit, happily reminiscing about their time together at the Lake Julia Tuberculosis Sanatorium.

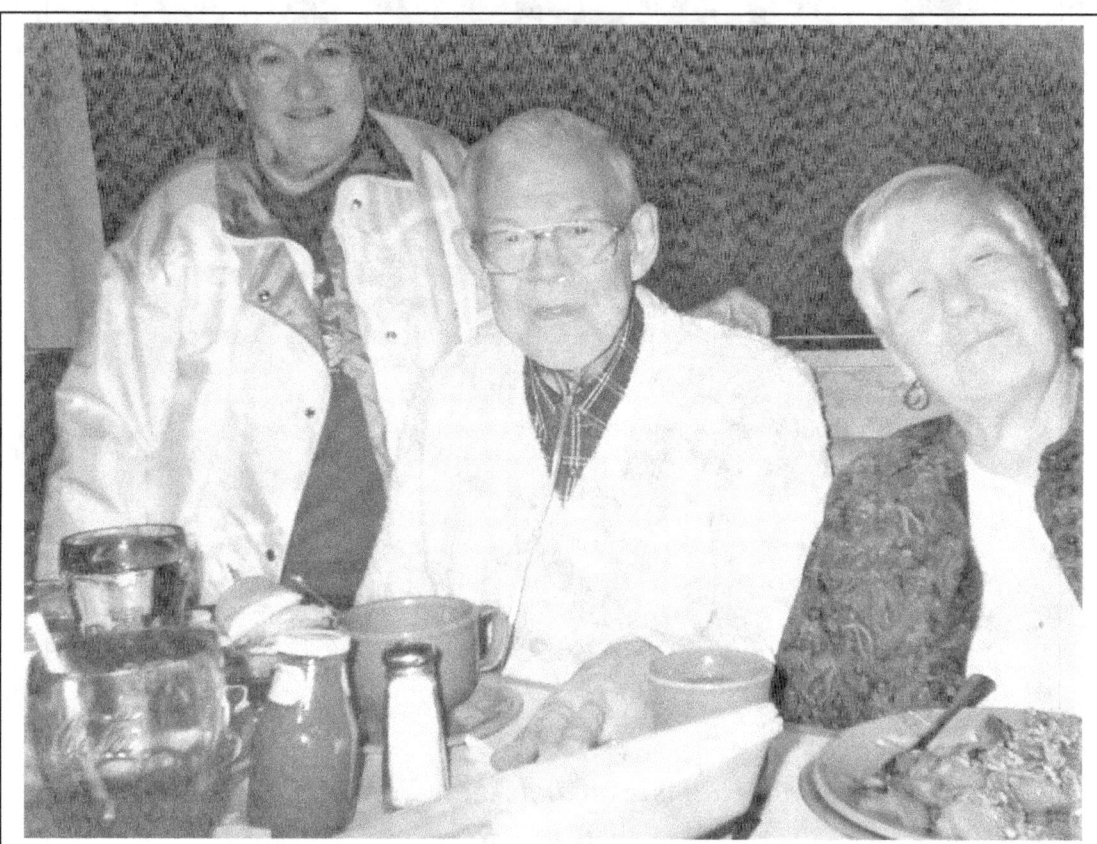

Annie Petersen, Art and Edith Holmstrom, 2008
Art and Annie hadn't seen each other since 1951.
Pat Nelson photo

Art Holmstrom died peacefully at home February 3, 2009, at the age of 83. He was a genealogist, historian, and fisherman, and he had enjoyed time at his cabin on Crow Lake, Ontario, Canada. He was a Sunday School teacher, he sang in the choir for 40 years, and he was a council member at First Lutheran Church as well as a member of the Koochiching County Historical Society.

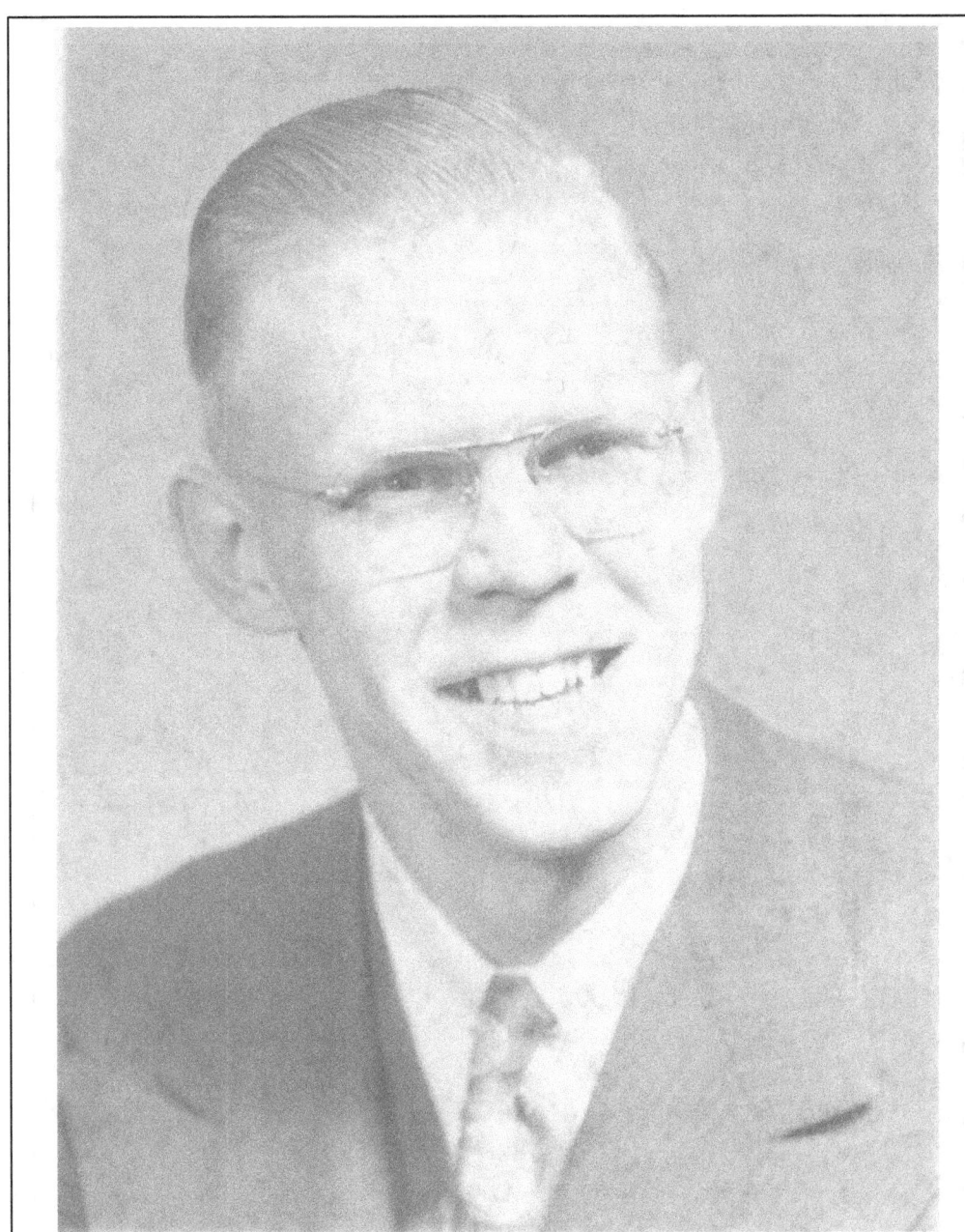

Art Holmstrom graduated in 1952 but received his diploma for 1944. He proved that he could live up to the rigors of life.
Art Holmstrom collection

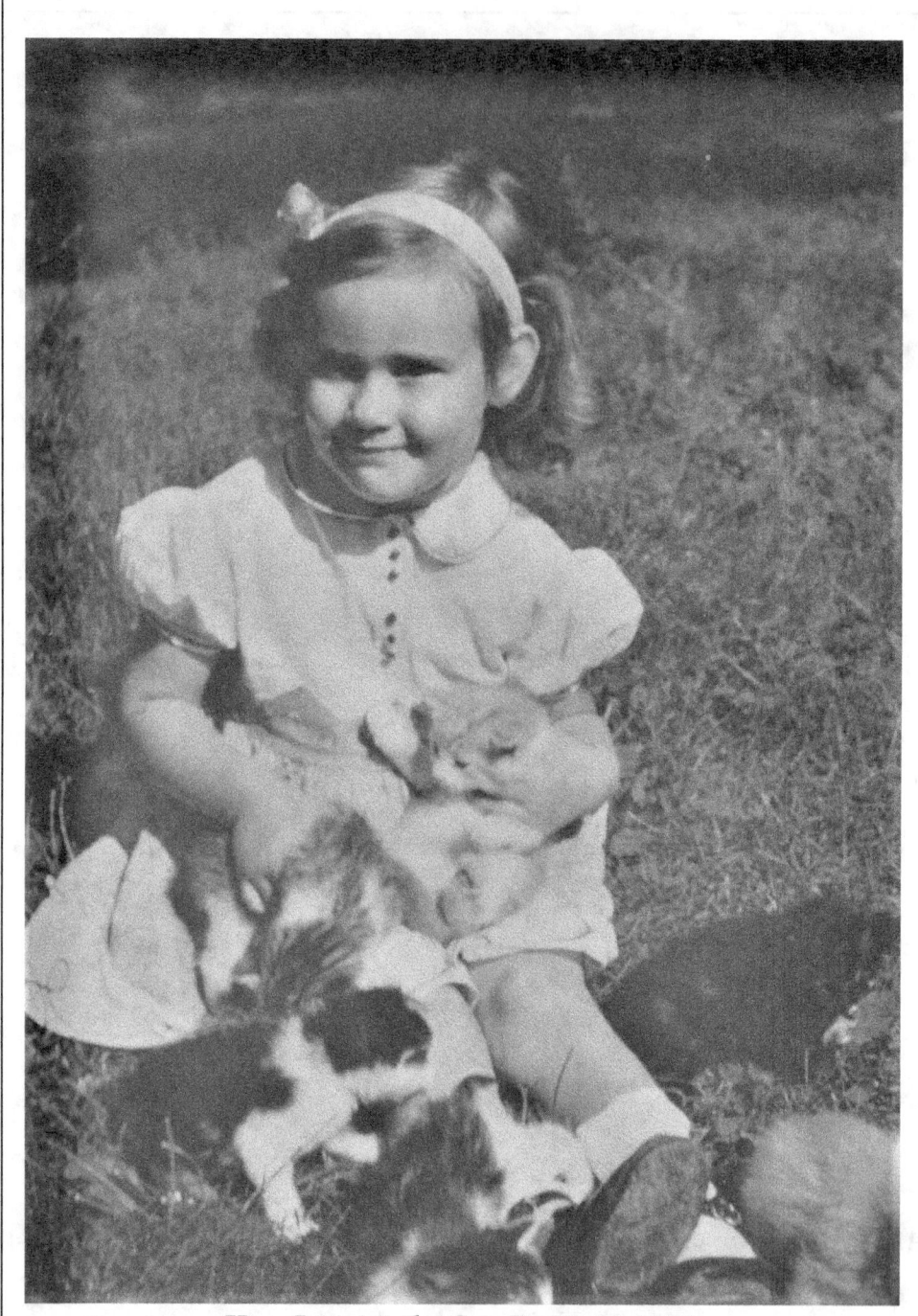
*Here I am at the San Dairy in 1950.
When I started writing this book, I didn't know it was
Art Holmstrom who had taken this photo.*

Chapter 44
My Surprise

After Art died, I received a letter from his wife, Edith. *"Thanks for celebrating with me a life well-lived, now safe in Heaven's keeping."* She spoke of Art's tenacity. *"Even when death was imminent, he was hesitant to sign a 'do not resuscitate' order because giving up was so contrary to his thinking."*

Two weeks before his death, he whispered to Edith, "I'm here today because I kept an optimistic outlook."

❦

As I worked on this book and reread my mother's notes, I received a surprise. I read, "Art Holmstrom, a patient at the San, snapped the picture of Patty and the kitties." I went to my study to get the framed picture, one of the few treasures we had brought when we moved from Minnesota. It had been on display wherever I had lived for most of my life. I carefully pulled the photo from its frame and read the note on the back, written in my mother's beautiful cursive: "Art Holmstrom took this picture, 1950."

Unbeknownst to either of us,
Art and I had met 55 years earlier,
and at the end of my search,
I had, indeed,
arrived where I had started.

Epilogue

Has tuberculosis returned ... or did it never really leave?

By the 1970s, many experts considered tuberculosis nearly eradicated. Then, in the United States during the 1970s and early 1980s, the country let its guard down, followed by an increase in the number of TB cases between 1985 and 1992. But with increased funding and diligence, the number of persons in the U.S. with TB has declined since 1993.[148]

Unfortunately, some countries lack the money and infrastructure to battle the disease. The World Health Organization estimates that today one in four in the world are infected with Mycobacterium tuberculosis.[149]

BCG, the vaccine for TB, is seldom used in the United States but is often given to infants and children in countries where tuberculosis is prevalent.[150]

After the discovery of medications to combat the disease, TB outsmarted us by becoming resistant to those drugs. Today, we battle multidrug-resistant TB (MDR TB) when the bacteria become resistant to two of the most important TB medicines, Isoniazid (INH) and Rifampin (RIF). Even more challenging to treat is extensively drug-resistant TB (XDR TB), a type of the disease that is resistant to nearly all medicines used to treat tuberculosis.

The bacteria can become resistant when the patient does not take the prescribed medications as directed. And those who spend time with someone who is ill with MDR TB or XDR TB are also at risk for becoming infected with the resistant bacteria. Those who develop tuberculosis again after having taken TB medicines previously, or those who are from areas where drug-resistant tuberculosis is common, are also at risk. Sometimes an adequate supply of the drugs is not available, allowing more tuberculosis.

Once drug resistance to the TB medicines occurs, there can be side effects and a higher risk of death.

By not being consistent with doses of medication, the patient risks allowing the disease to become drug-resistant. The best success in treating tuberculosis comes from directly observed therapy (DOT), under which the patient must be directly watched by a health-care worker when taking the medicines. Under the

---

[148] www.cdc.com

[149] www.who.int/tb/

[150] www.cdc.com

DOT program, a health-care worker meets with the patient daily several times a week for six or more months to watch the patient take the medicine.[151]

In 2018, the World Health Organization reported that there were an estimated 10 million new TB cases worldwide.

Each year on March 24, World TB Day commemorates the day in 1882 when Dr. Robert Koch announced that he had discovered the tubercle bacillus. "It's Time" is the theme for 2020.[152] Today, the disease is even more deadly than when our forbearers suffered from it. The goal of the United Nations is to end TB by 2030.[153]

---

[151] www.cdc.com
[152] www.who.int/tb/
[153] www.who.int/tb/

274

About the Author

Pat Nelson left Minnesota, "Land of 10,000 Lakes," when she was only five, but during that short time, she developed a love of the water. Today, she lives on a small lake in Washington State, where she swims in the summer. In any kind of weather, she is grateful for the serenity provided by her lake view. "If a natural body of water isn't available," she says, "I'll settle for a pool." She attends water aerobics three times a week. "Like many who have lived in Minnesota," she says, "I just love being near water. I hope one day to swim to Dr. Mary's rock in Rainy Lake, as she did."

She credits her mother with inspiring her to be a writer. "Mom wrote newsy letters to friends and family," she said, "and she encouraged me to write letters and stories. I first decided to become a writer when I was in sixth grade. I wrote a story for a class project, and I learned how much I enjoyed arranging words on paper."

Nelson wrote and self-published her first book when she was 29. "I guess I thought I was getting old because I was determined to write a book before I turned 30." She worked for a credit union and published "You … the Credit Union Member" to advise members on the best ways to use their credit unions. Though she wrote the book for members, it became a hit with credit unions as a training tool for employees and volunteers, and she sold 10,000 copies in a year. That was at a time when self-published books were not widely accepted, but she thought, "*I know how to reach my market, so why not?*"

Later, she wrote columns for *The Daily News* and *The Valley Bugler*, Longview, WA. She then started submitting stories to *Chicken Soup for the Soul*. That's how she got to know a couple of its co-creators who later established their own company, Publishing Syndicate. Nelson co-created two of Publishing Syndicate's books, *Not Your Mother's Book on Being a Parent* and *Not Your Mother's Book on Working for a Living*, and she proofread the 11 books in the series. In her retirement, she still occasionally edits manuscripts.

Nelson has a son, a daughter, a step-daughter, and four grandchildren. She enjoys traveling with her husband, Bob, (to places with water), and she likes to spend time with family, friends, and her spoiled Great-Dane/labradoodle mix named Brisa.

The Author's Bucket List

In 2021, my husband and I visited Bemidji, where I toured the San one last time. From there, we went to International Falls to view its excellent Dr. Mary Ghostley exhibit, then on to Rainy Lake, where Dr. Mary's cabin was located.

I went on the trip with the dream of fulfilling the one thing on my bucket list: to swim to "Dr. Mary's rock," as she had done so many times over the years. Her cabin had just been sold, so I decided to swim from nearby City Park. It was the farthest I had ever swum. The next day, to my disappointment, I learned I had swum to the wrong rock. After Dr. Mary's granddaughter got permission from the new owners, I tried again, swimming from their beach. I swam to the rock and back, as Dr. Mary had done, proud to have checked it off my bucket list. Not long after that trip, the old San was torn down, and now it truly is history.

Recommended Reading About Minnesota:

Interrupted Lives, the History of Tuberculosis in Minnesota and Glen Lake Sanatorium, by Mary Krugerud, North Star Press ©2017

Invited and Conquered by J Arthur Myers, Ph.D., M.D., Minnesota Public Health Association, 1949

Keeper of the Wild, The Life of Ernest Oberholtzer by Joe Paddock, Minnesota Historical Society Press ©2001

North Country History, anthology volumes edited by Hilda R. Rachuy, ©1970s-1990s. For information, contact Beltrami Historical Society, Bemidji, MN at depot@BeltramiHistory.org.

Taming the Wilderness by Hiram Drache, Interstate Publishers, Inc. ©1992

The Girl in Building C, edited by Mary Krugerud, Minnesota Historical Society Press ©2018

Gratitude

Many thanks to my husband, Bob Nelson, who urged me to travel to Minnesota to do research and who pushed me to "finish the book" when the task seemed daunting; to my cousin David Grande who shared his mother's and aunt's San memory books; and to Fred Hudgin, Kate Sherer, Jon P Langhout Jr., Nona Perry, Klazina Dobbe, and Dahlynn McKowen for their helpful advice. Sincere thanks, also, to the Beltrami History Center, the Minnesota History Center, and the Blackduck Area History and Arts Center, and to everyone who has helped me in so many ways with information and encouragement.

And special thanks to those who are no longer with us, without whom this book would not exist: Jim Ghostley, who shared his mother, Dr. Mary Ghostley, with me through memories, photos, conversations, and letters; my mother, Ella Grande Hedglin, who taught me to love to write and who left detailed notes of her time in Puposky and at the San—for whoever might someday want to read them (me!); my father, Lee Hedglin, for leaving precious memories; Art Holmstrom, a former patient at the Lake Julia Tuberculosis Sanatorium, for so willingly sharing his time, photos, memories, and support.; Edith Holmstrom, Art's wife, who continued to provide me with information even after Art's death; and most of all, thanks to Dr. Mary Ghostley for so generously giving her time, knowledge, compassion, and talent to others.

I thank you for your interest in the history of tuberculosis sanatoriums and for taking a closer look at the community created by the Lake Julia Tuberculosis Sanatorium.

Please share any additional information or photos with the Beltrami History Center, 130 Minnesota Avenue SW, Bemidji, MN 56601. With your help, we can make the history of the Lake Julia Tuberculosis Sanatorium even more complete. Identifying people in the photos and continuing to accumulate a history of the Lake Julia Tuberculosis Sanatorium will benefit family genealogists and historians for years to come.

Reviews

I hope you have enjoyed *Open Window*.
The best compliment you can give an author is a review at www.Amazon.com.

If you feel that "Open Window" is a worthwhile read, your genuine review at www.Amazon.com is the #1 way to let others know about the book. Can I count on your review while the book is still fresh in your mind?

I worked on "Open Window" for more than 15 years, during which time I passed from middle-aged to elderly. I want to be around to read your reviews, so please leave yours before I pass to the next stage. ☺

Please leave your review at: https://amazon.com *Just search for "Open Window Pat Nelson" and scroll down to the bottom of the "Customer Review" section where you will find the words "Write a customer review" in a box. Just click and enter your review. It need not be lengthy.*

Wondering how reviews work? See the explanation on the next page.

How Reviews Work

When you read a book that you enjoy or that you find to be valuable, you might want to leave a review of 4 or 5 stars. www.amazon.com or https://amzn.to/2WLjnSs.

To earn top reviews, a book should be well written and well edited.

It takes reviews of 4 or 5 stars to help propel a book into a position of selling well. The more positive reviews a book receives, the better it will rank. Your positive review helps increase the odds of people seeing and buying the book.

Besides reviews, what else can help increase the ranking of a book? When you read an Amazon review, you will be asked if the review was helpful. "Liking" a review by clicking that it was helpful will help boost the book's Amazon ranking.

A negative review is one of 3 or fewer stars. Negative reviews are harmful to writers and can significantly impact a book's sales and ranking, often making the difference between success and failure. For this reason, the decision to leave a review of three or fewer stars should not be treated lightly.

Thank you for taking the time to read and review *Open Window*.

In Memory of the Patients of the Lake Julia Tuberculosis Sanatorium

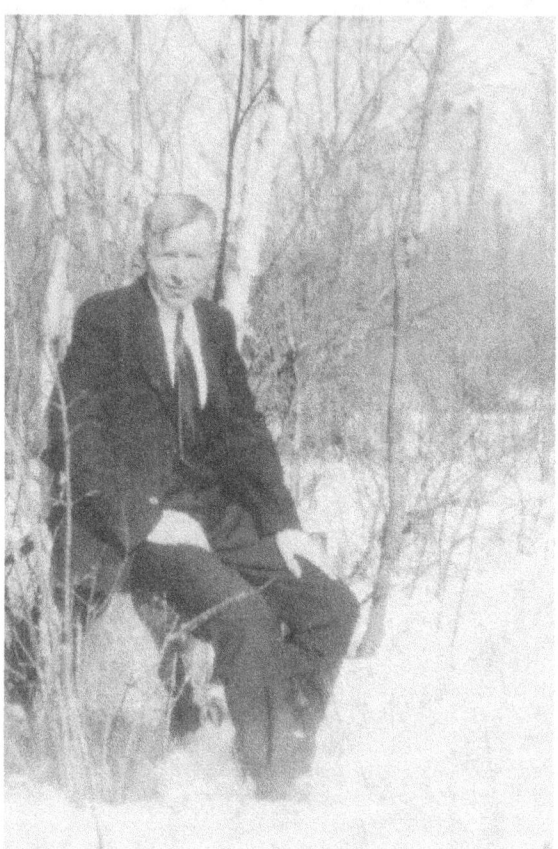

Andy Bohytari
Ella Hedglin photo collection

Andy Bohytari wanted to get well, but he wanted to be home even more. He was admitted to the San 10 times between May 1931 and July 1941. "One day," my mother said, "Andy just walked away and didn't come back."

One of the shortest stays at the San was that of 16-year-old patient Verlin Shockly who was admitted July 10, 1935. He was on his way to Ah-Gwah-Ching Sanatorium but was delivered by mistake to the Lake Julia Tuberculosis Sanatorium, where he died only two hours after his arrival.

Patient records, Minnesota History Center

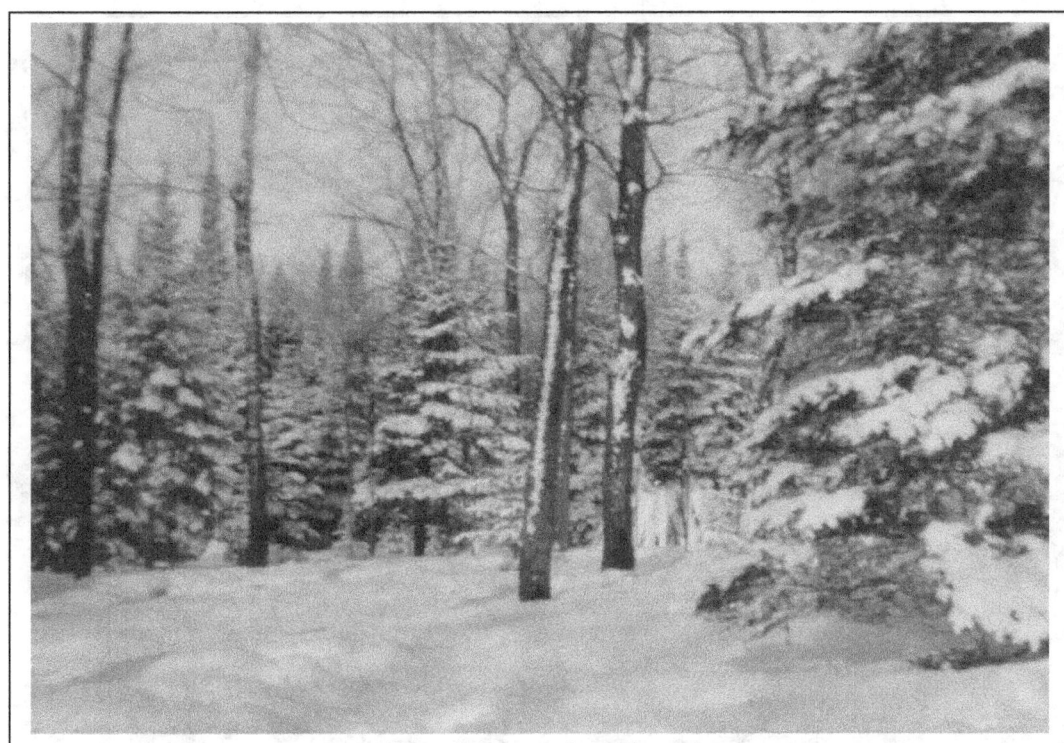

*The Sanatorium lawn
covered with snow
Art Holmstrom photo*

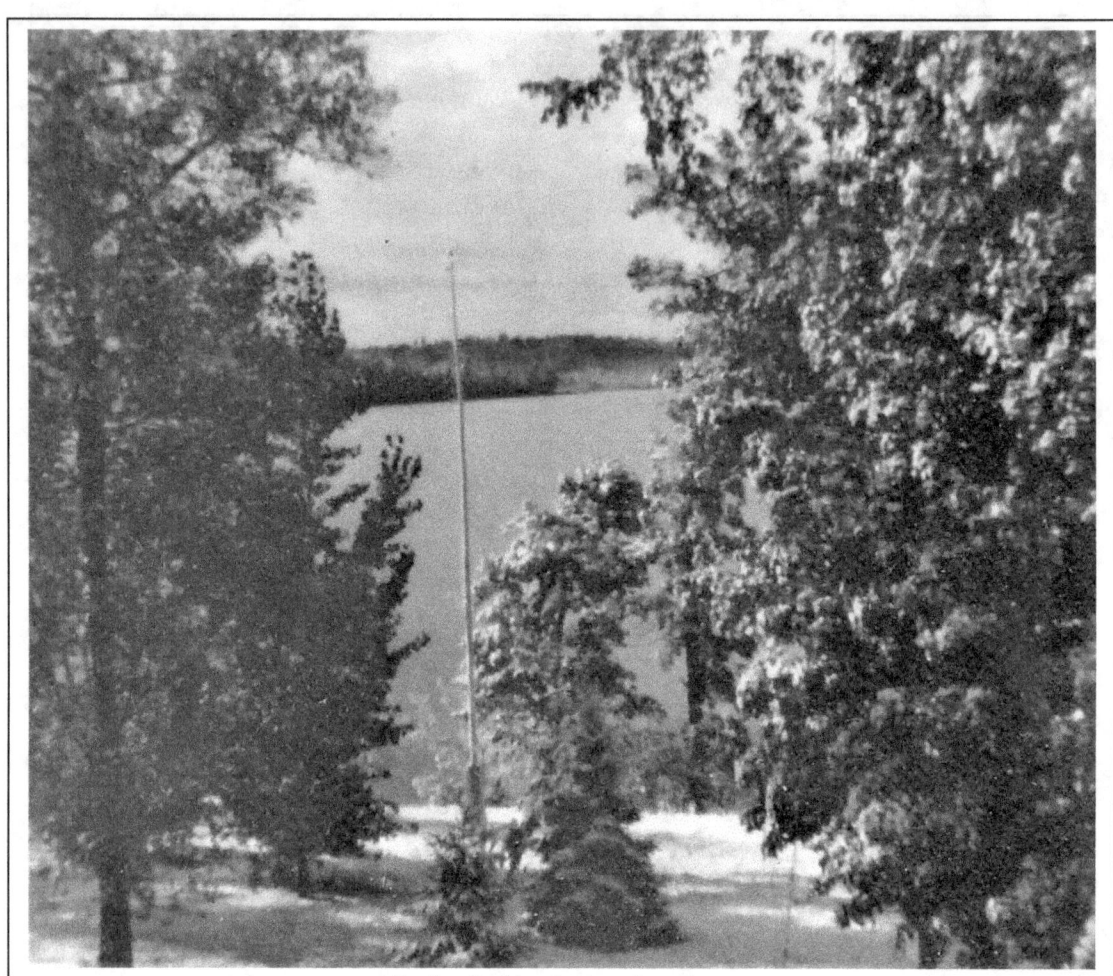

Lake Julia from the San
Art Holmstrom photo

www.ingramcontent.com/pod-product-compliance
Lightning Source LLC
Chambersburg PA
CBHW080451220526
45465CB00006B/2239